Medical Sciences at a Glance

Edited by

Michael D Randall

Professor of Pharmacology
School of Life Sciences
University of Nottingham
Nottingham, UK

WILEY Blackwell

This edition first published 2014 © John Wiley & Sons, Ltd

Registered Office
John Wiley & Sons Ltd, The Atrium, Southern Gate, Chichester, West Sussex, PO19 8SQ, UK

Editorial Offices
350 Main Street, Malden, MA 02148-5020, USA
9600 Garsington Road, Oxford, OX4 2DQ, UK
The Atrium, Southern Gate, Chichester, West Sussex, PO19 8SQ, UK

For details of our global editorial offices, for customer services, and for information about how to apply for permission to reuse the copyright material in this book please see our website at www.wiley.com/wiley-blackwell.

The right of Michael D Randall to be identified as the author(s) of the editorial material in this work has been asserted in accordance with the UK Copyright, Designs and Patents Act 1988.

Library of Congress Cataloging-in-Publication Data

Medical sciences at a glance / edited by Michael D. Randall.
    p. ; cm. – (At a glance series)
  Includes bibliographical references and index.
  ISBN 978-1-118-36092-7 (pbk. : alk. paper) – ISBN 978-1-118-36093-4 –
ISBN 978-1-118-36094-1 – ISBN 978-1-118-36095-8 (emobi) – ISBN 978-1-118-36096-5 (epub) –
ISBN 978-1-118-36097-2 (epdf)
  I. Randall, Michael D., editor of compilation. II. Series: At a glance series (Oxford, England)
  [DNLM: 1. Medicine. WB 100]
  R706
  610–dc23

2013026509

A catalogue record for this book is available from the British Library.

Cover image: iStock © BlackJack3D
Cover design by Meaden Creative

Set in 9/11.5 pt Times Roman by Toppan Best-set Premedia Limited
Printed and bound in Malaysia by Vivar Printing Sdn Bhd

1 2014

Contents

Preface

The *At a Glance* series provides brief summaries of the medical curriculum for medical, pharmacy and nursing students. Recent changes in curricula at medical schools have reduced the emphasis on students learning large amounts of factual detail and now focus more on core knowledge. Courses have also moved away from the traditional discipline-based approach of studying anatomy, physiology, biochemistry, pathology and pharmacology as distinct preclinical subjects, and many courses are now integrated. This provides a seamless study of the key physiological systems. The purpose of *Medical Sciences at a Glance* is to reflect the modernisation of medical courses and, as such, provides a single text to support students.

To understand and practise medicine the student needs to have a grasp of underlying biomedical sciences, and this book is intended for the early years' students. It should also help as a refresher of the medical sciences as students enter clinical phases of their courses, as a thorough knowledge of the medical sciences inevitably underpins clinical practice. For example, to understand the ECG in clinical practice one needs to understand the relevant anatomy, the underlying electrical events and the cardiac cycle.

By providing the background in biomedical sciences this edition feeds directly into *Medicine at a Glance* (Edited by Patrick Davey).

The aim of this book is to set out core material on which students can build a framework of learning and understanding. By using this book students should be able to define what they need to know and use the material as key summary points. It is all too easy for students to attempt to learn all lecture material superficially, but the key to medical studies is to *understand* the core material. We also feel that *Medical Sciences at a Glance* would be of use to students on the newer problem-based learning courses by setting a background against which students can define their own learning needs.

We hope that this text will help support early years' students getting to grips with physiological systems. We have deliberately limited the clinical content as this is the domain of the sister publication *Medicine at a Glance*, but have inevitably used some examples of diseases and treatment to place biomedical sciences in context.

The authors of *Medical Sciences at a Glance* are all from the University of Nottingham and all currently teach the relevant medical sciences to medical, science and pharmacy students.

Michael D Randall

Contributors

Dr Jane Arnold
University Teacher
School of Life Sciences
University of Nottingham

Dr Stuart Brown
Director of Biomedical Sciences Teaching
School of Life Sciences
University of Nottingham

Dr Steven Burr
Formerly University Teacher
School of Biomedical Sciences
University of Nottingham Medical School
Now Associate Professor in Physiology
Medical School
University of Plymouth

Dr Sue Chan
Lecturer in Cell Signalling
School of Life Sciences
University of Nottingham

Dr Chien-Yi Chang
Research Fellow
School of Life Sciences
University of Nottingham

Dr Fergus Doherty
Lecturer in Biochemistry
School of Life Sciences
University of Nottingham

Dr Lucy Fairclough
Lecturer in Immunology
School of Life Sciences
University of Nottingham

Dr James Lazenby
Research Fellow
School of Life Sciences
University of Nottingham

Dr Siobhan Loughna
Lecturer in Anatomy
School of Life Sciences
University of Nottingham

Dr Deborah Merrick
Lecturer in Anatomy
School of Life Sciences
University of Nottingham

Dr Ian Todd
Associate Professor and Reader in Cellular Immunology
School of Life Sciences
University of Nottingham

Prof Michael D Randall
Professor of Pharmacology
School of Life Sciences
University of Nottingham

Dr Sebastiaan Winkler
Associate Professor in Gene Expression
School of Pharmacy
University of Nottingham

Abbreviations

5-HT	5-hydroxytryptamine		CYP450	cytochrome P450
AI	angiotensin I		D	dopamine receptor
AII	angiotensin II		DCT	distal convoluted tubule
AC	adenylyl cyclase		DHAE	dehydroepiandrosterone
AcCoA	acetyl coenzyme A		DHAP	dihydroxyacetone phosphate
ACE	angiotensin-converting enzyme		DHFR	dihydrofolate reductase
ACh	acetylcholine		DM	diabetes mellitus
AChE	acetylcholinesterase		DPP-IV	dipeptidyl peptidase IV
ACTH	adrenocorticotropic hormone		DVT	deep vein thrombosis
ADCC	antibody-dependent cellular cytotoxicity		dUMP	deoxy uridine monophosphate
ADH	antidiuretic hormone		ECF-like	enterochromaffin-like cells
ADP	adenosine diphosphate		ECG	electrocardiogram
AIDS	acquired immune deficiency syndrome		EDHF	endothelium-derived hyperpolarising factor
ALT	alanine aminotransferase		EDV	end diastolic volume
AMP	adenosine monophosphate (AMP)		EGF	epidermal growth factor
			EPO	erythropoietin
ANP	atrial natriuretic peptide		EPPs	excitatory postsynaptic potentials
AP	action potential			
APCs	antigen-presenting cells		ER	endoplasmic reticulum
AST:	aspartate aminotransferase		ERV	expiratory reserve volume
AT$_1$	angiotensin II receptor type 1		ESV	end systolic volume
AV	atrioventricular		ETC	electron transport chain
AVP	arginine vasopressin		F	Faraday's constant
BNP	b-type natriuretic peptide		FCR	Fc receptors
BPH	benign prostatic hypertrophy		FDC	follicular dendritic cells
BSE	bovine spongiform encephalopathy		FEV$_1$	forced expiratory volume in the first second
CABG	coronary artery bypass graft		FSH	follicle-stimulating hormone
CAH	congenital adrenal hyperplasia		FVC	forced vital capacity
			G-CSF	granulocyte colony-stimulating factor
cAMP	cyclic adenosine monophosphate		GFR	glomerular filtration rate
CCK	cholecystokinin		GLP-1	glucagon-like peptide 1
CCRs	central chemoreceptors		GLUTs	glucose transporters
cGMP	cyclic guanosine monophosphate		GLUT2	glucose transporter 2
			GLUT5	glucose transporter 5
CHF	chronic heart failure		GnRH	gonadotrophin-releasing hormone
CJD	Creutzfeldt–Jakob disease			
CML	chronic myeloid leukaemia		GPCR	G-protein-coupled receptors
CNS	central nervous system		GTN	glyceryl trinitrate
CO	cardiac output		HAART	highly active antiretroviral therapy
COMT	catechol-O-methyltransferase			
COPD	chronic obstructive pulmonary disease		Hb	haemoglobin
			hCG	human chorionic gonadotrophin
Cox	cyclooxygenase			
CRH	Corticotropin-releasing hormone		HDL	high-density lipoprotein
			HER2	human growth factor receptor-2
CSF	colony-stimulating factors (e.g. G-CSF, granulocyte CSF)		HIV	human immunodeficiency virus
CSF	cerebrospinal fluid		HLA	human leucocyte antigens
CTLR	C-type lectin receptors		HMG-CoA reductase	hydroxyl-methylglutaryl coenzyme A reductase

hnRNA	heterogeneous nuclear RNA	P_ACO_2	arterial carbon dioxide
IC	immune complex	PCV	packed cell volume
IF	intrinsic factor	PCRs	peripheral chemoreceptors
I_f	'funny' current	PCT	proximal convoluted tubule
IFN	interferon	PDE	phosphodiesterase
IHD	ischaemic heart disease	PDH	pyruvate dehydrogenase
IMM	inner mitochondrial membrane	PE	phosphatidyl-ethanolamine
INR	international normalised ratio	PEF	peak expiratory flow
IPSP	inhibitory postsynaptic potential	PEFR	peak expiratory flow rate
		PFK-1	phosphofructokinase-1
IRV	inspiratory reserve volume	PGI_2	prostacyclin
JVP	jugular venous pressure	PI	phosphatidyl-inositol
K_d	dissociation constant	PIF	peak inspiratory flow
KIRs	killer cell immunoglobulin-like receptor	PL	phospholipase
		PPAR-γ	peroxisome proliferator-activated receptor-gamma
KLRs	killer cell lectin-like receptor	PPI	proton pump inhibitor
K_M	Michaelis-Menten constant	PRR	pathogen recognition receptor
LDL	low-density lipoprotein		
LH	luteinising hormone	PS	phosphatidyl-serine
LPS	lipopolysaccharide	PTH	parathyroid hormone
LTA	lipoteichoic acid	R	gas constant
LTD	long-term depression	RAAS	renin-angiotensin-aldosterone system
LT	long-term potentiation		
M-receptors	muscarinic receptors	RBC	red blood cell
MAO	monoamine oxidase	RER	rough endoplasmic reticulum
MAP	mean arterial pressure	RhD	rhesus antigen
MCV	mean corpuscular volume	RLRs	RIG-like helicase receptors
MDR1	multidrug resistance 1	rRNA	ribosomal RNA
mEPP	miniature end plate potential	SAN	sinoatrial node
MG	myasthenia gravis	SCID	severe combined immunodeficiencies
MHC	major histocompatibility complex		
		SCN	suprachiasmatic nucleus
MI	myocardial infarction	SIADH	syndrome of inappropriate antidiuretic hormone secretion
mRNA	messenger RNA		
MT	melatonin receptor		
NA	noradrenaline	sIg	surface immunoglobulin
nAChR	nicotinic acetylcholine receptor	SGLT1	the sodium-glucose transporter protein 1
NADP	nicotinamide adenine dinucleotide phosphate	SSRI	serotonin-selective reuptake inhibitor
NCR	natural cytotoxicity receptor	TAG	triacylglycerol
NLR	NOD-like receptor	Tc	T cytotoxic
NK	natural killer	TCA	tricyclic antidepressant
NMDA	N-methyl-D-aspartate	TCA cycle	tricarboxylic acid or Krebs cycle
NMJ	neuromuscular junction		
NO	nitric oxide	TCR	T cell receptor
NSAIDs	non-steroidal anti-inflammatory drugs	TIA	transient ischaemic attack
		Th	T helper
NTS	nucleus tractus solitarius (nucleus of the solitary tract)	TLC	total lung capacity
		TLR	toll-like receptors
PAMP	pathogen-associated molecular pattern	TNF-α	tumour necrosis factor-alpha
		TPR	total peripheral resistance
P_AO_2	arterial oxygen	tRNA	transfer RNA
PC	phosphatidyl-choline	TSG	tumour suppressor gene

V	rate of reaction	**V$_m$**	resting membrane potential
VC	vital capacity	**V$_{max}$**	maximum rate of reaction
VEGF	vascular endothelial growth factor	**VOCs**	voltage-operated channels
		V/Q	ventilation-perfusion
VIP	vasoactive intestinal polypeptide	**vWF**	Von Willebrand's factor
		UCP1	uncoupling protein 1
VLDL	very low-density lipoprotein	**UTI**	urinary tract infection

How to use your textbook

Features contained within your textbook

Each topic is presented in a double-page spread with clear, easy-to-follow diagrams supported by succinct explanatory text.

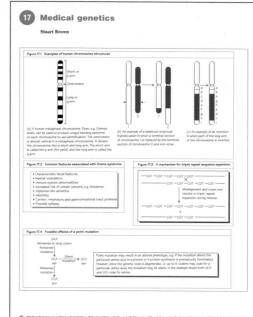

Your textbook is full of photographs, illustrations and tables.

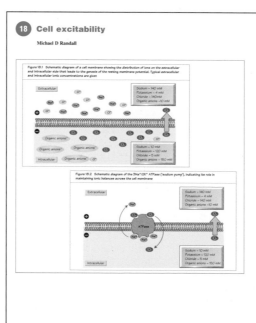

The anytime, anywhere textbook

Wiley E-Text

Your book is also available to purchase as a **Wiley E-Text: Powered by VitalSource** version – a digital, interactive version of this book which you own as soon as you download it.

Your **Wiley E-Text** allows you to:

Search: Save time by finding terms and topics instantly in your book, your notes, even your whole library (once you've downloaded more textbooks)

Note and Highlight: Colour code, highlight and make digital notes right in the text so you can find them quickly and easily

Organise: Keep books, notes and class materials organised in folders inside the application

Share: Exchange notes and highlights with friends, classmates and study groups

Upgrade: Your textbook can be transferred when you need to change or upgrade computers

Link: Link directly from the page of your interactive textbook to all of the material contained on the companion website

The **Wiley E-Text** version will also allow you to copy and paste any photograph or illustration into assignments, presentations and your own notes.

To access your Wiley E-Text:

• Visit **www.vitalsource.com/software/bookshelf/downloads** to download the Bookshelf application to your computer, laptop, tablet or mobile device.
• Open the Bookshelf application on your computer and register for an account.
• Follow the registration process.

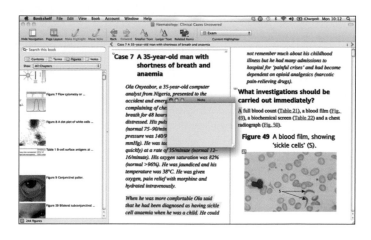

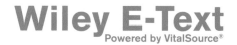

The VitalSource Bookshelf can now be used to view your Wiley E-Text on iOS, Android and Kindle Fire!

• **For iOS:** Visit the app store to download the VitalSource Bookshelf: **http://bit.ly/17ib3XS**
• **For Android:** Visit the Google Play Market to download the VitalSource Bookshelf: **http://bit.ly/ZMEGvo**
• **For Kindle Fire, Kindle Fire 2 or Kindle Fire HD:** Simply install the VitalSource Bookshelf onto your Fire (see how at **http://bit.ly/11BVFn9**). You can now sign in with the email address and password you used when you created your VitalSource Bookshelf Account.

Full E-Text support for mobile devices is available at: **http://support.vitalsource.com**

CourseSmart

CourseSmart gives you instant access (via computer or mobile device) to this Wiley-Blackwell e-book and its extra electronic functionality, at 40% off the recommended retail print price. See all the benefits at: **www.coursesmart.com/students**

Instructors . . . receive your own digital desk copies!

CourseSmart also offers instructors an immediate, efficient and environmentally-friendly way to review this book for your course.

For more information visit **www.coursesmart.com/instructors**.

With CourseSmart, you can create lecture notes quickly with copy and paste, and share pages and notes with your students. Access your **CourseSmart** digital book from your computer or mobile device instantly for evaluation, class preparation and as a teaching tool in the classroom.

Simply sign in at **http://instructors.coursesmart.com/bookshelf** to download your Bookshelf and get started. To request your desk copy, hit 'Request Online Copy' on your search results or book product page.

We hope you enjoy using your new book. Good luck with your studies!

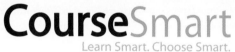

About the companion website

Don't forget to visit the companion website for this book:

 www.ataglanceseries.com/medicalsciences

There you will find valuable material designed to enhance your learning, including:
* Interactive multiple-choice questions
* Key summary points for each chapter

1 Cells

Sebastiaan Winkler

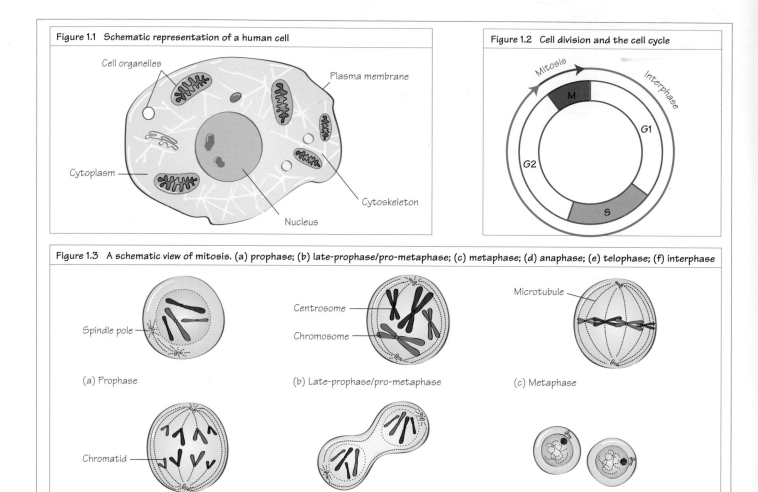

Figure 1.1 Schematic representation of a human cell

Cell organelles

Plasma membrane

Cytoplasm

Cytoskeleton

Nucleus

Figure 1.2 Cell division and the cell cycle

Mitosis

Interphase

M

G1

G2

S

Figure 1.3 A schematic view of mitosis. (a) prophase; (b) late-prophase/pro-metaphase; (c) metaphase; (d) anaphase; (e) telophase; (f) interphase

Spindle pole

(a) Prophase

Centrosome

Chromosome

(b) Late-prophase/pro-metaphase

Microtubule

(c) Metaphase

Chromatid

(d) Anaphase

(e) Telophase

(f) Interphase

 Medical Sciences at a Glance, First Edition. Edited by Michael D Randall. © 2014 John Wiley & Sons, Ltd. Published 2014 by John Wiley & Sons, Ltd.

A cell is the smallest functional and structural unit capable of replicating itself. As such, a cell is considered the basic unit of life. The boundary of a cell is the **plasma membrane** (see Chapter 2), while the **cytoskeleton** provides structural support (Figure 1.1). Cells of the human body have a characteristic nuclear compartment, which contains the genetic material, and are thus classified as **eukaryotic** cells as opposed to **prokaryotic** bacterial cells, which do not contain a nucleus. Cellular structures with specific functions, **organelles**, are discussed in Chapter 3.

Tissues

There are more than 200 different types of cells in the human body. These types are highly specialised (**differentiated**) to carry out specific functions. Groups of cells carrying out a similar function and forming a structure are called **tissue**. Different tissues combine to form organs. There are four main types of tissue.
• **Epithelial** tissue is found at the boundaries of structures in the body. The basal (**basolateral**) side faces the underlying tissue, which provides nutrients and support, while the **apical** side is exposed to a different environment. For instance, the apical side of intestinal epithelium faces the inside of the intestine and is exposed to constituents from (digested) food; the apical side of stomach epithelium is exposed to the acidic environment inside the stomach; lung and skin are exposed to air. Secreting glands are also formed by epithelial tissue. There are distinct types of epithelial structures:
– **stratified** epithelium: formed by layers of epithelial cells;
– **simple** epithelium: formed by a single layer of cells;
– **squamous** epithelium: formed by cells which are wider than tall;
– **columnar** epithelium: formed by cells which are taller than wide.
• Stratified squamous epithelium can be **keratinised**, forming a hard and dry layer as found in the skin, nails and hair, or **non-keratinised**, which is found in soft tissue such as the inside of the mouth. An example of simple columnar epithelium is the lining of the stomach.
• **Connective** tissue provides structure and rigidity. It is characterised by a large space between cells, which is filled with fibrous material that is part of the **extracellular matrix**. **Fibroblasts** are the most common cell type in connective tissue. **Adipose** tissue stores energy in the form of fat, but is also important for the protection and insulation of organs and is now recognised as having an endocrine role. Other types of connective tissue include blood, cartilage and bone.
• **Muscle** cells (**myocytes**) are characterised by their ability to contract when they receive appropriate signals. There are three different types of muscle tissue: skeletal muscle is directly attached to bones; cardiac muscle is the muscle of the heart; smooth muscle lines blood vessels and organs of the body.
• **Nerve cells** can sense stimuli and transfer electrical signals to chemical signals, which are sensed by surrounding cells. Nerve cells can have long extensions that are involved in the sensing and transmittance of signals (Chapters 18 and 19).

Cell division

The mass and volume of tissues can increase by **cell growth**, the increase of cell mass and volume by taking up nutrients and synthesising new cell structures, and **cell proliferation**, the increase of cell numbers by cell division. There are two types of cell division.
• **Mitosis**, in which each daughter cell acquires the same amount of genetic material as the parental cell.
• **Meiosis**, in which each daughter cell acquires half the amount of genetic material of the parental cell, only occurs in specialised germ tissue.

When cells receive signals to divide they progress through the cell cycle (Figure 1.2). In adult tissue, most cells reside in the **interphase**. The interphase can be further divided into three phases. In the **G1 phase** (first gap phase), cells prepare for the duplication of the genetic material. When cells start duplicating their DNA, they progress through the **S phase** (synthesis phase). Following the **G2 phase** (second gap), cells undergo mitosis (**M phase**). Compared with the interphase, the mitotic phase is very short. Mitosis (Figure 1.3) can be separated into the following distinct stages.
• **Prophase**: the DNA/chromatin condenses and the characteristic chromosomes become visible. The **mitotic spindle** starts to form outside the nucleus.
• In the **late prophase/pro-metaphase**, the nuclear membrane starts to degrade and the mitotic spindle body moves into the nuclear region. Regions in the chromosomes, **centrosomes**, are attached to the mitotic spindle.
• **Metaphase**: the chromosomes are aligned in the centre plane between the spindle poles.
• **Anaphase**: the chromatids of the sister chromosomes start to separate while the spindle poles move further apart.
• **Telophase**: the chromatids reach the spindle poles, which starts to disappear. The chromatids decondense and a nuclear membrane is formed around the chromatids.

During mitosis, the division of the cytoplasm between the two daughter cells is called **cytokinesis**. Cytokinesis starts during prophase, but is not completed until after the end of telophase when the two daughter cells have formed.

Stem cells

Stem cells are undifferentiated cells with two characteristics.
• **Self-renewal**: the ability to repeatedly divide while maintaining an undifferentiated state. Stem cells undergo **asymmetric cell division**: one of the daughter cells retains stem cell characteristics while the other daughter cell undergoes differentiation.
• The ability to differentiate into specialised cell types.
Stem cells are **pluripotent** if they retain the ability to differentiate into all cell types and tissues. For example, **embryonic stem cells** are pluripotent stem cells derived from early-stage embryos. **Adult stem cells** are not pluripotent, but are more specialised and can only form one or several tissues. For example, adult haematological stem cells isolated from the bone marrow can differentiate into the various cell types found in blood. Other adult stem cells are more specialised, e.g. skin stem cells found in the epidermis, which can only differentiate into skin cells. **Induced pluripotent** stem cells are derived from differentiated tissue that is genetically reprogrammed to return to their undifferentiated state.

2 Organisation of cell membranes

Sebastiaan Winkler

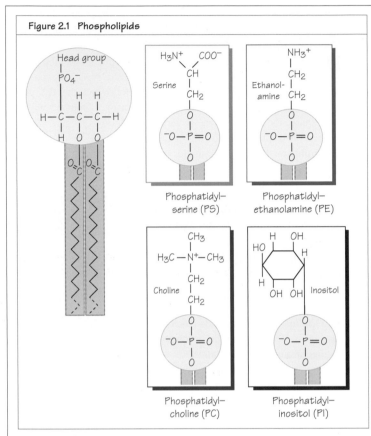

Figure 2.1 Phospholipids

Phosphatidyl–serine (PS)

Phosphatidyl–ethanolamine (PE)

Phosphatidyl–choline (PC)

Phosphatidyl–inositol (PI)

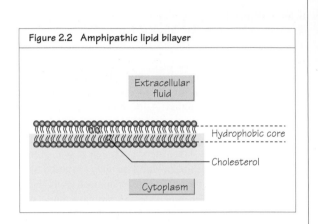

Figure 2.2 Amphipathic lipid bilayer

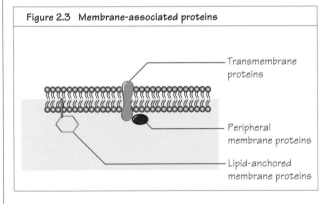

Figure 2.3 Membrane-associated proteins

Transmembrane proteins

Peripheral membrane proteins

Lipid-anchored membrane proteins

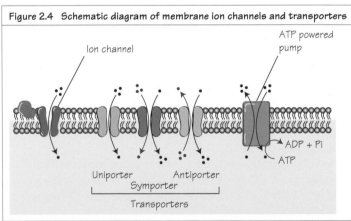

Figure 2.4 Schematic diagram of membrane ion channels and transporters

Ion channel

ATP powered pump

ADP + Pi

ATP

Uniporter

Antiporter

Symporter

Transporters

Cell membranes

Cell membranes are large cellular structures that constitute the boundary of a cell or a cell organelle. In contrast to proteins or nucleic acids, membranes are not made up of polymers, but a large number of diverse, relatively small molecules that form non-covalent interactions.

Phospholipids

The principal building blocks of cell membranes are a variety of compounds that are collectively known as **phospholipids**. Phospholipids are composed of three different parts: the backbone, a **polar head group** and a **fatty acid chain** (Figure 2.1). Different combinations of backbone, head groups and fatty acids result in a wide variety of phospholipids. In mammalian cells, glycerol is the backbone of the most abundant class of phospholipids, termed **phosphoglycerides**, although **sphingolipids** are also abundant. Backbone moieties have three hydroxyl groups, which are available for the conjugation of the polar head group, and two fatty acid chains. The polar head group is linked to the backbone via a phosphoester bond. In addition, two fatty acids are conjugated to the remaining hydroxyl groups of the backbone. The fatty acids can be broadly divided into two groups. The **saturated fatty acids** do not contain double bonds and always contains an even number of carbon atoms (usually 16–20). Due to the free rotation of the single carbon–carbon bonds, these lipid chains can adopt linear configurations. By contrast, the **unsaturated fatty acids** contain one or more double bonds. When the groups that lie on either side of the double bond are on opposite sides of the double bond (trans configuration) they are called **trans fatty acids** (Chapter 5). Like unsaturated fatty acids, trans fatty acids can adopt (near) linear configurations. However, when the groups next to the double bond are on the same side of the double bond (cis configuration) the fatty acids adopt very different shapes. The **cis fatty acids** have characteristic bends and cannot adopt linear configurations (Chapter 5).

A characteristic feature of the phospholipids is that they are **amphipathic**: they are both **hydrophilic** (due to the polar head group) and **lipophilic** (due to their fatty acid chain).

The lipid bilayer

Due to their amphipathic nature, phospholipids spontaneously organise in such a way that they form two sheets, with the polar head groups facing the aqueous exterior and the fatty acid chains forming a hydrophobic core (Figure 2.2). This structure is termed the **lipid bilayer**. Phospholipids can diffuse freely in the lipid bilayer, which behaves as a two-dimensional fluid. The lipid bilayer is **asymmetrical**, because phospholipids on one side of the bilayer do not freely flip to the other side. Thus, on the outside of cell membranes, phospholipids with PC head groups are enriched, while the cytoplasmic side is enriched with PE and PS lipids. The composition of the lipid bilayer is not homogeneous. The properties of cell membranes is influenced by the properties of the locally enriched phospholipids, e.g. the length of fatty acid chains influences the thickness of the lipid bilayer, and the presence of phospholipids containing cis fatty acids reduces the density of phospholipids in the lipid bilayer.

Sterols are another class of lipid components. **Cholesterol** is the most abundant sterol found in cell membranes (Chapter 5). Cholesterol impacts on the fluidity of the membrane: low concentrations of cholesterol can increase fluidity, whereas high concentrations of cholesterol can have the opposite effect.

Membrane proteins

Proteins are a third group of molecules found in cell membranes. There are three classes of membrane proteins (Figure 2.3).
- **Transmembrane proteins**: these traverse the lipid bilayer. In human cells, most integral membrane proteins contain a number of membrane-spanning **alpha helices**. In addition, the proteins may have extracellular and cytosolic domains. Examples of transmembrane proteins are **receptors**, proteins that mediate cell-cell interactions and transport proteins.
- **Lipid-anchored membrane proteins**: these contain lipid modifications, such as prenyl groups or fatty acids, that function as membrane anchors. Examples are proteins that mediate signals received by receptor proteins.
- **Peripheral (accessory) membrane proteins**: these proteins are not anchored in the membrane, but interact strongly with transmembrane proteins or proteins anchored in the lipid bilayer. As a consequence, these proteins do not diffuse freely in the cytoplasm. Similar to lipid-anchored membrane proteins, examples include proteins that mediate receptor signalling.

Membrane proteins do not diffuse freely in the lipid bilayer. Additional polar and non-polar interactions with phospholipids and cholesterol, as well as other membrane proteins, result in order around membrane proteins. These areas, which are more structured and packed compared with the lipid bilayer, are termed **lipid rafts**. Lipid rafts can diffuse freely in the lipid bilayer.

Transport across membranes

The lipid bilayer is a **semi-permeable** barrier that prevents the free diffusion of molecules. Gases, such as O_2, N_2 and CO_2, as well as small polar molecules, can diffuse through the membrane. In contrast, the lipid bilayer is impermeable to large polar molecules or charged molecules. Three types of membrane proteins facilitate and control the transport of ions and small molecules, including sugars and amino acids, across cell membranes (Figure 2.4).
- **Ion channels** facilitate the transport of small ions. The movement of ions is driven by a differential concentration on either side of the membrane.
- **Transporters** allow the transport of specific molecules and can be divided into three groups:
  - **uniporter**: facilitates the transport of specific molecules down its concentration gradient, for example the GLUT1 glucose transporter;
  - **symporter**: facilitates the transport of a specific molecules *against* its concentration gradient driven by the co-transport of one or more ions down their concentration gradient;
  - **antiporter**: facilitates the transport of a specific molecules *against* its concentration gradient driven by the movement in the opposite direction of one or more ions down their concentration gradient.
- **ATP-powered pumps** allow the transport of ions or specific small molecules against their electrochemical gradient by using energy released by the hydrolysis of ATP. Examples are the $3Na^+/2K^+$ ion pump (Chapter 18) and the H^+/K^+ gastric proton pump (Chapter 41).

3 Cell organelles

Sebastiaan Winkler

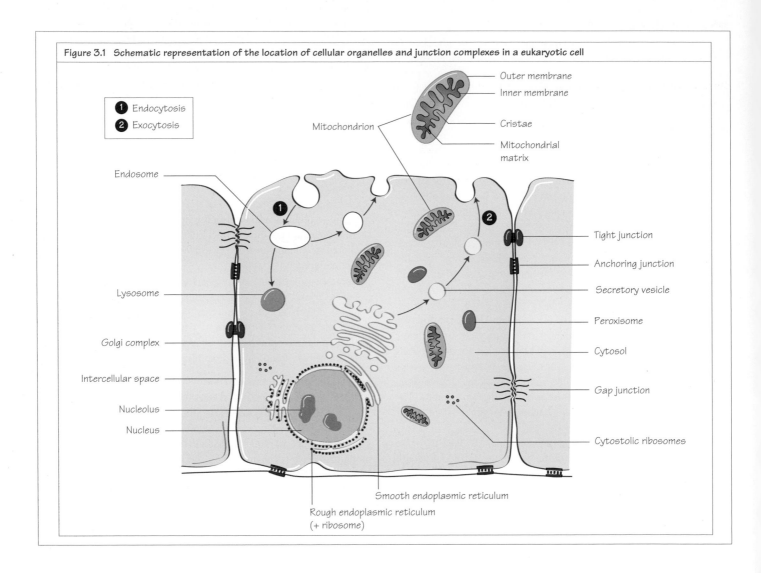

Figure 3.1 Schematic representation of the location of cellular organelles and junction complexes in a eukaryotic cell

1 Endocytosis
2 Exocytosis

Outer membrane
Inner membrane
Cristae
Mitochondrial matrix

Mitochondrion

Endosome

Tight junction
Anchoring junction
Secretory vesicle
Peroxisome
Cytosol
Gap junction
Cytostolic ribosomes

Lysosome

Golgi complex

Intercellular space

Nucleolus

Nucleus

Smooth endoplasmic reticulum
Rough endoplasmic reticulum
(+ ribosome)

Organelles (Figure 3.1) are most commonly defined as specialised structures within a cell that are enclosed by a membrane. The most prominent organelle of eukaryotic cells is the **nucleus**, which stores the maternally and paternally inherited **DNA**. The DNA in the nucleus is bound to proteins (**histones**) to form **chromatin** fibres, which help package the DNA into the nucleus. The DNA is used as a template for **messenger RNA** in a process called **transcription** (Chapter 16). The nucleus is separated from the **cytoplasm** by the **nuclear envelope**, a double membrane structure. Transport of proteins and nucleic acids (ribonucleic acid, **RNA**) between the nucleus and the cytoplasm is facilitated by the **nuclear pore complex**. The **nucleoskeleton** provides structure and rigidity to the nuclear compartment. One or several clearly distinct regions (**nucleoli**) are visible within the nucleus using light microscopy. The nucleoli are sites of ribosomal RNA production.

Mitochondria are the major sites of O_2 consumption. The majority of **ATP** (adenosine triphosphate), a central source of energy in cells, is produced by mitochondria. The outer membrane is smooth, while the inner membrane forms characteristic folds (**cristae**). While the initial stage of glycolysis, in which glucose is converted into pyruvate, takes place in the cytosol, mitochondrial enzymes associated with the cristae and present in the **mitochondrial matrix** transfer energy present in pyruvate and fats to ATP via the **tricarboxylic acid (TCA) cycle** and the **electron transport chain** (Chapter 10). Mitochondria contain specialised enzymes encoded by **mitochondrial DNA**, which resides in the mitochondrial matrix. Because mitochondria in the embryo are derived from the egg cell, mitochondrial DNA is **maternally inherited**.

The **endoplasmic reticulum (ER)** is membrane-containing structure surrounding the nucleus and attached to the nuclear envelope. Based on its appearance on electron micrographs, the endoplasmic reticulum is divided into the **smooth endoplasmic reticulum** and **rough endoplasmic reticulum**. The smooth endoplasmic reticulum is associated with phospholipid biosynthesis, storage of Ca^{2+} ions and other processes. The **rough endoplasmic reticulum** is associated with many **ribosomes**. Whereas **ribosomes** present in the cytosol produce soluble proteins that will function in the cytosol, ribosomes associated with the RER are involved in the synthesis of three classes of proteins.

• **Membrane proteins**, which contain hydrophobic regions and are inserted into the ER membrane during translation.

• Soluble proteins that contain a sorting signal resulting in the release of the protein into the **lumen** of the ER. These proteins will eventually be secreted into the extracellular space (**secretory proteins**).

• Proteins of other organelles.

Many proteins undergo **post-translational modifications** in the lumen of the ER. Branched sugar chains are attached to serine and asparagine residues (**glycosylation**). The formation of the covalent bond between two cysteine residues (**disulfide bond**) also occurs in the lumen of the ER.

Proteins synthesised by the RER are transported in **transport vesicles** to the **Golgi complex**, a network of membrane-enclosed compartments. Both proteins inserted in the ER membrane as well as proteins present in the lumen of the ER are transported in this manner to the **cis-Golgi** network. The proteins in the Golgi continue to be transported in membrane-enclosed vesicles to the **trans-Golgi** network. At least two processes are carried out in the Golgi network.

• **Glycosylation** initiated in the ER is modified and completed in the Golgi complex, where both addition and removal of sugar moieties take place.

• **Protein sorting**: membrane and soluble proteins are sorted into membrane-enclosed vesicles. During **exocytosis**, these vesicles will travel from the trans-Golgi network and fuse with the plasma membrane, resulting in the release of secretory proteins and the delivery of trans-membrane proteins to the plasma membrane. Vesicles with specific signals will not travel to the plasma membrane, but target specific organelles. The signals required for sorting to specific organelles may be sugar moieties (lysosome) or short amino acid sequences (peroxisome).

Endosomes are formed from **endocytic vesicles**, which are pinched off from the plasma membrane facilitating transport from the plasma membrane into the cell (**endocytosis**). Often, membrane receptors bound to their ligands are involved. The lumen of endosomes gradually becomes more acidic and the contents of endosomes are finally delivered to lysosomes.

The **lysosome** is a membrane-enclosed organelle specialised in the degradation and recycling of proteins, lipids, polysaccharides and nucleic acids. Many lysosomal enzymes catalyse hydrolysis reactions. The products of these reactions, such as simple sugars and amino acids, are re-used in the cytosol.

Peroxisomes are enclosed by membranes and consume significant amounts of O_2, which is used to form hydrogen peroxide (H_2O_2). The enzyme catalase uses H_2O_2 for oxidative degradation of diverse substrates, including large fatty acids and ethanol. Peroxisomes are also important for the synthesis of the main phospholipid components of myelin. This role of peroxisomes is especially relevant for the function of nerve cells.

The system containing the numerous vesicles involved in transport between the ER, Golgi, endosomes, lysosomes and peroxisomes is collectively referred to as the **membrane trafficking network**.

In addition, there are a number of structures that are not enclosed by membranes, but which have clearly identified roles. These structures are sometimes classified as non-membrane organelles.

• The **cytoskeleton**: structural support is provided by a network of filaments. This results in a shape characteristic for a specific cell type. The main kinds of filaments are:

– **actin filaments** play a particularly important role in cellular movement (**motility**);

– **microtubules** are formed by tubulin and are important for cell movement as well as the movement of vesicles inside the cell;

– **intermediate filaments** are made from a collection of different proteins. These filaments are important for the basic shape of cells and provide mechanical strength.

• **Cell junctions** are involved in the organisation of cells in tissues. The main types are:

– **desmosomes**, which are multi-protein complexes that join cells (e.g. connect epithelial cells) and lead to integrity. Hemidesmosomes adhere the basal membranes of epithelial cells to the basement membrane;

– **tight junctions**, which prevent passage of small molecules and fluid between cells;

– **anchoring junctions**, which are linked to cytoskeletal structures (mostly intermediate filaments) and provide rigidity in a group of cells;

– **gap junctions**, which provide channels between cells thereby facilitating movement of small molecules between neighbouring cells.

4 Protein biochemistry

Fergus Doherty

Figure 4.1 The hierachy of protein structure

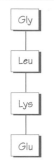 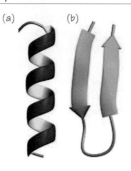 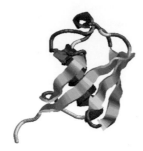 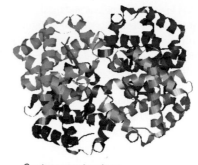

Primary structure
The linear sequence of amino acids joined by peptide bonds

Secondary structure
Regions of regular polypeptide structure: α-helix (a), β-sheet (b) and β-turn

Tertiary structure
How secondary structure is arranged in space. Soluble, globular proteins generally hide hydrophobic residues in the interior

Quaternary structure
This is only found in proteins of more than one polypeptide chain (subunit) and describes how these are arranged

---

Figure 4.2 Protein secondary structure

(a) The right-handed α-helix with 3.6 residues per turn and an H-bond between every fourth residue. Side chains protrude from the helix
(b) A type 1 β-turn, there are two types of these turns

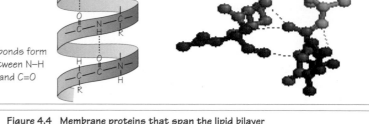
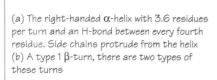
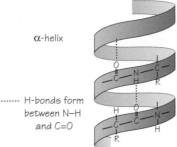

α-helix

-------- H-bonds form between N–H and C=O

Figure 4.3 A slice through the soluble, globular protein, haemoglobin

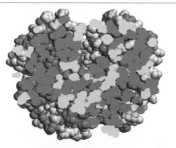

Shows hydrophobic amino acids (green) largely in the interior of the protein away from the aqueous environment

---

Figure 4.4 Membrane proteins that span the lipid bilayer

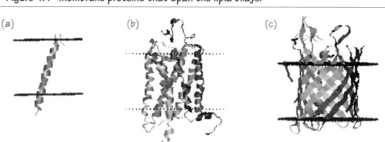

Membrane spanning regions may be single (a) or many (b) α-helices of about 20 residues. Some membrane proteins (e.g. the porins) consist of 'barrel' structures composed of β-strands (c)

Proteins are polymers of the 20 common L-amino acids and constitute about 16% of the body weight of the average adult. Proteins have a wide range of functions in the human body, including as enzymes, motors, transporters, receptors and other signalling factors; components of the immune system; as well as structural components of cells and the extracellular matrix. Proteins do not serve as a primary energy store, although during starvation protein is degraded, especially in skeletal muscle, to release amino acids, the carbon skeletons of which can be used for **gluconeogenesis** in the liver (Chapter 12).

Structure

L-amino acids are combined in proteins by the formation of a bond between the carbon atom of the α-carboxyl group of one amino acid and the nitrogen of the α-amino group of the next. This is the **peptide bond**. A small number of amino acids (residues) joined in this way are called a peptide, a larger number a polypeptide. The electrons of the double bond of the carbonyl group are delocalised, giving the C–N peptide bond a partial double bond character, which restricts rotation about this bond and influences how polypeptides fold in space. The sequence of amino acids joined by peptides in a polypeptide, the primary sequence or structure, is determined by the sequence of the gene coding for that polypeptide, and in turn determines how the polypeptide folds in three-dimensional space (Figure 4.1). **Primary sequence** is always written from the free amino terminus on the left to the free carboxyl terminus on the right, which is the direction of protein synthesis. The structure of polypeptides exhibits a hierarchy, with the primary structure being the first level.

The next level of polypeptide or protein structure is the **secondary structure** (Figure 4.2), which describes some of the folding of the polypeptide in 3D space. Regions of polypeptides can adopt three types of secondary structure determined by the amino acid sequence. The **α-helix** (Figure 4.2a) has a right-handed thread with 3.6 amino acids per turn and is stabilised by hydrogen bonds between every fourth amino acid formed by the carbonyl and NH groups of peptide bonds. Amino acid side chains point out from the helix. **β-strands** are pleated structures that hydrogen bond together to **form β-sheets** with amino acids side chains positioned above or below the plane of the sheet, while the strands can run in the same (parallel) or opposite (anti-parallel) directions. Secondary structure also includes **β-turns** (Figure 4.2b), consisting of about 4–7 amino acids, which introduce a turn into the backbone of the polypeptide (e.g. between two anti-parallel β-strands). Polypeptides can also include regions lacking in the clearly defined secondary structures described, such as various loops, random coils, or disordered regions. An example of a polypeptide containing mostly α-helix is **myoglobin**, while some **membrane channel proteins** contain extensive β-sheets that form a barrel-like structure.

Tertiary structure describes how secondary structures are arranged in space with respect to each other and the overall 'fold' of the polypeptide, and is stabilised mainly by hydrophobic interactions. Soluble proteins (Figure 4.3) generally fold to hide hydrophobic amino acid side chains in the interior away from water, while polypeptides resident in membranes (Figure 4.4) tend to have hydrophobic amino acids in the membrane-spanning regions, with side chains facing the interior of the membrane. Many polypeptides fold to create distinct domains, which are associated with a particular function, for example binding ATP, and similar domains can be found in different polypeptides with this function. The final level of protein structure is **quaternary** and describes how many polypeptide chains are grouped together in the functional protein, held together largely by non-covalent interactions, although inter-chain disulfide bonds between cysteine residues can play a role. Individual polypeptides in proteins are called subunits; although many proteins will have only one subunit many have two, four, or more.

Life cycle

Proteins are synthesised (**translated**) from amino acids on ribosomes using the information transcribed from DNA on to mRNA (Chapters 15 and 16). Following translation, covalent modification may occur (proteolytic processing, formation of disulfide bonds, or modification of some amino acid side chains, e.g. hydroxylation of proline in collagen). Some proteins will be secreted from the cell (e.g. extracellular matrix proteins). Intracellular proteins are subjected to degradation to amino acids at various rates, depending on the protein, so different proteins have different half-lives. Degradation is carried out by the **ubiquitin-proteasome system**, which regulates the concentration of many regulatory proteins, or in lysosomes. Proteins that have become damaged or fail to fold correctly are rapidly degraded to prevent their accumulation. The accumulation of undegraded 'abnormal' proteins can be lead to disease, for example prion proteins in the transmissible encephalopathies (BSE in cows, CJD in humans) and amyloid in Alzheimer's disease.

Jane Arnold

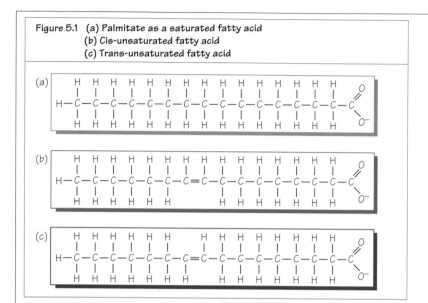

Figure 5.1 (a) Palmitate as a saturated fatty acid
(b) Cis-unsaturated fatty acid
(c) Trans-unsaturated fatty acid

Figure 5.2 Triacylglycerol (TAG)

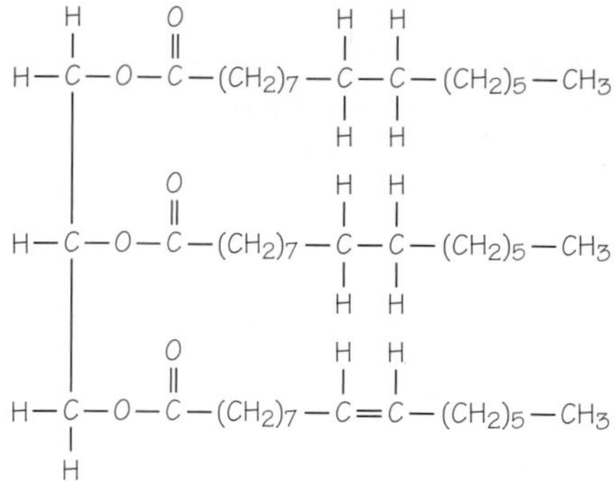

Figure 5.3 Cholesterol and an esterified cholesterol with RO-added

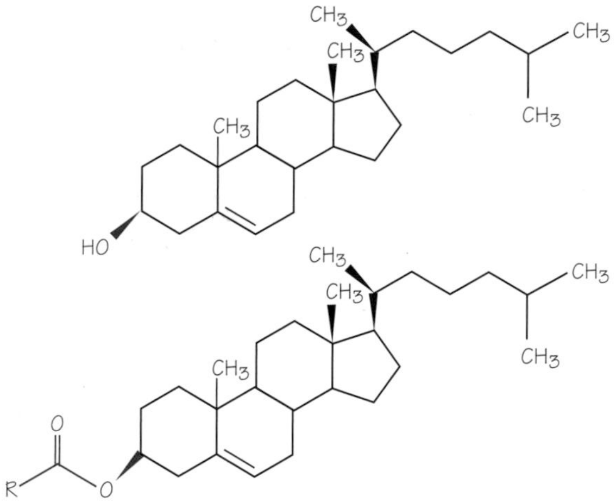

Table 5.1 Different fatty acids

Saturated		
Fatty acid	Formula	symbol
Palmitate	$CH_3(CH_2)_{14}COO^-$	16:0
Stearate	$CH_3(CH_2)_{16}COO^-$	18:0
Arachidate	$CH_3(CH_2)_{18}COO^-$	20:0
Unsaturated		
Fatty acid	Formula	
Palmitoleate	$CH_3(CH_2)_5CH=CH(CH_2)_7COO^-$	16:1
Oleate	$CH_3(CH_2)_7CH=CH(CH_2)_7COO^-$	18:1
Linoleate	$CH_3(CH_2)_4CH=CHCH_2CH=CH(CH_2)_7COO^-$	18:2
Linolenate	$CH_3CH_2CH=CHCH_2CH=CHCH_2CH=CH(CH_2)_7COO^-$	18:3
Arachidonate	$CH_3(CH_2)_4(CH=CHCH_2)_4(CH_2)_2COO^-$	20:4

Lipids are defined as organic molecules that share the property of being water insoluble but are highly soluble in organic solvents. They are structurally diverse and have many different functions, including:

- components of cell membranes (Chapter 2)
- fuel molecules (Chapter 11)
- signalling molecules.

Some of the most important biological lipids include fatty acids, triglycerides and cholesterol.

Fatty acids
Structure
Fatty acids are composed of a long hydrocarbon chain with a terminal carboxylic acid. They normally contain between 14 and 24

carbon atoms and have the general formula $CH_3(CH_2)_nCOOH$ (Figure 5.1a). They exist in a **saturated** (no double bonds in hydrocarbon chain), **monounsaturated** (one double bond) and **polyunsaturated** (two or more double bonds) form. Most of the double bonds in naturally occurring unsaturated fatty acids exist in a **cis configuration** (same side of the double bond) (Figure 5.1b). A **trans configuration** (opposite sides of the double bond) can also occur (Figure 5.1c). The addition of the double bond causes a bend or kink in the hydrocarbon chain, which impacts on the packing of these molecules and causes a reduction in the melting point of the molecule. For example, stearate, an 18C saturated fatty acid has a melting point of 69°C, while oleate, a monosaturated 18C fatty acid, has a melting point of 13°C. This is important when considering the role of fatty acids in cell membrane structure (Chapter 2). The chain length also affects the melting point; the longer the chain length, the higher the melting point.

Nomenclature

The naming of fatty acids is slightly confusing, as while systematic names exist, naturally occurring fatty acids are generally called by their common names. A numbering system is also used, whereby the left-hand number depicts the number of carbon atoms and the right hand number reflects the number of double bonds in the hydrocarbon chain. Table 5.1 lists some of the naturally occurring common fatty acids. Normally the name of the fatty acid ends in '**oic acid**', but most fatty acids are ionised at physiological pH (COO^- instead of $COOH$) and end in '**ate**'. For example, palmitic acid ($CH_3(CH_2)_{14}COOH$) will occur physiologically as palmitate ($CH_3(CH_2)_{14}COO^-$).

Sources

Most fatty acids are ingested in the diet in the form of triglycerides. However, there is a *de novo* pathway of fatty acid synthesis in the liver where **acetyl coenzyme A (acetylCoA)** is used as the building block to produce long-chain fatty acids. Two important fatty acids, however, cannot be synthesised in the body and must be taken in the diet. These are linoleate and linolenate (Table 5.1), which are collectively called the omega fatty acids. Linoleate (omega 6) is a precursor to a family of signalling molecules known as prostaglandins, while linolenate (omega 3) is an important constituent of some specialised membranes (e.g retinal cell membranes).

The majority of trans fatty acids are produced as a product of hydrogenation of vegetable oils (e.g. in margarine production). Ingestion of trans fatty acids is of concern as they have been linked to an increased risk of coronary heart disease.

Functions

Component of cell membranes – fatty acids and modified forms of fatty acids are an important component of the lipid bilayer of membranes (Chapter 2).

In metabolism – fatty acids can either be obtained from the diet or can be synthesised from AcCoA. These can then be stored as triglycerides in adipose tissue (see below). The energy stored in these molecules can then be released by beta oxidation to produce large quantities of ATP (see Chapter 11).

In cell signalling – fatty acids are used in a number of ways in cell signalling.
- Linoleate is metabolised to arachidonic acid, which is an important precursor in prostaglandin synthesis.
- Some derivatives of fatty acids (e.g inositol phosphate) are important in signal transduction pathways.
- Some fatty acids can be attached to proteins (post-translational modification) to activate specific proteins.

Triglycerides

Triglycerides are a major fuel source for the body and are commonly referred to as fats (if solid at room temperature) or oils (if liquid at room temperature). **Triacylglycerol** (TAG) contains a glycerol backbone to which three fatty acids chains are attached by an ester linkage. The three fatty acids can be identical (simple TAG) or different (mixed TAG) (see Figure 5.2). As both the chain length and level of saturation affect the melting point of the fatty acid, the composition of the fatty acids in the TAG will determine whether the TAG is a fat (longer chain lengths and/or saturated C-bonds, e.g. lard) or an oil (shorter chain lengths and/or mono- or polyunsaturated, e.g. one of the major TAGS of olive oil contains two oleic and one palmitic acid).

TAGS can be obtained through the diet or made from de *novo* fatty acids and will be stored in the cytoplasm of adipose cells. As these molecules are hydrophobic, they contain very little water and so are an efficient way of storing energy. They can be mobilised to break down and produce ATP under the appropriate hormonal signals (see Chapter 10).

Cholesterol

Despite elevated plasma cholesterol being linked to increased risk of coronary heart disease, cholesterol performs some essential functions in the body.

Structure

Cholesterol is structurally very different to the other lipids already discussed. It is a 27-carbon molecule containing four fused hydrocarbon rings. A branched eight-carbon chain is attached to the C17 of the D ring (Figure 5.3). Cholesterol is the major sterol in animal cells.

Cholesterol also exists in an esterified form where the OH at C3 is esterified with a long-chain fatty acid. This makes the cholesterol molecule even more hydrophobic.

Sources

Cholesterol can be taken up from the diet but there is an active *de novo* synthesis pathway in the liver.

Lipoproteins and cholesterol transport
- **Low-density lipoprotein (LDL)** ('bad cholesterol') is cholesterol rich and is taken up by the liver and tissues, and this involves the LDL receptor. LDL provides cholesterol for cell membranes, steroid synthesis and the production of bile acids. Its uptake into arterial walls is associated with atherogenesis.
- **High-density lipoprotein (HDL)** ('good cholesterol') takes up cholesterol from cellular breakdown and prevents its deposition.

Functions
- Component of cell membranes (Chapter 2).
- Precursor to bile acids.
- Precursor to steroid hormones.
- Precursor to vitamin D.

Carbohydrate biochemistry

Fergus Doherty

Figure 6.1 Simple carbohydrates

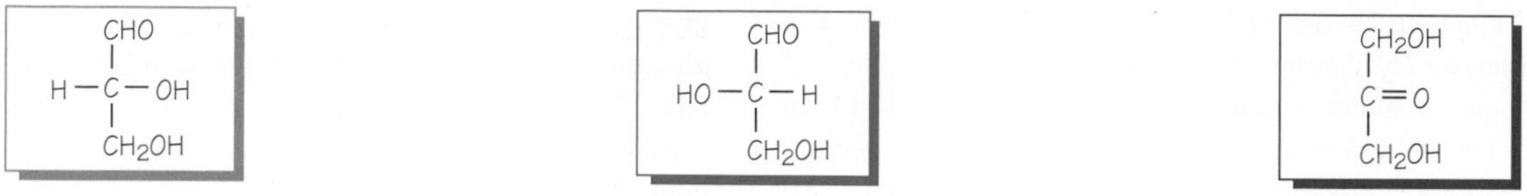

$$
\begin{array}{c}
\text{CHO} \\
| \\
\text{H} - \text{C} - \text{OH} \\
| \\
\text{CH}_2\text{OH}
\end{array}
$$

D-glyceraldehyde

$$
\begin{array}{c}
\text{CHO} \\
| \\
\text{HO} - \text{C} - \text{H} \\
| \\
\text{CH}_2\text{OH}
\end{array}
$$

L-glyceraldehyde

$$
\begin{array}{c}
\text{CH}_2\text{OH} \\
| \\
\text{C} = \text{O} \\
| \\
\text{CH}_2\text{OH}
\end{array}
$$

Dihydroxyacetone

The simplest carbohydrates are the trioses glyceraldehyde (an aldose) and dihydroxyacetone (a ketose). Glyceraldehyde has an asymmetric carbon at position two, which means there are two optically active mirror images molecules possible (enantiomers), D- and L-glyceraldehyde

---

Figure 6.2 Glucose

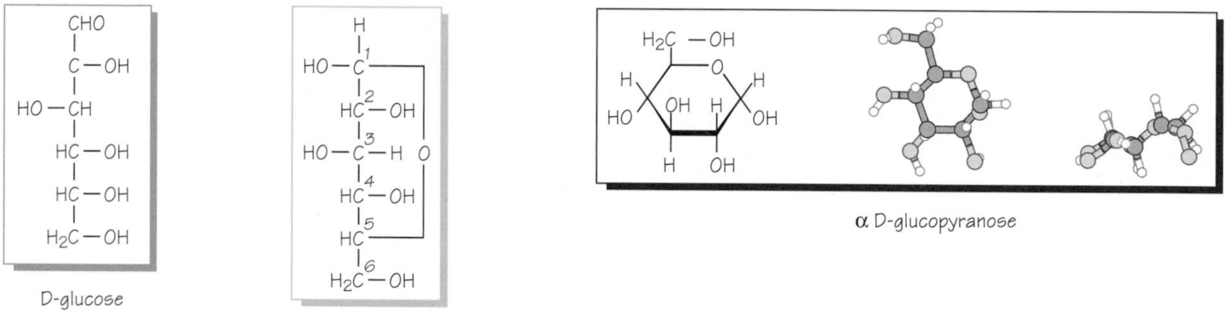

$$
\begin{array}{c}
\text{CHO} \\
| \\
\text{C} - \text{OH} \\
| \\
\text{HO} - \text{CH} \\
| \\
\text{HC} - \text{OH} \\
| \\
\text{HC} - \text{OH} \\
| \\
\text{H}_2\text{C} - \text{OH}
\end{array}
$$

D-glucose

$$
\begin{array}{c}
\text{H} \\
| \\
\text{HO} - \text{C}_1 \\
| \\
\text{HC}_2 - \text{OH} \\
| \\
\text{HO} - \text{C}_3 - \text{H} \quad \text{O} \\
| \\
\text{HC}_4 - \text{OH} \\
| \\
\text{HC}_5 \\
| \\
\text{H}_2\text{C}_6 - \text{OH}
\end{array}
$$

D-glucopyranose

α D-glucopyranose

Glucose, the most abundant carbohydrate in humans, is a six-carbon (hexose) monosaccharide with an aldehyde group (aldose) at carbon atom 1. Carbon 4 is asymmetric so there are two enantiomers of glucose, D- and L-glucose. D-glucose is the metabolically active enantiomer in humans. Glucose readily forms six-membered oxygen-containing ring structures (a pyranose) in solution. This produces an anomeric carbon at position 1, so two forms α and β exist. α D-glucopyranose is the building block for glycogen

---

Figure 6.3 Glycogen

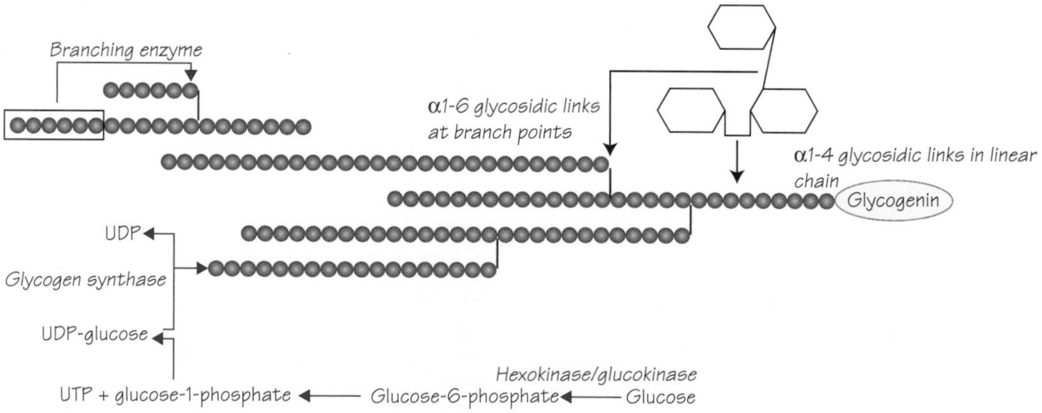

Glycogen is the storage form of glucose in animals and is a highly branched polymer of α-D-glucopyranose units joined by α1-4 glycosidic bonds to form linear chains, with α1-6 glycosidic bonds forming branch points every 5–8 glucose units. Glycogen is built up on a glycogen fragment ('seed') or on the protein glycogenin by the enzyme glycogen synthase, which transfers glucose from UDP-glucose to the end of a glycogen chain to form the α1-4 glycosidic bond. Branching enzyme transfers a string of glucose units from the end of a chain to an internal glucose to form the α1-6 branch point

---

 Medical Sciences at a Glance, First Edition. Edited by Michael D Randall. © 2014 John Wiley & Sons, Ltd. Published 2014 by John Wiley & Sons, Ltd.

Carbohydrates (CHOs) are probably the most abundant organic molecules in living organisms and serve a variety of roles. Carbohydrates provide about 55% of dietary calories for a healthy human, so they are our major fuel. Humans store some carbohydrate, in the form of glycogen, in tissues such as skeletal muscle and liver. Carbohydrates are also found as structural components of membranes, mostly attached to membrane proteins, and the carbohydrates on these proteins can have a role in cell-to-cell signalling.

Carbohydrate structure

As their name implies, carbohydrates are molecules made up of 'hydrated carbon', containing many hydroxyl groups, plus an aldehyde or a keto group, and can be represented by the simple empirical formula CH_2O_n. Simple carbohydrates (or **monosaccharides**) consist of a single carbohydrate unit, the smallest of which is glyceraldehyde. This has three carbons and is therefore classed as a triose. Typically, carbohydrates in humans range from three to nine (**nonose**) carbon atoms, with many abundant and important carbohydrates containing six carbons (**hexoses**). Monosaccharides with an aldehyde group are classed as aldoses (e.g. glyceraldehyde), while those with keto groups are ketoses (e.g. dihydroxyacetone).

Glyceraldehyde (Figure 6.1) has an asymmetric carbon atom at position 2 (the four groups attached to it are different) and therefore can exist in two conformations that are mirror images of each other (**enantiomers**). These are known as the D and L forms. The majority of carbohydrates in humans are in the **D-form**. Enzymes are stereospecific and will only act on the correct enantiomer of a carbohydrate.

Glucose

The most abundant carbohydrate in the human body is glucose, with the empirical formula $C_6H_{12}O_6$, which can be represented as a linear chain of carbon atoms with an aldehyde group at one end (designated carbon atom 1) and hydroxyl groups attached to the other carbons (Figure 6.2). Other **hexoses** share the same empirical formula as glucose but differ in the arrangement of the various hydroxyl and aldehyde groups and are therefore isomers. Epimers differ in the arrangement of groups around a single carbon, e.g. glucose and mannose. In solution, monosaccharides rapidly cyclise by reaction of the aldehyde (e.g. C6 in an aldohexose) or keto (e.g. C5 in ketohexose) to form ring structures resembling a chair. A pyranose is a six-membered ring and a furanose a five-membered ring. Formation of a ring creates an anomeric carbon (which carried the aldehyde or keto group), and two isomers (diastereomers) are possible, α and β. Glucose exists in both forms in solution, but these rapidly interconvert; however, enzymes are specific for a particular diastereomer. Glucose also exists as enantiomers, but it is the D form that is metabolically active in humans.

Polysaccharides

Monosaccharide units can be joined together to form polymers of various lengths, e.g **disaccharides** such as lactose in milk (galactose and glucose) and sucrose in fruit (glucose and fructose). Larger polymers are called oligosaccharides and very large polymers are called polysaccharides. Monosaccharide units are joined together via **glyco-sidic bonds**, named after the carbon atoms involved and the configuration of the **anomeric carbon**, e.g α1-4 in the polymer of glucose known as glycogen.

Glycogen

Glucose cannot be stored in cells as it is osmotically active, and at high intracellular concentrations would lead to osmotic lysis. The supply of glucose in the diet is intermittent, so to overcome these problems glucose is stored as an insoluble polysaccharide known as glycogen. Glycogen is composed of linear chains of α1-4 linked glucose units with an α1-6 linked branch point every 8–10 glucose units. To this branch is added more α1-4 linked glucose units, creating a very large (molecular weight approximately 10^8 Daltons), highly branched structure.

Skeletal muscle, which comprises a large proportion of the body weight of a human, is approximately 2% by weight glycogen, and liver is about 10% by weight glycogen. Glycogen is found in cytoplasmic granules associated with the enzymes of glycogen metabolism. Synthesis of glycogen occurs when glucose is abundant, after feeding, and starts with glucose-6-phosphate, which is formed when glucose enters the cell and can be converted to glucose-1-phosphate. This is followed by the transfer of the glucose moiety to UTP (a high-energy phosphate compound) to form UDP-glucose, which serves as the donor of glucose for elongation of the glycogen chain by glycogen synthase from a small glycogen 'seed' (Figure 6.3). Alternatively, the glycogen may be built on a protein, **glycogenin**. A separate branching enzyme transfers 5–8 glucosyl residues from the end of the chain to a branch point. The highly branched structure of glycogen allows for its rapid breakdown when glucose is needed (e.g. during fasting or exercise).

Structural carbohydrates

As well as being important fuels, carbohydrates serve as structural components of the body. **Glycosaminoglycans** are long unbranched chains of monosaccharide units, including monosaccharide units with amino groups (e.g. glucosamine or galactosamine). These are often further modified by N-acetylation or sulfation. Glycosaminoglycans associate with small amounts of protein and are found in the extracellular matrix where, with their affinity for water, they form a jelly-like substance. Glycosaminoglycans can also act like lubricants and are known as **mucopolysaccharides**. Inherited deficiencies in the lysosomal enzymes that degrade glycosaminoglycans/mucopolysaccharides result in accumulation of these molecules, leading to skeletal muscle problems and mental retardation.

Many secreted or cell-surface proteins are modified (glycosylated) by the addition of relatively small, branched, heterogeneous carbohydrate chains. Glycosylated proteins at the cell surface can act as important signal molecules between adjacent cells and between cells and the extracellular matrix. Glycosylation of proteins occurs in the endoplasmic reticulum and Golgi apparatus.

Prolonged, high levels of glucose in the circulation, for instance in uncontrolled diabetes, leads to non-enzymatic modification of protein by glucose (glycation). High levels of glycation of blood proteins is a major contributor to diabetic pathology and is associated with increased morbidity.

7 Basic mechanisms of drug action

Michael D Randall

Figure 7.1 A schematic diagram of a G-protein coupled receptor

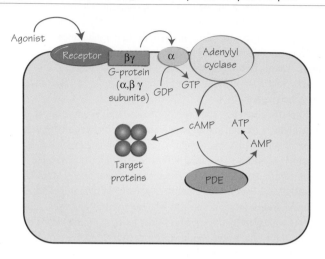

A G-protein coupled receptor (such as the β-adrenoceptor) in which agonist binding leads to the exchange of GDP with GTP on the α-subunit of the G-protein which disassociates from the βγ subunits and activates the adenylyl cyclase, leading to an increase in cAMP. The cAMP interacts with target proteins and is also broken down (and recycled) by the phosphodiesterase (PDE) enzyme

Figure 7.2 A schematic diagram of 3 different receptor-transduction mechanisms

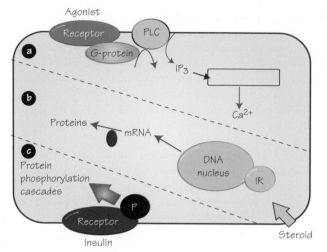

a) G-protein coupling of receptor to phospholipase C activation (PLC), leading to the release of inositol 1,4,5-trisphosphate (IP_3) and calcium release b) an intracellular receptor (IR) which regulates DNA transcription and protein synthesis c) a catalytic receptor (such as the insulin receptor) which undergoes autophosphorylation (P), which initiates an intracellular cascade

Figure 7.3 A ligand-gated ion channel

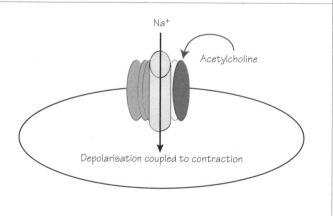

This case shows the nicotinic receptor at the neuromuscular junction, which is opened by acetylcholine binding, which leads to cellular depolarisation

Figure 7.4 A log concentration-response curve

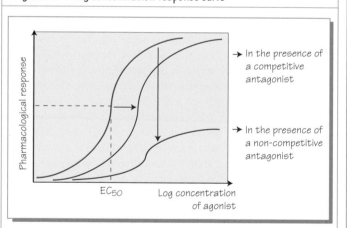

A log concentration-response curve to an agonist, which undergoes a rightward parallel shift in the presence of a competitive antagonist and suppression of the maximal response in the presence of a non-competitive antagonist

---

Drugs interact with their specific target, which may be coupled to a second messenger and/or effector system, leading to a cellular response.

Pharmacological targets
Receptors

Receptors are proteins that are targets for drug action and are located in the membrane or intracellularly. Many receptor classes have sub-types with different locations and physiological roles. For example, **noradrenaline** acts at:

- α_1-adrenoceptors (e.g. vascular smooth muscle)
- α_2-adrenoceptors (e.g. CNS, presynaptically)
- β_1-adrenoceptors (e.g. heart)
- β_2-adrenoceptors (e.g. airways).

Acetylcholine acts at **nicotinic (N)** receptor subtypes at autonomic ganglia and neuromuscular junctions, and in the parasympathetic nervous system at **muscarinic (M)** receptors.

7-transmembrane receptors: many receptors are transmembraneous and are coupled to G-proteins (**G-protein-coupled receptors**, GPCR). For example, β-adrenoceptors following activation are coupled via a **G-protein**, which leads to activation of **adenylyl cyclase**, and the formation of **cAMP**, which leads to a pharmacological response. These receptors are referred to as **metabotropic** (Figure 7.1).

G-proteins: heterotrimeric proteins (α, β and γ subunits), and at rest the α subunits bind GDP, but following coupling to an activated receptor a conformation change results in exchange of GDP for GTP and the α-GTP subunit dissociates. This leads to the α-GTP subunit interacting with coupled enzymes such as adenylyl cyclase and phospholipases (releasing membrane-derived second messengers) or ion channels. There are many subtypes and they can be stimulatory or inhibitory. They undergo a cycle such that activated α-GTP has intrinsic GTPase activity, and when α-GDP is formed the subunit can reassociate with the β and γ subunits (Figure 7.2).

Intracellular or nuclear receptors: located within the cell and are activated by lipophilic molecules such as steroids, which pass through the membrane and enter the cytoplasm. Once the receptor is activated the resulting complex influences DNA transcription, resulting in the production or suppression of mRNA and target proteins, and so their effects are delayed.

Receptors coupled to enzymic activity (catalytic receptors): activation of these receptors results in activation of enzymic activity. For example, an insulin receptor has intrinsic tyrosine kinase activity, such that activation leads to autophosphorylation of tyrosine residues on the receptor, which is coupled to the cellular responses.

Receptors linked to ion channels (ligand-gated ion channels): these are **ionotropic** receptors and activation leads to altered channel function. For example, at neuromuscular junctions (NMJs) acetylcholine activates N receptors and this leads to channel opening (Chapter 22). This is part of the receptor complex and results in ion (predominantly Na$^+$) influx and depolarisation of the skeletal muscle, which ultimately leads to contraction (Figure 7.3).

Responses linked to ionotropic receptors can be inhibitory. For example, in the central nervous system (CNS) the inhibitory neurotransmitter gamma-amino butyric acid (GABA) acts at the GABA$_A$ receptor and causes activation of its chloride channel. This results in the influx of Cl$^-$ and hyperpolarisation, which reduces cell excitability. Benzodiazepines (e.g. diazepam) modulate the GABA$_A$ receptor and augment the actions of GABA.

Drug–receptor interactions

Agonists: cause receptor activation and a response, which may be either excitatory or inhibitory. A **full agonist** causes a maximum response (Figure 7.4).

Antagonist: binds to a receptor. While not causing a direct response, it prevents the receptor activation by an agonist.

Competitive antagonism: the antagonist binds at the same site as the agonist and so reduces the action of the agonist by competition. The competition may be overcome by increasing the concentration of the agonist (Figure 7.4).

Non-competitive antagonism: the antagonist binds at a site distinct from the agonist and prevents its action. For example, it might block the channel associated with the receptor or interfere with the transduc-

tion mechanism. The effects of the antagonist cannot be overcome by increasing the concentration of the agonist (Figure 7.4).

Irreversible antagonism: often due to the antagonist chemically modifying the receptor so that it prevents the action of an agonist; this cannot be reversed.

Partial agonist: causes a response but cannot elicit a full response even at its highest concentration.

Spare receptors: a full agonist can cause a maximum response without needing to occupy all receptors, and the unoccupied receptors are 'spare'. A partial agonist, even when it occupies all of its receptors, cannot elicit the maximum response and it does not have a receptor reserve of 'spare' receptors.

Inverse agonism: the drug binds to a receptor which itself has intrinsic activity, i.e. in the resting state the receptor is causing a basal response. When the drug binds it reduces the intrinsic activity and may cause a response that is opposite to that caused by an agonist.

Receptor desensitisation: repeated exposure of a receptor to an agonist may lead to a reduction in responses.

Description of drug actions

Pharmacological effects are described as concentration-dependent, with increasing concentrations causing a larger response until a maximum is achieved. The log concentration-response curve is usually sigmoidal (Figure 7.4).

EC$_{50}$: the agonist concentration that yields the half-maximal response, where the maximum is the maximal response caused by the specific agonist (Figure 7.4). It is a measure of **potency**.

Affinity: this is a measure of how well a drug binds to a receptor. The affinity constant is K$_A$ (molar^{-1}), and 1/K$_A$ is the dissociation constant, K$_d$, the concentration at which the drug occupies half of the receptor population. A high-affinity drug will have a low K$_d$.

Efficacy: how effective an agonist is at causing a response. A full agonist has high efficacy, an antagonist has zero efficacy and a partial agonist is intermediate.

Drugs can also act at other sites, which include the following.

Pumps and transporters: in the cell membrane, these systems are responsible for influx or efflux of ions, transmitters or substrates (e.g. glucose).
• Proton pump inhibitors suppress acid production from parietal cells and are used in peptic ulceration (Chapter 42).
• Inhibitors of neurotransmitter transporters are antidepressants, e.g. serotonin-selective reuptake inhibitors (SSRIs) (Chapter 57).

Ion channels: voltage-operated ion channels may be activated or inhibited by drugs, e.g. Calcium channel blockers (Chapter 32), local anaesthetics (Chapter 19).

Extracellular enzymes: usually specifically inhibited by drugs, either competitively or irreversibly, e.g. ACE inhibitors (Chapter 32).

Intracellular enzymes: usually specifically inhibited by drugs, either competitively or irreversibly, and alter enzymic activity associated with cellular processes such as synthesis or degradation, e.g. statins (Chapter 35).

DNA: anticancer drugs target rapidly dividing cells by interfering with purine/pyrimidine synthesis, chemically modifying or damaging DNA or the spindle fibres involved in mitosis (Chapter 65).

Bacterial cells and organelles: antibiotics target cellular processes such as protein synthesis (e.g. erythromycin) or bacterial structures such as the cell wall (e.g. penicillins).

Fergus Doherty

Figure 8.1 An overview of metabolism. Metabolism can be divided into energy-producing (largely in the form of ATP) catabolism and energy-consuming (largely as ATP) anabolism

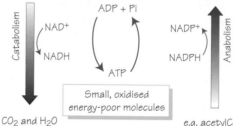

Larger, more reduced energy rich molecules, e.g. complex lipids, carbohydrates, proteins

Catabolism

Anabolism

ADP + Pi

NAD⁺

NADH

ATP

NADP⁺

NADPH

Stage 1: breakdown of complex molecules to building blocks, e.g. polysaccharides to monosaccharides

Stage 2: conversion of building blocks to acetate (as acetylCoA) – involves oxidation generating NADH and sometimes FADH$_2$

Stage 3: oxidation of acetate (acetylCoA) to CO_2 and H_2O (citric acid cycle)

Anabolism involves the formation of building blocks, e.g. amino acids, fatty acids, in reactions often involving reduction with NADPH, and the incorporation of the building blocks into large molecules, e.g. proteins, complex lipids

Small, oxidised energy-poor molecules

CO_2 and H_2O (and NH_3 from amino acids)

e.g. acetylCoA, pyruvate, amino acids, fatty acids, monosaccharides

Note: the reducing power in NADH, formed from NAD⁺ in catabolism, can be transferred to NADP⁺ to give NADPH used in anabolic pathways. Some of the ATP generated in catabolism can be used to drive anabolic reactions

---

Figure 8.2 The 'energy currency' of the cell is ATP. Energy released during catabolism is used to drive the synthesis of ATP and this ATP can be hydrolysed to release energy to drive anabolic processes

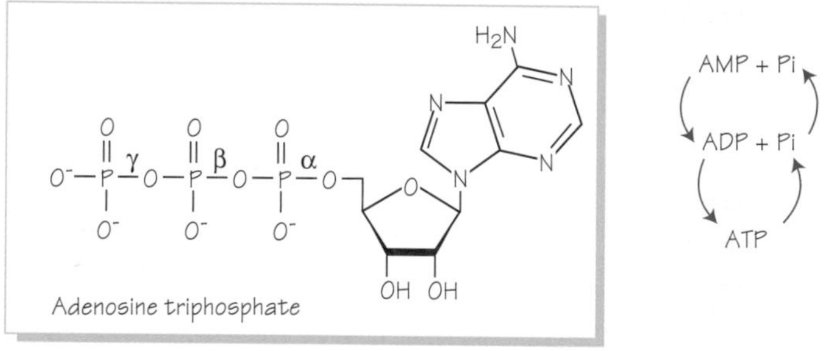

H_2N

γ   β   α

Adenosine triphosphate

AMP + Pi

ADP + Pi

ATP

The last two O–P bonds are 'high-energy' bonds. Hydrolysis of ATP to ADP and Pi (inorganic phosphate) releases energy (35.7 kJ/mol) as does hydrolysis of ADP to AMP and Pi. ADP can be formed from AMP by phosphorylation and ADP further phosphorylated to ATP, both energy-requiring steps

---

Figure 8.3 Enzymes involved in metabolism are often subject to regulation by covalent modification by the addition or removal of phosphate groups. The resulting change in enzyme activity can alter the rate of the metabolic pathway involved

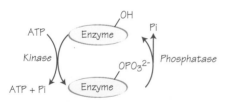

ATP

Kinase

Enzyme

OH

Pi

Phosphatase

ATP + Pi

Enzyme

OPO_3^{2-}

Enzymes that regulate metabolic pathways are often themselves regulated by addition (phosphorylation) or removal (dephosphorylation) of phosphate groups, by kinases and phosphatases respectively, on hydroxyl-containing amino acids (usually serine or threonine). ATP is the phosphate donor. The activity of the modified enzyme may increase or decrease. Phosphorylation/dephosphorylation in turn is often regulated by signalling pathways starting at the cell surface with hormone binding to a receptor. Signalling pathways may contain 'cascades' of different kinases, one phosphorylating many molecules of the next to amplify the original signal and produce a large metabolic effect

---

Metabolism can be described as the sum of the chemical reactions in an organism that produce and maintain its molecular structure, and the chemical reactions that make energy available for those processes. Metabolism can therefore be divided into anabolism and catabolism.

Anabolism

This is the production of complex molecules from more simple precursors, e.g. the synthesis of amino acids from simpler carbon skeletons and a source of amino groups, the synthesis of proteins from amino acids. These are energy-requiring processes where energy is usually consumed in the form of adenosine triphosphate (ATP). The end products are often more reduced than the simple precursors, and so reducing power, in the form of NADPH, is often required (Figure 8.1).

Catabolism

This is the destruction or disassembly of complex molecules, often ultimately leading to the release of chemical energy, which is usually stored in the form of ATP (Figure 8.1). Examples of catabolism include the breakdown of complex lipids (fats) to glycerol and fatty acids, and the oxidation of the resulting fatty acids in mitochondria (**β-oxidation**) to acetyl coenzyme A, which in turn can be further oxidised to carbon dioxide and water (**TCA cycle**). Both processes lead to the reduction of NAD^+ to NADH, which in turn can be used to drive the formation of ATP.

Energy requirements

It follows from the above that to maintain cells and, in addition, to support cell growth and division, energy is continually required. Note that many key molecules, especially proteins, once made do not last forever but rather are subject to turnover, that is continual synthesis and degradation back to amino acids. This turnover requires energy, therefore simply to maintain the normal complement of cellular proteins, outside of growth, requires energy input. The average daily energy requirement of a sedentary women is just under 2000 kcal/day, rising to 3080 kcal/day for a very active person. This energy is supplied by the oxidation of fuel molecules: carbohydrates, fats (lipids) and proteins, with carbohydrate being the major fuel for most humans. To sustain growth or support pregnancy, the calorific requirement will rise. If the calorific intake does not match the demands made on the organism then mechanisms will be invoked to try and match those demands by utilising stored fuels, such as fat reserves, and even by the breakdown of body proteins and oxidation of the resulting amino acids. It is recommended that human calorific intake should be 55% from carbohydrates, 30% from fats (lipids) and 15% from protein.

High-energy phosphates

Cellular oxidation releases some energy as heat but most is trapped in the form of a 'high-energy' molecule. These high-energy molecules include ATP (and also adenosine diphosphate, ADP) and creatine phosphate. ATP consists of an adenine base attached to a ribose sugar (adenosine) (Figure 8.2a). Three phosphate groups are attached sequentially to carbon atom 5 of the ribose (Figure 8.2b). To add a phosphate to adenosine monophosphate (AMP) to form ADP requires more energy than for most covalent bonds. This may be explained in a simple way as being necessary to overcome the resistance of AMP (already negatively charged due to the phosphate) to the addition of another negative charge. To add yet another phosphate requires even more energy because of the two phosphate groups on ADP. It follows that more energy is released when these bonds between the phosphates are broken. ATP, therefore, can serve as a short-term energy 'store' and is referred to as the 'energy currency' of the cell. The oxidation of fuels ultimately leads to phosphorylation of ADP to ATP and the ATP is used to drive energy-requiring processes as the hydrolysis of ATP to ADP is linked to an energy-requiring reaction. Another important high-energy phosphate is creatine phosphate, which is abundant in muscle. When ATP is used to support muscle contraction the resulting ADP is phosphorylated to ATP by transfer of the high-energy phosphate from creatine phosphate.

How is ATP generated? The oxidation reactions in cells, which are exergonic (release energy), are coupled to the reduction of a small molccule, most often nicotinamide adenine dinucleotide or NAD^+ to NADH, i.e. an electron is transferred from the molecule oxidised to NAD^+. Under aerobic conditions NADH is then re-oxidised by the electron transport chain in mitochondria, which pumps protons across the **inner mitochondrial membrane** (IMM). The subsequent flow of these protons back across the IMM drives the phsophorylation of ADP by inorganic phosphate to form ATP. The electrons are ultimately transferred to molecular oxygen to form water.

Enzymes and regulation (Chapter 9)

Metabolic reactions, like all biological reactions, are catalysed by enzymes. Organisms need to regulate these metabolic pathways to match the supply of energy (catabolism) with their requirements (anabolism). Regulation of these enzymes is therefore key to regulating the pathway. Enzyme activity responds to changes in substrate concentration, but enzymes may also be regulated by changes in the concentration of small molecules that may not be the substrate but, for example, the end product of a pathway. As the concentration of the end product increases this will inhibit the activity of an early enzyme in that pathway, thus preventing an unwanted build-up of end product and wastage of the starting material. This is an example of 'end product inhibition or 'negative feedback'. Enzymes may also be regulated by covalent modification, especially addition of a phosphate to the protein, known as phosphorylation. This modification may activate or inhibit the enzyme. **Phosphorylation** and **dephosphorylation** of specific enzymes, by **kinases** and **phosphatases**, is often in turn regulated by hormone signals and in this way hormones can regulate metabolic pathways (Figure 8.3).

9 Enzymes

Michael D Randall

Figure 9.1 Rate of reaction plot for enzymic reactions that obey Michaelis-Menten kinetics

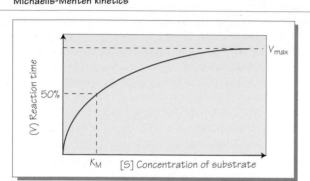

Figure 9.2 The double reciprocal or Lineweaver-Burke plot

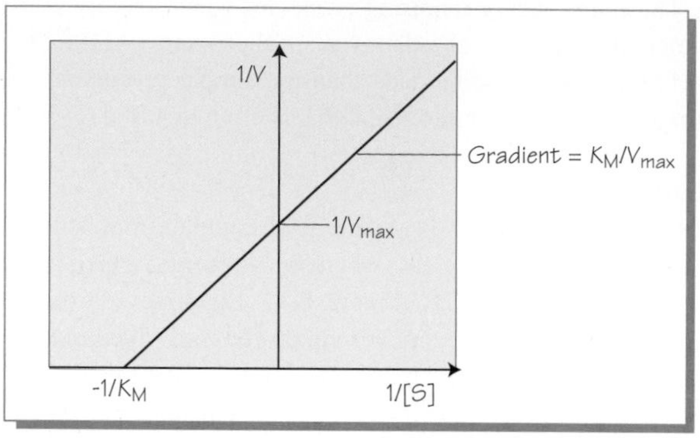

Figure 9.3 The characteristic effects of a competitive and a non-competitive inhibitor on enzymic activity as shown on the Lineweaver-Burke plot

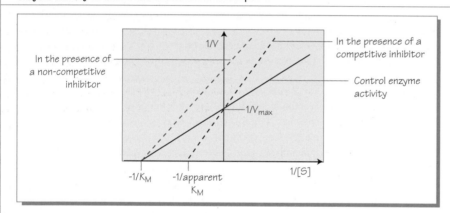

Medical Sciences at a Glance, First Edition. Edited by Michael D Randall. © 2014 John Wiley & Sons, Ltd. Published 2014 by John Wiley & Sons, Ltd.

Enzymes are biological catalysts that are involved in most biochemical reactions. As with catalysts in chemistry, they speed up chemical reactions and this is achieved by lowering the activation energy for a chemical reaction. Most enzymes are proteins, an important exception being rRNA, which has peptidyl transferase enzyme activity (Chapter 15).

Characteristics of enzymes

The proteinacious nature of enzymes means that they often show:

Activation: many enzymes are released as inactive precursors that can be activated, for example by hydrolysis, which then liberates the active enzyme. An example of this is the coagulation cascade in blood, in which the activation of a coagulation factor from its precursor involves cleavage.

pH dependence: changes in pH can affect the protein structure and function. For example, gastric enzymes such as **pepsins** are activated at acidic pH in the stomach but inactivated as they enter the small intestine at pH 5.3.

Temperature sensitivity: many enzymes show temperature dependence and undergo substantial increases in activity with small increases in temperature. Enzymic activity is usually optimal at the physiological temperature of 37°C. Increasing temperature can destroy the protein structure and lead to **denaturation**.

Enzyme kinetics
Michaelis-Menten kinetics

This is a relatively simple model that accounts for enzyme kinetics. It takes account of the substrate concentration in relation to the rate of reaction.

The Michaelis-Menten equation is summarised:

$$V = \frac{V_{max}[S]}{[S] + K_M},$$

where V = rate of reaction (number moles produced per unit time), V_{max} = maximum rate of reaction, [S] = concentration of substrate, K_M = Michaelis constant.

The K_M is defined as the concentration of substrate at which the rate of reaction (V) is half of the maximal reaction (V_{max}). The K_M value is typically in the range of 10^{-1}–10^{-6} M, where a low concentration indicates high affinity of the enzyme for the substrate. As it is the concentration at which half of the enzyme's active sites are occupied by substrate, it is affected by factors such as pH and temperature. The V_{max} occurs when all of the active sites are occupied and the enzyme is **saturated**, and is therefore dependent on the quantity of enzyme present.

Figure 9.1 summarises the plot reaction for an enzyme that obeys Michaelis-Menten kinetics.

Enzyme inhibition

Enzymes can be inhibited by **competitive** and **non-competitive inhibitors**. Competitive inhibitors literally compete with the substrate for the active site and so the inhibition can be overcome by increasing the concentration of the substrate. Generally, the competitive inhibitor is similar to the substrate but unreactive. An example of this are the statins, which inhibit the HMG CoA reductase enzyme in cholesterol synthesis.

A non-competitive inhibitor may bind at a site distinct from the active site and decreases enzymic activity. In contrast to competitive inhibitors, the effects of non-competitive inhibitors cannot be overcome by increasing the concentration of the substrate. Examples include heavy metals such as Pb^{2+} binding to enzymes and reducing their activity.

Irreversible inhibitors bind to the enzyme and this interaction is irreversible and the enzymic activity is blocked. An example of this is the interaction between penicillins and the transpeptidases responsible for cross-linking peptidoglycans in the bacterial cell wall.

Characteristically, a competitive inhibitor does not affect V_{max}, but there is an apparent decrease in K_M, whereas a non-competitive inhibitor decreases V_{max} and K_M remains unchanged. The effects of inhibitors can be analysed by the double reciprocal plot (1/V vs 1/[S]; the Lineweaver-Burke plot) (Figures 9.2 and 9.3).

Allosteric modulation

As enzymes are invariably proteins with quaternary structures, the binding of modulatory molecules can lead to conformational changes, which can result in increased or decreased enzymic activity. This allows physiological control of enzymic activity in relation to the body's needs. A key example of this is phosphorylation of pyruvate dehydrogenase, which reduces activity, whereas dephosphorylation increases activity.

Key enzymic activities

The suffix '-ase' usually indicates an enzyme, here are some key terms and enzymes.

ATPase: involved in ATP dephosphorylation to provide energy, e.g. to drive pumps (e.g. $3Na^+/2K^+$ ATPase) (Chapter 18).

Cofactors: these are non-protein components that are required for correct enzymic activity. Examples include ions such as Zn^{2+}, haem groups and coenzyme A. A prosthetic group is present when the cofactor is bound and a coenzyme is a more loosely associated.

Cyclases: these lead to formation of cyclic structures via cyclisation, e.g. adenylyl cyclase leads to the formation of cAMP as a second messenger from ATP (Chapter 7).

Isomerases: lead to isomerisation.

Kinases: phosphorylate targets, e.g. tyrosine kinases leads to phosphorylation of kinases in cell signalling (Chapter 7).

Ligases: connect molecules via covalent bonds.

Lipases: breakdown lipids, e.g. breakdown of lipids in digestion (Chapter 43).

Oxidases: lead to oxidation.

Phosphatases: dephosphorylate targets.

Proteases: break down proteins. Involved in protein digestion, and many coagulation factors when active are serine proteases, which cleave at serine residues.

Reductase: lead to reduction, e.g. dihydrofolate reductase involved in folate metabolism in purine synthesis (Chapter 65).

Synthase: a synthetic enzyme, e.g. nitric oxide synthase (Chapter 31).

Transferases: transfer a functional group, e.g. choline acetyltransferase in the synthesis of acetylcholine (Chapter 20).

Fergus Doherty

Figure 10.1 The formation of acetylCoA

AcetylCoA is formed by the β-oxidation of fatty acids and the oxidative decarboxylation of pyruvate, following transport across the inner mitochondrial membrane, by pyruvate dehydrogenase (PDH), a multi-enzyme complex in the mitochondrial matrix. PDH is regulated by phosphorylation (inactivates) and dephosphorylation (activates) by a kinase and phosphatase, which are in turn allosterically and hormonally regulated. The reverse reaction is catalysed by a separate enzyme in gluconeogenesis–pyruvate carboxylase

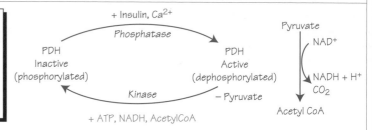

Figure 10.2 The TCA cycle

The TCA cycle takes place in mitochondria and starts with the condensation of the two carbon acetyl CoA with oxaloacetate to form citrate. Two carbon atoms are lost as CO_2 for each round of the cycle, which generates NADH and $FADH_2$, which yield ATP via oxidative phosphorylation, and a molecule of GTP, which can be used to phosphorylate ADP to ATP. The acetylCoA can come from the PDH reaction (above) or from the β-oxidation of fatty acids

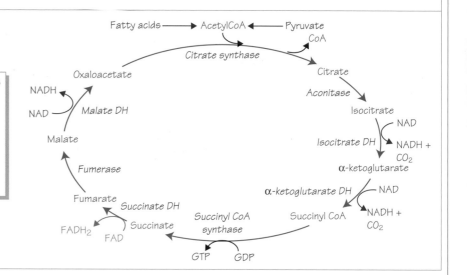

Figure 10.3 Oxidative phosphorylation

ATP is generated from reduced co-enzymes NADH and $FADH_2$ via the electron transport chain on the inner mitochondrial membrane and the activity of ATP synthase. The flow of electrons from along the chain drives the pumping of protons from the matrix to the intermembrane space to create an electrochemical gradient. The flow of these protons through the ATP synthase back into the matrix drives a conformational change in the synthase, which in turn leads to the phosphorylation of ADP to ATP. An ATP/ADP exchanger in the inner membrane allows ATP to cross out of the matrix in exchange for ADP

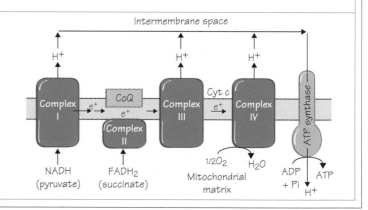

Catabolism of lipids, carbohydrates and the carbon skeletons of some amino acids converge on acetylCoA. **AcetylCoA** is a precursor for ketone bodies (acetoacetate and β-hydroxybutyrate) and for the biosynthesis of fatty acids (under anabolic conditions), and is also fed into the tricarboxylic acid cycle (**TCA cycle, citric acid cycle, Krebs cycle**), which generates substantial amounts of energy in the form of ATP and reduced co-factors (**NADH, FADH$_2$**) which in turn generate ATP via the electron transport chain.

The Link Reaction – pyruvate dehydrogenase

Pyruvate, generated by the **glycolytic pathway** or from **amino acid metabolism**, can be transported across the inner mitochondrial membrane into the matrix and oxidatively decarboxylated to acetylcoenzyme A (acetylCoA) by the multi-enzyme complex **pyruvate dehydrogenase** (PDH). The product of the reaction, acetylCoA, can enter the TCA cycle. Pyruvate dehydrogenase is regulated by phosphorylation and dephosphorylation by a dedicated kinase and phosphatase. Phosphorylation by the kinase, which is allosterically activated by high levels of 'high-energy' molecules (ATP, acetylCoA, NADH, inactivates PDH (Figure 10.1). In this way, PDH responds to the energy needs of the cell, only producing acetylCoA when energy, generated from the TCA cycle, is required. In skeletal muscle, calcium ions, which increase during muscle contraction, also stimulate the PDH phosphatase, which in turn activates PDH by dephosphorylation. The phosphorylation status of PDH is also regulated in the liver by the hormones insulin and glucagon. During the fed state (high blood glucose) the high insulin:glucagon ratio activates PDH phosphatase and PDH is dephosphorylated and active, the resulting acetylCoA being used in the TCA cycle or for fatty acid synthesis. During fasting/starvation the high glucagon:insulin ratio favours PDH phosphorylation and inhibition, therefore sparing pyruvate for gluconeogenesis.

The TCA cycle

In many tissues, the major fate for acetylCoA will be oxidation via the TCA cycle to CO_2 and H_2O (Figure 10.2). Most of these reactions take place in the mitochondrial matrix and start with condensation of acetylCoA with oxaloacetate to form citrate (citrate can act as a source of acetylCoA for fatty acid synthesis), which is then isomerised to isocitrate. The oxidative decarboxylation of isocitrate to α-ketoglutarate generates CO_2 and NADH (+ H$^+$) and the α-ketoglutarate is oxidatively decarboxylated to succinylCoA and produces another molecule of NADH. SuccinylCoA is cleaved to succinate, yielding the high-energy phosphate molecule GTP (which subsequently generates ATP), and then oxidised to fumarate, yielding FADH$_2$. Fumarate is hydrated to form malate, which is oxidised to oxaloacetate, producing another NADH, and the oxaloacetate can accept another acetylCoA to repeat the cycle. In this way, oxaloacetate acts as a 'carrier' for acetate, which is completely oxidised to CO_2 and H_2O yielding 3 x NADH, 1 x FADH$_2$ and 1 x GTP (=ATP). Each NADH generates around 3 ATP and the FADH$_2$ 1 ATP via the electron transport chain, so there is a yield of 12 ATP for each acetate oxidised.

The electron transport chain (ETC) and oxidative phosphorylation

Reduced coenzymes, NADH and FADH$_2$, produced by the TCA cycle, the PDH reaction, oxidation of fatty acids and other reactions, can be oxidised in mitochondria via the electron transport (respiratory chain) to reduce oxygen to water and phosphorylate ADP to ATP (oxidative phosphorylation) (Figure 10.3). The **electron transport chain**, located in the convoluted inner mitochondrial membrane, which is impermeable to most ions, comprises **Complexes I-IV** of various proteins and coenzyme Q (ubiquinone). A hydride (H$^-$) from NADH and a proton (H$^+$) are transferred to Complex I (NADH dehydrogenase) to reduce the coenzyme FMN to FMNH$_2$. Hydrogens from the coenzyme FADH$_2$ (e.g. from the oxidation of succinate) are transferred to Complex II. The hydrogens from both Complex I and Complex II are transferred to coenzyme Q, which transfers electrons to Complex III (cytochrome bc$_1$). Complex III donates electrons to cytochrome c and from there they are transferred to Complex IV (cytochromes a + a$_3$). Cytochrome a$_3$ is then able to donate the electrons to O_2, which combines with H$^+$ in solution to form water. As oxygen is required as the final electron acceptor this is aerobic respiration and the ETC is also called the respiratory chain.

It is thought that the flow of electrons along the ETC drives the **pumping of protons** out of the mitochondrial matrix and into the inter membrane space to create a proton (charge and pH) gradient (the **chemiosmotic hypothesis**). The inner mitochondrial membrane is impermeable to protons except for Complex V (ATP synthase). Flow of protons down the concentration gradient through ATP synthase results in a conformation change (rotation) in the protein, which in turn provides the energy for phosphorylation of ADP to ATP by the synthase.

Oligomycin is a small molecule that blocks the proton channel in Complex V (ATP synthase), thus preventing the flow of protons into the matrix and the production of ATP. The build up of the proton gradient prevents any further electron flow along the ETC – electron transport and phosphorylation are coupled. These processes can be uncoupled by molecules that allow the protons to flow back across the inner mitochondrial membrane without passing through Complex V, such as 2,4-dinitrophenol, when the energy is dissipated as heat. Toxic doses of salicylate (aspirin) have the same effect. Uncoupling proteins (e.g. **UCP1** or thermogenin) are found in brown adipose tissue and therefore lead to heat generation (non-shivering thermogenesis), although humans have little brown adipose tissue.

Fergus Doherty

Figure 11.1 Low blood glucose leads to release of fatty acids acids from adipose to the circulation

TAG = triacylglycerol
FFA = free fatty acids

Low blood glucose in fasting/starvation leads to increased glucogon, which activates hormone-sensitive lipase of adipocytes leading to TAG hydrolysis. Free fatty acids are carried in the plasma bound to albumin and taken up by tissues (e.g. skeletal muscle, liver), where they are oxidised in mitochondria to acetylCoA

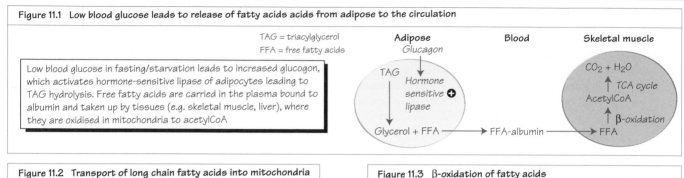

Adipose   **Blood**   **Skeletal muscle**

Glucagon

TAG

Hormone
sensitive ⊕
lipase

Glycerol + FFA ⟶ FFA-albumin ⟶ FFA

$CO_2 + H_2O$
↑ TCA cycle
AcetylCoA
↑ β-oxidation

Figure 11.2 Transport of long chain fatty acids into mitochondria

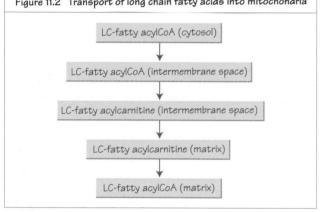

LC-fatty acylCoA (cytosol)

↓

LC-fatty acylCoA (intermembrane space)

↓

LC-fatty acylcarnitine (intermembrane space)

↓

LC-fatty acylcarnitine (matrix)

↓

LC-fatty acylCoA (matrix)

Figure 11.4 Ketone body metabolism

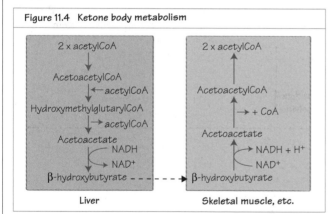

2 x acetylCoA

↓

AcetoacetylCoA
← acetylCoA

HydroxymethylglutarylCoA
← acetylCoA

Acetoacetate
↘ NADH
↘ NAD+

β-hydroxybutyrate ⇠ ⇠ ⇢ β-hydroxybutyrate

Liver

2 x acetylCoA

↑

AcetoacetylCoA
↗ + CoA

Acetoacetate
↗ NADH + H+
↗ NAD+

β-hydroxybutyrate

Skeletal muscle, etc.

Figure 11.3 β-oxidation of fatty acids

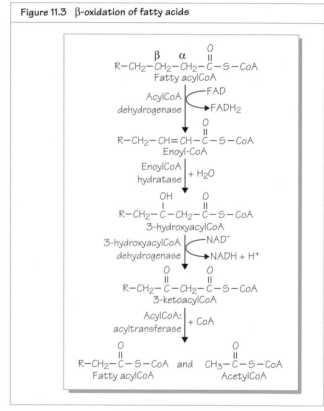

$$R-CH_2-CH_2-CH_2-\overset{\overset{O}{||}}{C}-S-CoA$$
(β   α)
Fatty acylCoA

AcylCoA
dehydrogenase ⟩ FAD → FADH₂

$$R-CH_2-CH=CH-\overset{\overset{O}{||}}{C}-S-CoA$$
Enoyl-CoA

EnoylCoA
hydratase | + H₂O

$$R-CH_2-\overset{OH}{\underset{|}{C}}-CH_2-\overset{\overset{O}{||}}{C}-S-CoA$$
3-hydroxyacylCoA

3-hydroxyacylCoA
dehydrogenase ⟩ NAD⁻ → NADH + H⁺

$$R-CH_2-\overset{\overset{O}{||}}{C}-CH_2-\overset{\overset{O}{||}}{C}-S-CoA$$
3-ketoacylCoA

AcylCoA:
acyltransferase | + CoA

$$R-CH_2-\overset{\overset{O}{||}}{C}-S-CoA \quad and \quad CH_3-\overset{\overset{O}{||}}{C}-S-CoA$$
Fatty acylCoA   AcetylCoA

Lipids (fats and oils) are a high-energy source yielding twice the energy per gram of protein and carbohydrate. Around 30% of calorific intake by humans is currently recommended, as an upper limit, to be in the form of lipid. Lipids are utilised as a fuel during fasting, starvation and stress, when fatty acids are mobilised from the storage lipid triacyglycerol, stored in adipose tissue, and are metabolised by tissues such as skeletal muscle and liver, but not by the brain or erythrocytes. Fatty acid oxidation yields energy and **acetylCoA (acetylCoA)**, which feeds into the **tricarboxylic acid (TCA) cycle** or in the liver is used to make **ketone bodies**.

Lipolysis

Low blood glucose concentrations trigger the release of glucagon by the pancreas, which in turn activates a hormone-sensitive lipase in adipose cells (adipocytes), which in turn hydrolyses triacyglycerol to free fatty acids and glycerol (Figure 11.1). **Glucagon** binding to its cell-surface receptor leads to an increase in intracellular cAMP, which activates **protein kinase A**, which phosphorylates and activates **hormone-sensitive lipase**. The resulting free fatty acids are released to the circulation, bound to the plasma protein albumin, from where they can be taken up by other tissues. Fatty acids freely pass the plasma membrane into the cytosol but cannot cross the blood–brain barrier. The glycerol, released from triacyglycerol breakdown, is transported to liver, phosphorylated to glycerol 3-phosphate and converted to **dihydroxyacetone phosphate** (DHAP). DHAP can be used in glycolysis or more likely converted to glucose via gluconeogenesis to provide glucose for glucose-dependent tissues.

Metabolism of fatty acids
Activation of fatty acids and transport into mitochondria

Long-chain (>12 C) fatty acids are activated in the cytosol by esterification to **coenzyme A (CoA)**, an ATP-consuming process, to form acylCoA esters (Figure 11.2). Oxidation of fatty acids occurs in the mitochondria, but the inner membrane is impermeable to acylCoA. Consequently the acyl group is transferred to carnitine and the acylcarnitine is transferred to the matrix using a shuttle system. Once in the matrix the long-chain acyl group is transferred to CoA and the carnitine exported to the cytosol via the shuttle. Short (2–4 C) and medium-chain (6–10 C) fatty acids pass directly into the mitochondrial matrix and form acylCoA there.

Oxidation of fatty acids

Fatty acids are oxidised in the mitochondria by **β-oxidation**, which cleaves two carbons off the fatty acid from the carboxyl end, as acetylCoA, for each round of oxidation (Figure 11.3). First the fatty acyl CoA is oxidised by a family of **acylCoA dehydrogenases** to yield $FADH_2$ and an enoylCoA with a double bond between carbon atoms 2 and 3 (the β-carbon). This is then hydrated to form a hydroxyl group at position 3 and further oxidised to yield a carbonyl group at position 3 (a ketoacylCoA) and NADH (and H^+). The ketoacylCoA is cleaved between carbons 2 and 3 to yield acetylCoA and a fatty acylCoA shortened by two carbons. The shortened fatty acylCoA enters β-oxidation again until it is all converted to acetylCoA. The $FADH_2$ and NADH produced can be oxidised via the electron transport chain (ETC) to generate 2 and 3 ATP. Each acetylCoA generates 12 ATP via the TCA cycle and the electron transport chain, so large amounts of ATP are generated from the complete oxidation of fatty acids. Very-long-chain fatty acids are first subject to β-oxidation in peroxisomes until short enough to be oxidised in mitochondria. Various additional enzymatic steps are also available to allow the oxidation of unsaturated and odd-numbered fatty acids. ω-oxidation (from the methyl end) occurs in the endoplasmic reticulum, especially if there is a problem with β-oxidation, and leads to the excretion of dicarboxylic acids.

Ketone bodies

In the initial stages of starvation, fatty acids are mobilised from adipose and oxidised in liver and skeletal muscle (low insulin results in low glucose uptake by muscle), sparing glucose for glucose-dependent tissues. The brain and red blood cells cannot utilise fatty acids. From about three days of starvation the high levels of acetylCoA in the liver from fatty acid oxidation cannot all be consumed in the TCA cycle and are surplus to the liver's energy needs. The acetylCoA is diverted to the formation of the ketone bodies, acetoacetone and β-hydroxybutyrate (Figure 11.4), and individuals are said to be **ketotic**. β-hydroxybutyrate is formed from the reduction of acetoacetate resulting from the high levels of NADH generated by fatty acid oxidation. The ketone bodies are released to the circulation and utilised by the kidneys and then the brain, so that eventually 75% of the brain's energy needs are met by ketone bodies. The liver cannot utilise ketone bodies, which in other tissues are converted to acetylCoA which enters the TCA cycle. High levels of ketone bodies reduce skeletal muscle breakdown during starvation. When the ketone body concentration in the plasma reaches 7 mM the tissues are saturated and ketones appear in the urine (ketonuria). Very high levels of plasma ketones reduce blood pH, leading to a form of metabolic acidosis – **ketoacidosis** – which can be life threatening and can occur in uncontrolled diabetes.

12 Glucose metabolism

Fergus Doherty

Figure 12.1 Hormonal changes in response to glucose ingestion

Following a meal containing carbohydrate, glucagon levels fall and insulin levels rise, which promotes insulin uptake by tissues and therefore a drop in blood glucose. The fall in blood glucose eventually leads to a drop in insulin and a rise in glucagon, which triggers glucose release from the liver, therefore these hormone help to maintain glucose homeostasis

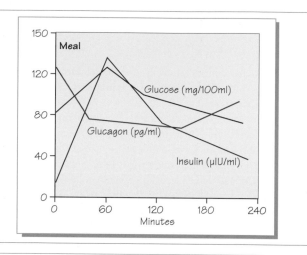

Figure 12.2 Glucose metabolism

Glycolysis and gluconeogenesis showing key enzymes (italics). Glycolysis is an energy-yielding pathway ending in pyruvate, found in all cells. In aerobic conditions pyruvate is oxidatively decarboxylated to acetate (as acetylCoA), which can then enter the TCA cycle. In anaerobic conditions pyruvate is reduced to lactate to regenerate NAD^+, tissues such as skeletal muscle release lactate, which can be utilised by the heart after conversion back to pyruvate and then to acetylCoA, or converted to pyruvate and then to glucose (gluconeogenesis) in the liver

Gluconeogenesis occurs in the liver when blood glucose is low and is the formation of glucose from amino acids via pyruvate, or glycerol (from triacylglycerol) via dihydroxyacetone phosphate. Much of gluconeogenesis is the reverse of glycolysis except for the steps shown in green. Removal of the phosphate from glucose by glucose-6-phosphatase allows the glucose to be released from the liver to the blood

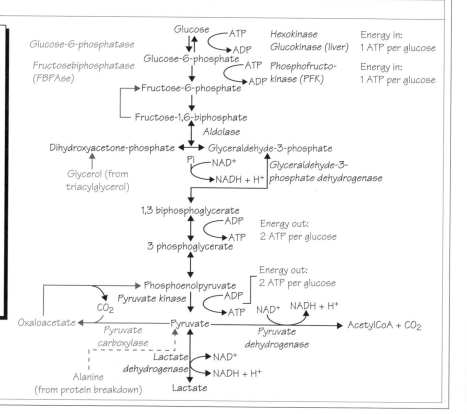

Approximately 55% of the energy needs of the average human are met by the metabolism of carbohydrates, of which the major component is glucose. The glucose concentration in the blood is maintained at 4–8 mmol/L (glucose homeostasis) largely by the action of hormones such as **insulin** and **glucagon** (Figure 12.1 and Chapter 46). The majority of carbohydrates in the diet are polysaccharides, which are digested in the gastrointestinal tract to mono- and disaccharides by amylases and other enzymes.

Glucose uptake

Glucose is transported into the enterocytes of the gastrointestinal tract by an energy-requiring process against a concentration gradient and then passes down a concentration gradient into the plasma (Chapter 43). Uptake of glucose from the plasma into tissues is mediated by a family of **glucose transporters (GLUTs)**. GLUT4 in adipose and skeletal muscle is dependent on insulin for activity, while GLUT 1 and 3 (brain, erythrocytes) are not. GLUT2 in liver and kidney is insulin independent and can also transport glucose out to the plasma. On entry into the cell, glucose is phosphorylated by **hexokinase** (all tissues) or **glucokinase** (liver) to **glucose-6-phosphate**, which traps it in the cell. Glucokinase is only active at high glucose concentrations.

Glucose metabolism (Figure 12.2)

Glycolysis

All cells are capable of glycolysis. The first stage of glycolysis consumes ATP due to glucose phosphorylation, and then as **glucose-6-phosphate** is converted to fructose-6-phosphate and then phosphorylated by the regulatory enzyme of glycolysis, **phosphofructokinase-1** (PFK-1), to fructose-1,6-bisphosphate. PFK-1 is activated by low ATP concentrations and high ADP and AMP concentrations, as the purpose of glycolysis is to produce ATP. Fructose-1,6-bisphosphate is cleaved to two three-carbon glyceraldehyde-3-phosphate, which is subject to oxidation, generating two molecules of NADH in total, and phosphorylation (not requiring ATP) before 4 ATP is generated for every glucose molecule in energy-yielding steps, leading to the formation of the end product pyruvate. The net yield is 2 ATP for each molecule of glucose, but a further 6 ATP can be generated from the oxidation by the electron transport chain of the 2 NADH produced, and in aerobic conditions the pyruvate can be converted to acetylCoA, which enters the TCA cycle (Chapter 10) to generate more ATP. Under anaerobic conditions, e.g. in skeletal muscle or in erythrocytes (without mitochondria), NADH cannot be oxidised in this way, but instead pyruvate is reduced to lactate to regenerate NAD^+ to allow glycolysis to continue. Lactate from these tissues is released to the plasma and converted back to pyruvate in the heart, which respires aerobically, or the liver, where the pyruvate is used to synthesise glucose (**gluconeogenesis**), which is released back to the circulation (the **Cori cycle**).

Pentose phosphate pathway

In some tissues (adipose, liver), when glucose concentrations are high glucose-6-phosphate is fed into the pentose phosphate pathway. This pathway generates NADPH, a co-factor used in the biosynthesis of fatty acids which is important in both these tissues, and ribose-5-phosphate used in nucleotide biosynthesis.

Glycogen metabolism

Glucose comes not only from the diet but also from body stores of glycogen, a glucose polymer, in particular in the skeletal muscle and liver. When blood glucose levels are low, glucagon released from the pancreas causes the activation of **glycogen phosphorylase**. This breaks down glycogen to glucose-1-phosphate, which is converted to glucose-6-phosphate, which in turn can enter glycolysis. Low cellular concentrations of ATP and high AMP in muscle also activate this enzyme. While muscle utilises the glucose-6-phosphate, in liver much of this will be converted to glucose by glucose-6-phosphatase and the resulting glucose will be released to the circulation to maintain glucose homeostasis.

Gluconeogenesis

The liver is capable of producing glucose, not just from glycogen but also from other, non-carbohydrate, sources (gluconeogenesis). Alanine, produced in skeletal muscle from amino acids released following protein degradation during fasting/starvation (low blood glucose, low insulin, high glucagon), is taken up by the liver, deaminated (to form urea) and the resulting pyruvate can be converted back to glucose by gluconeogenesis and released to the plasma.

Glucose utilisation and homeostasis

Following ingestion of carbohydrate the plasma concentration rises to 7–8 mmol/L, triggering the release of insulin from the pancreas, which stimulates glucose uptake into muscle and adipose as well as glycogen synthesis in liver and muscle. The result is a lowering of blood glucose concentration. During fasting, blood glucose levels drop to about 4 mmol/L, triggering glucagon release and a fall in insulin. This stimulates glycogen breakdown, allowing the liver to release glucose to the blood, while gluconeogenesis in the liver increases and glycolysis decreases. In this way blood glucose levels are kept from falling too low, as the brain and erythrocytes are dependent on glucose as a fuel.

Amino acid metabolism

Jane Arnold

Figure 13.1 The fate of amino acids

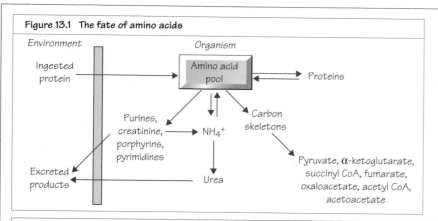

Table 13.1 Glucogenic and ketogenic amino acids

Ketogenic	Both	Glucogenic	
Leu	Iso	Ala	Cys
Lys	Trp	Gly	Ser
	Phe	Asp	Asn
	Tyr	Met	
	Thr	Val	Glu
		Gln	His
		Pro	Arg

Figure 13.2 Transamination and deamination reactions

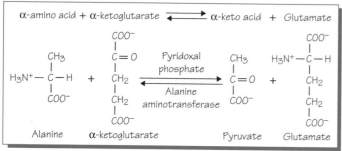

(a) Transamination reaction

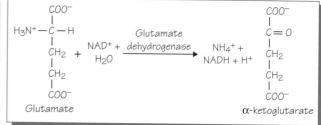

(b) Oxidative deamination of glutamate

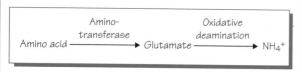

(c) Overall reaction of ammonium ion production

Figure 13.3 The urea cycle

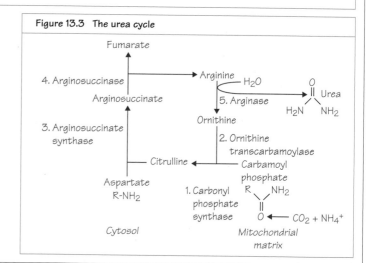

Medical Sciences at a Glance, First Edition. Edited by Michael D Randall. © 2014 John Wiley & Sons, Ltd. Published 2014 by John Wiley & Sons, Ltd.

Amino acid synthesis

Of the 20 amino acids needed for protein synthesis, humans are only able to make 11. These are termed the **non-essential amino acids** and are made by either *de novo* pathways or by conversion from existing amino acids. These pathways involve, in the first instance, the addition of an amino group to a carbon skeleton via a **transaminase reaction**. The other nine amino acids are termed **essential amino acids** and have to be obtained from the diet. In a well-nourished adult approximately 50 g of dietary protein is required daily.

The amino acid pool and protein turnover

A major source of amino acids is from the hydrolysis of dietary protein as well as from the breakdown of cellular protein. These sources, in addition to synthesised amino acids, give rise to a pool of free amino acids within the body (Figure 13.1). Cellular protein is continuously undergoing synthesis and breakdown in a process known as **protein turnover**, which allows damaged or abnormal proteins to be removed from the body. This is a highly regulated process and approximately 400 g of cellular protein is degraded and re-synthesised each day. In a well-nourished adult the rate of protein synthesis is equal to the rate of protein degradation.

Formation of nitrogen-containing molecules

Amino acids are precursors to a number of important nitrogen-containing molecules. These include **porphyrins** (e.g. heme groups), **purines** and **pyrimidines** (e.g. nucleotides for DNA synthesis; Chapter 15), **neurotransmitters** (e.g. dopamine, noradrenaline) and **creatine** (found in muscle as the high-energy molecule creatine phosphate) (Figure 13.1).

Catabolism of amino acids

Unlike fatty acids and carbohydrate, amino acids cannot be stored in the body. Consequently any surplus amino acids have to be broken down. This involves the removal of the α-amino group to form an ammonium ion, which will in turn be converted to urea via the urea cycle. The remaining carbon skeletons are then further metabolised to form intermediates used in energy production. The main reactions are are as follows.

Removal of the α-amino group via transamination

The α-amino group of the amino acid is removed by an enzyme reaction known as **transamination** and is catalysed by an **aminotransferase** enzyme (also called a transaminase). Two of the most important aminotransferases are alanine aminotransferase (ALT) and aspartate aminotransferase (AST), which are highly expressed in the liver (Chapter 44). In this reaction the α-amino group of the amino acid is transferred to α-ketoglutarate to produce the corresponding α-keto acid and glutamate, e.g. alanine aminotransferase transfers the amino group of alanine to α-ketoglutarate to form glutamate and its corresponding α-keto acid, pyruvate (see Figure 13.2a). Similarly, aspartate aminotransferase catalyses the deamination of aspartate to form glutamate and its corresponding α-keto acid, oxaloacetate. All aminotransferases require pyridoxal phosphate (derived from vitamin B6) as a cofactor. These reactions are near equilibrium, so they can also be used to synthesise amino acids, e.g. alanine will be produced when levels of pyruvate and glutamate are high and alanine levels are low.

Formation of the ammonium ion via oxidative deamination

Following on from transamination, the enzyme glutamate dehydrogenase releases the amino group from glutamate to form the ammonium ion and α-ketoglutarate (Figures 13.2b and 13.2c). This enzyme can use either NAD^+ or $NADP^+$ as a coenzyme.

Formation of urea

A series of reactions known as the urea cycle takes place in the liver, where the highly toxic ammonium ion is converted into urea (Figure 13.3). The first two reactions of the urea cycle occur in the mitochondria to produce citrulline, which is then transported into the cytosol, where the remaining reactions occur. Urea is then transported in the blood to the kidneys, where it is excreted as urine. The two nitrogen atoms in urea come from one **ammonium ion** and one molecule of **aspartate.**

Metabolism of the remaining carbon skeletons

The carbon skeletons of amino acids are an important energy source and are used under certain metabolic conditions, e.g. short-term starvation, for energy production. Amino acids are defined as being glucogenic or ketogenic (Table 13.1). Glucogenic amino acids are those that will form pyruvate, or the TCA cycle intermediates α-ketoglutarate, oxaloacetate, succinyl CoA, or fumarate. They will primarily be used in gluconeogenesis to form glucose (in the liver) and are an important source of glucose in short-term starvation. Ketogenic amino acids form acetylCoA or the ketone body acetoacetate. Leucine and lysine are the only two amino acids that are purely ketogenic. The ability of amino acids to be converted into these metabolic intermediates means that amino acids, when in excess, have the ability to form **glucose, fatty acids** (from acetylCoA) and **ketone bodies**.

Aminoacidopathies

There are more than a hundred genetic defects in amino acid metabolism. One of the most clinically important is phenylketonuria. This is due to a defect in the enzyme phenylalanine hydroxylase.

14 Principles of molecular genetics

Stuart Brown

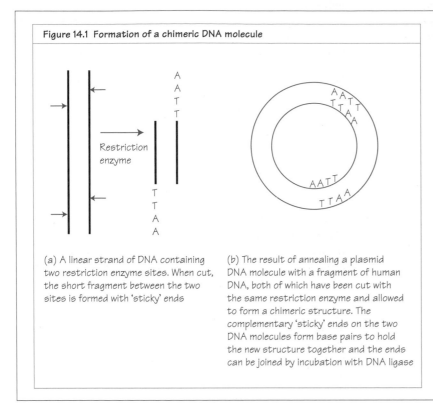

Figure 14.1 Formation of a chimeric DNA molecule

(a) A linear strand of DNA containing two restriction enzyme sites. When cut, the short fragment between the two sites is formed with 'sticky' ends

(b) The result of annealing a plasmid DNA molecule with a fragment of human DNA, both of which have been cut with the same restriction enzyme and allowed to form a chimeric structure. The complementary 'sticky' ends on the two DNA molecules form base pairs to hold the new structure together and the ends can be joined by incubation with DNA ligase

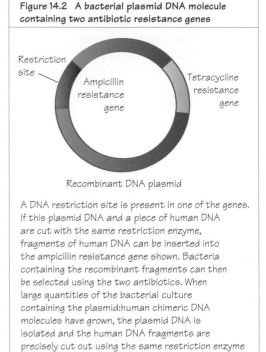

Figure 14.2 A bacterial plasmid DNA molecule containing two antibiotic resistance genes

Restriction site

Ampicillin resistance gene

Tetracycline resistance gene

Recombinant DNA plasmid

A DNA restriction site is present in one of the genes. If this plasmid DNA and a piece of human DNA are cut with the same restriction enzyme, fragments of human DNA can be inserted into the ampicillin resistance gene shown. Bacteria containing the recombinant fragments can then be selected using the two antibiotics. When large quantities of the bacterial culture containing the plasmid:human chimeric DNA molecules have grown, the plasmid DNA is isolated and the human DNA fragments are precisely cut out using the same restriction enzyme

Prior to the development of molecular genetic techniques our understanding of genetic disease and potential treatments was based on the analysis of pedigrees and studying abnormal proteins. The knowledge gained from understanding the structure of a gene and gene cloning techniques has revolutionised knowledge of the cause of genetic diseases and potential treatments, including gene therapy.

Gene cloning

The basis of gene cloning technology owes its origins to the realisation that two different practical techniques (the use of **restriction enzymes** and the use of **bacterial plasmids**) could be utilised to generate **chi-** **meric DNA** molecules in large quantities. Restriction enzymes are **endonucleases** that recognise and cut DNA at specific sequences within the molecule (Figure 14.1a). They recognise short four- or six-base pair sequences and either cut at opposite ends of these sequences, generating overlapping ends known as **'sticky' ends** because they can reanneal using allowed base pair rules, or they cut both strands at the same site to generate 'blunt' ends.

Plasmids are small circular DNA molecules that can be present in a bacterial cell and replicate along with the bacterial genome (Figure 14.1b). They can code for proteins such as antibiotic-resistance proteins (Figure 14.2) and are responsible for creating many multi-drug-resistant bacteria.

 Medical Sciences at a Glance, First Edition. Edited by Michael D Randall. © 2014 John Wiley & Sons, Ltd. Published 2014 by John Wiley & Sons, Ltd.

The combination of these two technologies led to the production of **recombinant DNA molecules**. If a plasmid preparation is cut with a particular restriction enzyme, small lengths of DNA with identical sticky ends will form. Similarly, if a piece of human DNA is cut with the same restriction enzyme, short sequences of DNA will result with the same sticky ends. The two sets of DNA pieces can be incubated together and allowed to reanneal. The annealed DNA pieces can then be covalently joined *in vitro* using DNA ligase. The result will be a mixture of reformed plasmid molecules in addition to some plasmids into which human DNA sequences have been inserted. It is now possible to use selection techniques to select for only the chimeric human/plasmid molecules. These chimeric DNA molecules will be replicated by the host bacteria. The plasmid acts as the **vector**, to produce large quantities of the human molecules. The human DNA sequences can then be extracted using the same restriction enzyme that was used to cut the DNA initially.

Libraries

If a sample of total human DNA is treated with a restriction enzyme and the fragments are inserted into a vector, the **chimeric molecules** generated will contain the sum total of all the DNA sequences present in the human genome. The product of this process has been called a **human genomic library**. It can be prepared from the DNA of human tissue or human cell lines and will not be dependent on the source of DNA. Much of our understanding of the sequences in human genes has come from studies on human DNA libraries. However, these sequences cannot be used to generate human proteins in a bacterial protein synthesising system because bacterial cells cannot process the complex intron/exon structure of human genes.

If the total mRNA is isolated from a specific human tissue or cell line it can be **reverse transcribed** into **complementary DNA** *in vitro* using the RNA virus enzyme reverse transcriptase. The complementary DNA sequences can be ligated into a particular vector. The vector will then contain DNA copies of all the mRNA molecules present in that tissue. This is known as a **complementary DNA (or cDNA)** library. Unlike the genomic library, a cDNA library will be specific to the tissue used to isolate the mRNA because different tissues express different genes at different times. cDNA libraries can be used to produce large quantities of proteins.

Isolation of a specific DNA sequence

If cellular DNA is isolated from human tissue and treated with a restriction enzyme, thousands of fragments result. These can be separated on a polyacryamide gel. The different size fragments will migrate to different positions in the gel based on their molecular weights. A specific fragment can be identified using a specific 'probe' for that fragment. Probes are any molecule that can be used to detect a specific polynucleotide or polypeptide sequence. For example, a small piece of radioactively labelled DNA complementary to the sequence to be isolated can be used to detect the required DNA fragment. It can be incubated with the gel containing all the human fragments and it will specifically bind to the complementary sequence and can be detected using autoradiography. Once detected, the DNA fragment can be cut from the gel, ligated into a plasmid and grown in a suitable bacterial host to produce large quantities of the DNA sequence. Similar strategies are now used to detect RNA and peptide sequences on gels.

The use of a DNA probe to detect a DNA sequence on a gel is called a **Southern blot**. A **Northern blot** is used to detect RNA sequences on a gel and the use of an antibody to probe a gel containing a mixture of polypeptides is called a **Western blot**.

DNA sequencing

It is possible to sequence DNA molecules to test whether the sequence isolated from a Southern blot or a DNA library is the correct one. **DNA polymerases** replicate DNA by adding new deoxyribonucleotides at the 3′ end of the growing DNA chain. If a dideoxynucleotide, i.e. one with no 2′ or 3′ hydroxyl group on the deoxyribose ring, is used as a substrate in a DNA synthesis reaction the incorporation of a dideoxynucleotide will terminate DNA synthesis, as there will be no 3′ hydroxyl group to accept a new deoxynucleotide. To sequence a DNA strand a mixture of deoxynucleotides and dideoxynucleotides is added to the reaction mixture. DNA synthesis will terminate at random when a dideoxynucleotide is inserted, producing many DNA strands of different length. Careful analysis of these fragments allows the sequence to be determined. Automation of this process has finally led to techniques able to sequence the complete three billion bases in the human genome.

Practical applications
Gene mapping

In order to attempt to correct genetic disease it is necessary to know the location of the defective gene. Prior to the development of modern recombinant DNA technology this used to be performed by extensive analysis of a set of hybrid cells. For example, when human and mouse cells are fused the resulting hybrid cell is viable and gradually loses human chromosomes. It was possible to map a human gene to a human chromosome using these cells. This technique was limited. The gene to be mapped not only had to produce a protein that could be detected in the cells but also be different from the mouse counterpart. With modern technology it is now possible to use molecular probes for specific genes to locate the gene on a specific human chromosome using Southern blot analyses without any knowledge of the gene product. In addition, the automation of DNA sequencing has finally led to the sequencing of the complete human genome.

Protein synthesis

Using a cDNA library it is now possible to generate human proteins in large quantities for research purposes or for treatment of human diseases. This has been especially important in the production of proteins that are only present in very small quantities in cells and hence are very difficult to purify by conventional techniques. It is now possible to produce proteins for treatment of disease, such as insulin, human growth hormone and interferon, or for diagnostic purposes, such as HIV detection, in large quantities.

Prenatal diagnosis of disease

It is now possible to use Southern blotting techniques to analyse a chorionic villus sample or amniotic fluid for the presence of an abnormal gene in a fetus. Sickle cell anaemia and cystic fibrosis are just two diseases that can be detected using this new technology.

The ultimate goal of the new technology is to be able to replace a missing gene in order to correct a genetic disease. It is now possible to clone a gene such as adenosine deaminase or the cystic fibrosis transmembrane conductance regulator gene and, using a suitable vector such as a viral vector or a liposome, introduce the synthetic gene back into the patient's cells. Although still in its infancy this technology is showing great promise.

Stuart Brown

Figure 15.1 DNA and chromatin structures

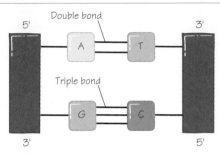

(a) A diagram of a DNA double helix showing the base pairs that form perpendicular to the direction of the helix. Adenine pairs with thymine: forms two hydrogen bonds, while guanine pairs with cytosine: forms three hydrogen bonds. The two phosphodiester backbone strands consist of alternating deoxyribose and phosphate molecules and are shown running antiparallel, i.e. one strand runs 5' to 3' and the other runs 3' to 5'

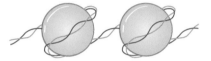

(b) In mammalian cells DNA does not exist without being combined with proteins. Two copies of histone proteins H2a, H2b, H3 and H4 form spherical structures around which DNA can wrap. In this way the strand of DNA is more condensed. Histone H1 attaches to the DNA linker region between the histone octamers to protect the DNA from degradation. This 'beads-on-a-string'-type structure then coils in several further modification steps until a chromosome is formed

Figure 15.2 A DNA replication fork

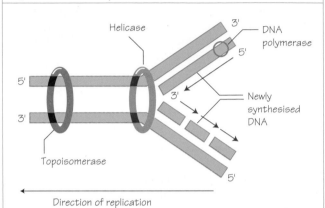

The double-stranded DNA unwinds to expose the two separate DNA strands. DNA polymerases then copy the template strands to form two new daughter DNA strands. DNA polymerases can only travel in the 5' to 3' direction and thus a complex series of events has to occur to copy both template strands. The 3' to 5' template strand can be copied continuously by a DNA polymerase travelling in the 5' to 3' direction. The other template strand has to be unwound to allow a DNA polymerase to attach and synthesise short DNA sequences in the opposite direction to the direction of replication. These short sequences, known as Okazaki fragments, are then joined together by a DNA ligase to form the new DNA molecule

Deoxyribonucleic acid (DNA)

DNA is the hereditary material in prokaryotic and eukaryotic cells. It consists of four nitrogenous bases, **adenine (A), guanine (G), cytosine (C)** and **thymine (T)**, attached to deoxyribose (a pentose sugar) molecules (Figure 15.1a). The deoxyribose molecules are linked by covalent ester bonds to phosphate molecules to produce a long thin polymer. The monomeric units of this polymer are known as **nucleotides**. A single nucleotide consists of a base bound to a deoxyribose molecule with a phosphate attached. Since the polymer is made up of nucleotides, DNA is called a polynucleotide. In prokaryotes such as *Escherichia coli*, there is a single DNA polynucleotide chain consisting of 4×10^6 bases. This DNA is known as the genome. In humans,

there is a separate DNA molecule in each of the 46 chromosomes. The total number of bases in the human genome is 3×10^9.

DNA polymers can be described in terms of the position of the chemical bonds joining the sugar and the phosphate. The five carbon atoms in deoxyribose are numbered 1' to 5' (the primes are added to differentiate the carbon atoms in the sugar from those in the base). In a DNA polymer, phosphate molecules are attached at the 5' and 3' carbons of a deoxyribose. Thus at the ends of the polymer there will be a deoxyribose with either a free 3' hydroxyl group or a free 5' phosphate group. The ends are known as the 5' or 3' ends and the polymer can be described as having a direction, i.e. 5' to 3' or 3' to 5'.

DNA sequence

Each nucleotide in the DNA helix can be described by the letter representing the specific base it contains. By convention the base sequence is written in the 5′ to 3′ direction. Thus the sequence AATTGCC would represent a base sequence with an adenine base at the 5′ end and a cytosine base at the 3′ end.

The DNA double helix

DNA strands in human cells are wound around each other to form a **double helix** with the deoxyribose–phosphate hydrophilic backbone on the outside and the bases on the inside. The strands run in an antiparallel direction, i.e. one strand runs 5′ to 3′ and the other 3′ to 5′. Thus the DNA helix is asymmetric. The bases are attached at the 1′ position on the sugar. The bases on opposite strands of the helix form hydrogen bonds with each other and the numerous hydrogen bonds formed in the base pairs contribute to the force stabilising the helix structure. The hydrogen-bonded base pairs are known as base pairs and can only form in certain specific combinations: A pairs with T via two hydrogen bonds and G with C via three hydrogen bonds. The base pairs are perpendicular to the direction of the helix. The base pairs are hydrophobic and stack on top of each other. This '**hydrophobic stacking force**' provides another main source of force holding the DNA helix together.

In the most common form of DNA, known as the B form, the helix is a right-handed double helix with 10 bases per turn, i.e. the angle of rotation between base pairs is 36°. Although the B form of DNA is the most common form found, DNA can form an A form right-handed helix in which the base pairs are tilted with respect to the helix direction or even a Z form left-handed helix. The Z form is thought to exist in cells but its role is still not totally understood.

DNA organisation in human cells

Double-stranded DNA does not exist alone in human cells. Two molecules of histone proteins H2A, H2B, H3 and H4 form a cylindrical structure around which the DNA strand is wrapped (Figure 15.1b). Two turns of DNA (147 base pairs) are wrapped around each octamer and the DNA linking these structures is protected by binding a histone H1 molecule. This fundamental form of DNA wrapped around the histones is known as the 'beads-on-a-string' structure. It represents the most uncondensed form of DNA in a cell. Higher-order structures in which the DNA is gradually more and more condensed form by the coiling of the 'beads-on-a-string' structure into a coil and then a coiled coil and ultimately into the highly condensed form known as the chromosome. Only the most condensed form of DNA and histone is called a chromosome. The other forms are called chromatin. **Chromatin** can exist in a cell in two forms: heterochromatin, which is highly condensed; and euchromatin, which is less condensed and is the form that would be present during transcription. This condensation process is the means by which the vast amount of DNA, approximately 2m in total length, can be contained in the nucleus of a human cell, with a diameter of only approximately 10 μm.

DNA replication

Watson and Crick deduced the structure of DNA in 1953. They postulated that the helix structure would enable the molecule to be replicated by unwinding the helix and producing new copies using the separate strands of the parent helix as a template. This is indeed the case. Each strand of the DNA molecule contains the genetic information and thus can act as a template for the synthesis of two new daughter DNA strands each containing the same genetic information as the parental strand (Figure 15.2).

DNA polymerases are the enzymes responsible for replication. There are several different DNA polymerases found in bacterial and human cells. *E. coli* contains five different DNA polymerases known as **pol I, II, III, IV** and **V**. Although all possess similar properties, pol III is the main replication enzyme. The others have roles in DNA repair. In humans, there are 15 DNA polymerases. DNA pol α, δ and ε are involved in nuclear DNA replication, and pol γ is responsible for replication of mitochondrial DNA. Several others are involved in DNA repair and not too well understood.

Despite the fact that several forms of DNA polymerase exist they have similar properties:
• they require all four deoxyribonucleotide triphosphates as substrates;
• they require a divalent cation, e.g. magnesium ions;
• they cannot initiate DNA synthesis without a primer;
• they cannot join two DNA molecules together;
• most of them have endonuclease activity.

Several of these properties are to ensure the great accuracy required to copy such large sequences of nucleotides faithfully, without making errors. The accuracy of human DNA replication is estimated at one error for every 10^{10} bases copied. This is essential to avoid the introduction of mutations that could lead to genetic disease.

Due to the restrictions on the properties of DNA polymerases, several other proteins and enzymes are required to completely replicate a DNA molecule:
• **RNA primase** to generate the RNA primer
• **DNA ligase** to join single DNA strands together
• **helicases** and **topoisomerases** to wind or unwind the helix when required
• *single-stranded binding proteins* to protect the unwound single stranded DNA strands.

In humans, the process is complicated further by the fact that the DNA is in the form of chromatin. The chromatin must be unwound before replication starts and rewound after replication.

Ribonucleic acid (RNA)

RNA has a very similar structure to DNA, except that:
• it is usually single stranded;
• it contains ribose sugars instead of deoxyribose;
• it contains uracil as a base instead of thymine.

There are three different major types of RNA in a cell:
• **messenger RNA (mRNA)**
• **ribosomal RNA (rRNA)**
• **transfer RNA (tRNA)**.

All three forms are coded for by genes in DNA and are required for protein synthesis.
• mRNA is the RNA copy of a gene that is used to code for proteins.
• rRNA, together with several proteins, forms the small and large subunits of the ribosome, which is used in protein synthesis.
• tRNA is responsible for delivering the correct amino acid to the ribosome for protein synthesis to occur.

Stuart Brown

Figure 16.1 Transcription of a eukaryotic gene

RNA polymerase recognises a promoter region in DNA and binds upsteam of the transcription start site. It moves to the start site and transcribes the whole length of the gene, including exon and intron regions, until it recognises a stop signal in the DNA. The introns are spliced out and the exons are joined together. This is a very carefully controlled process. Despite this control errors can occur and it is estimated that up to 15% of genetic diseases are caused by splicing errors. For example, in the cystic fibrosis gene there are 26 introns to be spliced out. The hnRNA is 250 000 bases long, whereas the mRNA is only 6129 bases long. Most of the sequence in a eukaryotic gene is intron sequence. A cap is attached to the 5' end. This refers to an extra guanine (often methylated) nucleotide attached to the 5' end of the hnRNA via a 5' to 5' linkage. This serves to protect the end of the mRNA from degradation and also serves a role in ribosome binding during protein synthesis. At the 3' end a poly A tail is added. Up to 300 adenine nucleotides are added by poly A polymerase. The tail again serves to protect the mRNA structure from degradation and is also involved in the movement of the mRNA into the cytosol. The mature mRNA enters the cytosol through a pore in the nuclear membrane

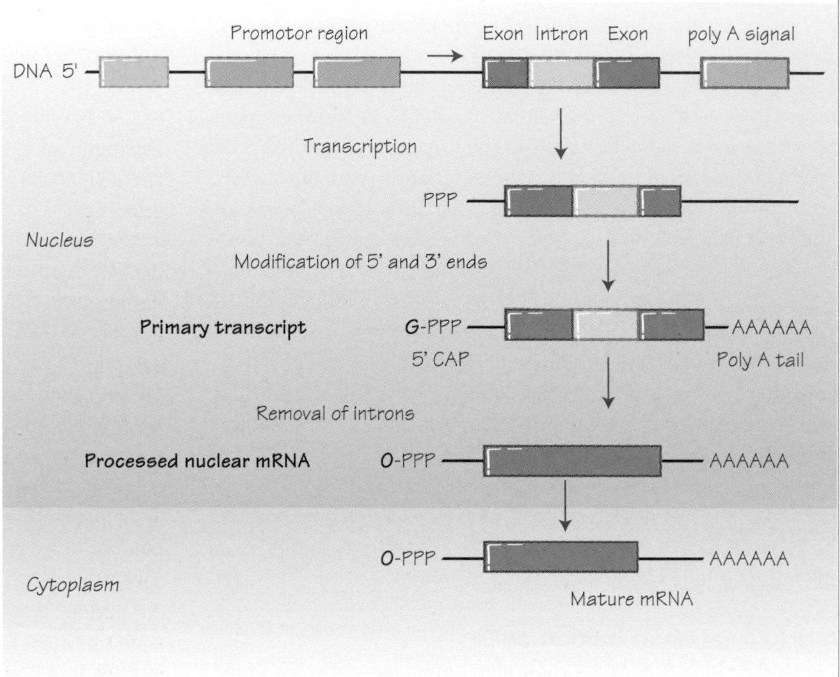

Gene sequences occupy only about 2% of the human genome. Following the successful genome project that enabled the sequence of bases in the human genome (3 billion) to be elucidated, it is now thought that there are only approximately 20–25 000 genes in the human genome. The term **genotype** is used to describe the genes present in a genome. However, in different cells and tissues not all the same genes will be expressed. The term **phenotype** is used to describe which genes are expressed in different cells or tissues. **Gene expression** refers to the processes in which the information in a gene in DNA is used to produce the corresponding protein in a cell. It involves the **transcription** of the DNA sequence into RNA and then the **translation** of RNA into proteins. Gene expression is very carefully regulated in order to control not only how much of a protein is made but also when particular proteins are synthesised, e.g. during development or differentiation of cell types. Although cells can control transcription and translation, the major control of gene expression is at the level of transcription.

Transcription (Figure 16.1)

Cells contain three different types of RNA molecules: **mRNA, rRNA** and **tRNA** (Chapter 15). All three types of RNA are transcribed from genes present in DNA. Only mRNA, however, is used as a template for new protein synthesis. rRNA and tRNA are used in the translation process. In eukaryotic cells, transcription is carried out by three different **DNA-dependent RNA polymerases**:

- **pol I** transcribes rRNA genes and is located in the nucleolus;
- **pol II** transcribes mRNA genes;
- **pol III** transcribes tRNA genes and other small RNA molecules.

Pol II and III are found in the nucleus. RNA polymerase enzymes are multisubunit structures containing approximately 16 subunits and are more complex than the single RNA polymerase enzyme found in bacteria.

To understand the series of events that produce an mRNA molecule from a gene it is necessary to understand the eukaryotic gene structure. Eukaryotic genes are made up of **exons**, regions of DNA that will code for the mature mRNA, and **introns**, regions of DNA that will be transcribed into RNA but later removed during post-**transcriptional processing**. RNA polymerase II will transcribe the full length of the gene using the template strand as a template so that the mRNA sequence is the same as that in the DNA-coding strand. Only one DNA strand is copied. This initial product is called heterogeneous nuclear RNA (**hnRNA**). Three important post-transcriptional processing events occur while the hnRNA is still in the nucleus (see Figure 16.1).

Following completion of these events the product is mRNA. It now moves out of the nucleus, through the nuclear pores, and is located in the cytosol where translation occurs.

Control of transcription

As mentioned above, transcription is very well regulated, specifically transcription initiation. This regulation is exerted through a combination of special DNA sequences and proteins known as transcription factors, which recognise and bind to the control elements in DNA. One major DNA control element is the **promoter** situated at the 5′ end of the gene. Eukaryotic promoters have several features in common. The promoter sequence will allow the polymerase to bind and start transcription at the correct base. A specific conserved sequence was identified approximately 25–35 bases upstream of the transcription start site. This sequence is rich in A and T bases and is known as the **TATA box**. There are other special DNA sequences up to 200 bases upstream of the transcription start site that also help regulate the level of gene transcription, and even others that can be many hundreds or thousands of bases upstream of the gene. The latter are known as **enhancers or silencers** because they can increase or decrease the frequency of transcription.

The DNA-controlling elements at the 5′ end of the gene bind other proteins known as transcription factors. The initiation of transcription can be controlled by many of these proteins forming a multisubunit transcription complex at the promoter site. These will form in some cell types but not others, or at different times during development, and hence control transcription. Transcription factors have several distinctive protein motifs that enable them to bind to DNA and to other proteins in the complex. These motifs include zinc fingers, helix loop helix motifs and leucine zippers.

A recent development has been the discovery of **alternative splicing**. During the removal of introns from a hnRNA the exons may be spliced in different ways in different tissues. This increases the diversity of proteins that can be made from the relatively small number of genes present in the human genome. An example of this phenomenon is **tropomyosin**. This is used in different contractile systems in different cells and the specific form required is produced by alternative splicing of the single hnRNA rather than having different tropomyosin genes in the different cell types.

Translation

The final stage in gene expression is translation. Translation is the term used for the process of translating mRNA into protein. In a eukaryotic cell, this can occur in the cytosol when synthesising soluble proteins destined for use in that cell, or at the endoplasmic reticulum membrane when synthesising proteins destined for secretion from the cell or ones that will be membrane bound. Note the information instructing the protein to its final destination was originally in the DNA.

Translation requires the use of all three RNA species: the mRNA is used as the template for protein synthesis; rRNA, together with many proteins, forms the complex ribosomes that carry out the synthesis reactions; and the tRNA is responsible for selecting the correct amino acid and placing it at the ribosome for incorporation into the growing peptide.

Like DNA replication and transcription, translation occurs in three stages: initiation, elongation and termination. Each stage is well controlled by protein factors and each requires GTP as an energy source. During initiation a ribosome assembles at the start site on the mRNA and tRNA brings the first amino acid, usually methionine, to the growing complex. A second amino acid is attached to the ribosome and a **peptidyl transferase enzyme** activity, unusually present in the rRNA molecule, forms the first peptide linkage. This completes the initiation reactions. The ribosome begins to translocate along the mRNA in the 5′ to 3′ direction as tRNA molecules bring more amino acids to join the growing chain. These are the elongation reactions. Finally, the ribosome reaches a stop or termination signal in the mRNA and the complex stops and releases the complete peptide. Several **post-translational modifications** can occur to produce the mature protein: the peptide may be gylcosylated, phosphorylated or acetylated; it may be present in the form of a proprotein or prepeptein that is cleaved to produce the smaller mature proteins as in the case of insulin; or it may carry a signal peptide that will direct it to the site or organelle in the cell where it will function. Finally, the signal peptide may direct it to the endoplasmic reticulum and it may be used as a membrane protein or even be secreted from the cell.

The genetic code

An mRNA molecule is translated into a peptide using the genetic code. This is a triplet code in which three bases in RNA, i.e. originally in DNA and called a codon, code for a specific amino acid. The four bases in DNA can code for 64 different codons. Three of these are called termination or nonsense codons (UAG, UGA and UAA) and do not code for amino acids. One is the initiation codon (AUG) and codes for methione. Other important features of the genetic code are:
• it is degenerate: up to six different codons may code for the same amino acid;
• it is not ambiguous: a particular codon always codes for a particular amino acid;
• apart from the start and stop signals there is no other punctuation.
Thus when a ribosome starts synthesising a peptide at the first AUG codon in the mRNA it sets the reading frame: the next three bases will be the second codon and so on. Point mutations that add or delete one or two bases in a gene will alter the reading frame of a gene and alter the peptide sequence synthesised. This type of mutation is called a frameshift mutation. If three bases are deleted, the reading frame may not be altered but the peptide will be missing one amino acid; this is one of the common mutations responsible for cystic fibrosis.

The fact that the code is degenerate is an advantage to the cell. Some point mutations in DNA may result in an altered codon in the mRNA, but this new codon may also code for the same amino acid as the non-mutated codon: thus a normal protein is synthesised. This type of mutation is called a silent mutation.

17 Medical genetics

Stuart Brown

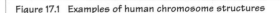

Figure 17.1 Examples of human chromosome structures

Short or
p arm
Centromere
Long or
q arm
2
1
1
2
a
b
c
d
e
f
g
h
i
a
b
h
g
f
e
d
c
i

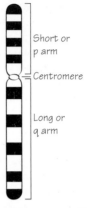

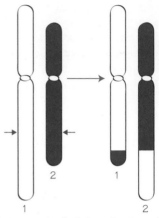

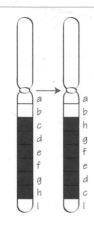

(a) A human metaphase chromosome. Dyes, e.g. Giemsa stain, can be used to produce unique banding patterns on each chromosome to aid identification. The centromere is almost central in a metaphase chromosome. It divides the chromosome into a short and long arm. The short arm is called the p arm (for petit) and the long arm is called the q arm

(b) An example of a balanced reciprocal translocation in which a terminal section of chromosome 1 is replaced by the terminal section of chromosome 2 and vice versa

(c) An example of an inversion in which part of the long arm of the chromosome is inverted

Figure 17.2 Common features associated with Down's syndrome

- Characteristic facial features
- Mental retardation
- Immune system abnormalities
- Increased risk of certain cancers, e.g. leukaemia
- Alzheimer-like dementia
- Infertility
- Cardiac, respiratory and gastrointestinal tract problems
- Possible epilepsy

Figure 17.3 A mechanism for tripet repeat sequence expansion

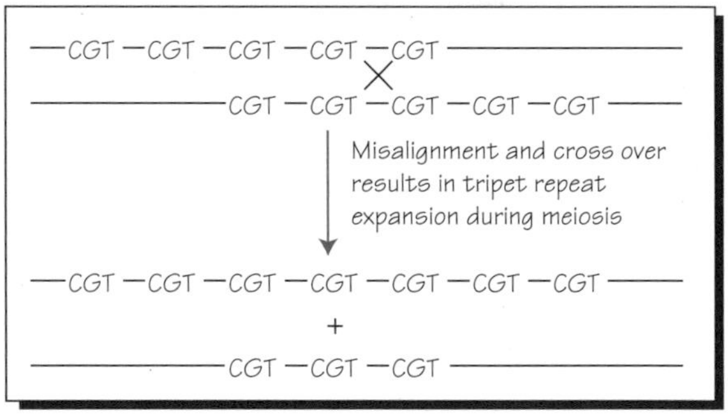

—CGT —CGT —CGT —CGT —CGT
—CGT —CGT —CGT —CGT —CGT
Misalignment and cross over results in tripet repeat expansion during meiosis
—CGT —CGT —CGT —CGT —CGT —CGT —CGT
+
—CGT —CGT —CGT

Figure 17.4 Possible effects of a point mutation

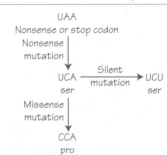

UAA
Nonsense or stop codon
Nonsense mutation
UCA
ser
Silent mutation
UCU
ser
Missense mutation
CCA
pro

Point mutation may result in an altered phenotype, e.g. if the mutation alters the particular amino acid in a protein or if protein synthesis is prematurely terminated. However, since the genetic code is degenerate, i.e. up to 6 codons may code for a particular amino acid, the mutation may be silent. In the example shown both UCA and UCU code for serine

 Medical Sciences at a Glance, First Edition. Edited by Michael D Randall.

Genetic disease is a common cause of illness and even death. Approximately 3% of babies are affected by a genetic disease. Genetic diseases can be considered to be caused by chromosomal defects or single or multiple gene defects. One per cent of children admitted to hospitals suffer from chromosomal defects, 5–10% from single gene defects and 35–45% from multi-gene defects. Chromosomal defects are relatively common, with 15% of all conceptions affected, and if severe they usually result in miscarriage.

Chromosome structure

Human cells are **diploid**, i.e. there are two copies of each chromosome. They are the result of an 8000-fold condensation of chromatin during mitosis. The human genome consists of 23 pairs of chromosomes: 22 pairs of autosomes and a pair of sex chromosomes, XX for a female and XY for a male. The chromosome content of a cell is known as the **karyotype**. Each cell in an individual contains the same genome, known as the genotype. The expression of certain genes in different tissues refers to the phenotype.

Cytogenetic analysis shows that humans contain metaphase chromosomes (Figure 17.1).

Sources of genetic variation

• During reproduction the fertilisation of an ovum of one individual by the sperm of another.

• Human genes are inherited according to Mendelian laws. Offspring inherit one chromosome from each parent.

• During meiosis crossing-over of DNA between two chromatids occurs.

Mutations

A mutation is any permanent heritable change in DNA sequence. A mutagen is an agent that increases the mutation rate. There are two major types of mutation.

Chromosomal defects

During cell division the following changes in chromosome structure or content can occur.

• Gain of a whole set of chromosomes to form a tetraploid.

• Changes in the number of copies of a single chromosome arising from non-disjunction during meiosis, a failure to separate chromosomes correctly; the resulting cells are aneuploid, e.g. the gain of a chromosome results in a triploid cell. Triploidy is deleterious to the cell. Down syndrome results from the presence of three copies of chromosome 21. Fewer than 30% of Down fetuses survive to birth (Figure 17.2). For trisomy 18 (Edward's syndrome) and trisomy 13 (Patau syndrome) fewer than 10% survive to birth. Sex chromosomes are an exception to this. Aneuploidy is usually much less severe if a cell contains 47XXX, 47XXY, or 47XYY. This is as a result of the inactivation of all but one X chromosome in a somatic cell during the early stages of embryogenesis (known as the Lyon hypothesis) or the small number of genes on the Y chromosome.

Changes in chromosome structure can occur (Figure 17.1).

• Triplet repeat sequences occur in normal chromosomes. For example, the normal myotonin gene contains between five and 35 copies of a CTG sequence. The number of these repeats can increase during meiosis (Figure 17.3). In patients suffering from myotonic dystrophy, the number of these repeat sequences increases to greater than 50 and may be over 1000. A similar situation occurs in a number of other diseases, including Huntington's disease. It is possible to estimate in which generation a future offspring will inherit sufficient triplet repeats to be affected by the disease. This phenomenon is known as anticipation.

Point mutations

A **point mutation** is the alteration of a single base in DNA. Point mutations can be caused by the following

• Spontaneous changes in DNA structure:
  – a defective DNA polymerase may introduce errors during replication;
  – a nucleotide may be in the incorrect tautomeric (isomeric) form such that it pairs with the wrong base.

• Chemicals can alter the H-bonding capacity of DNA bases.

• Physical agents such as X-rays or UV light can interact with DNA to cause breaks or cross-links.

Point mutations can have various effects on cells (Figure 17.4).

• They may have no effect. Following completion of the Human Genome Project in 2003 the 4 billion bases that make up the human genome have been sequenced and the number of genes present is estimated to be between 20 000 and 25 000. Thus genes occupy less than 10% of the genome. Mutations in the majority of DNA will not affect cell behaviour.

• In addition, the mutation may be **silent**.

• The mutation may be a **missense mutation**. This may have a range of effects on the host. For example, sickle cell anaemia is caused by a single base change resulting in a glutamate residue being replaced by valine at position 6 in the beta chain of haemoglobin. This substitution of a non-polar amino acid for a polar amino acid causes the red cells to 'sickle'. Sickle cell anaemia was the first haemoglobinopathy to be discovered and although more than 4000 are now known, it is still the most serious.

• The mutation may be a **nonsense mutation**. If the mutation results in the formation of a nonsense codon, no amino acid is inserted into the protein and the synthesis is prematurely terminated.

Treatment of genetic disease

The treatment of genetic disease has usually concentrated on the manipulation of the environment rather than genetic manipulation. The emphasis has been on prevention rather than cure. It is possible to avoid genetic disease by screening and prenatal diagnosis. It is also possible to reduce the effects of a genetic disease on an individual by altering the diet, e.g. for phenylketonuria or familial hypercholesterolemia. It is possible to replace certain materials or even organs in an individual, e.g blood transfusions in haemophilia patients or even liver transplants for patients with familial hypercholesterolemia. Cancer can be considered a genetic disease and great emphasis has been placed on avoiding the mutagens present in sunlight or cigarette smoke.

More recently considerable effort has been placed on **gene therapy**, the introduction of genetic material into a patient to replace the absent or damaged gene. Numerous trials have been undertaken and although progress has been slow, it is possible to treat diseases such as cystic fibrosis by introducing copies of the normal gene into the lungs of affected individuals. Viral and liposome vectors have been developed to deliver the new gene sequences and long-term success in the near future is possible.

18 Cell excitability

Michael D Randall

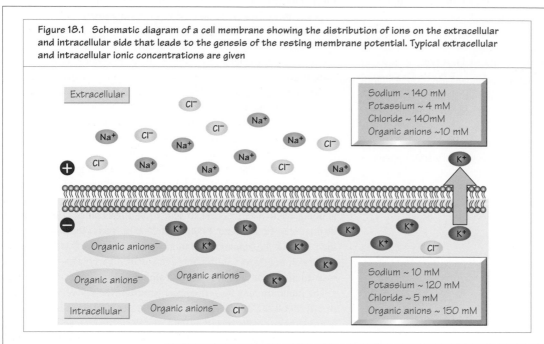

Figure 18.1 Schematic diagram of a cell membrane showing the distribution of ions on the extracellular and intracellular side that leads to the genesis of the resting membrane potential. Typical extracellular and intracellular ionic concentrations are given

Extracellular
Sodium ~ 140 mM
Potassium ~ 4 mM
Chloride ~ 140mM
Organic anions ~10 mM
Cl⁻
Na⁺
K⁺
Organic anions⁻
Intracellular
Sodium ~ 10 mM
Potassium ~ 120 mM
Chloride ~ 5 mM
Organic anions ~ 150 mM

Figure 18.2 Schematic diagram of the $3Na^+/2K^+$ ATPase ('sodium pump'), indicating its role in maintaining ionic balances across the cell membrane

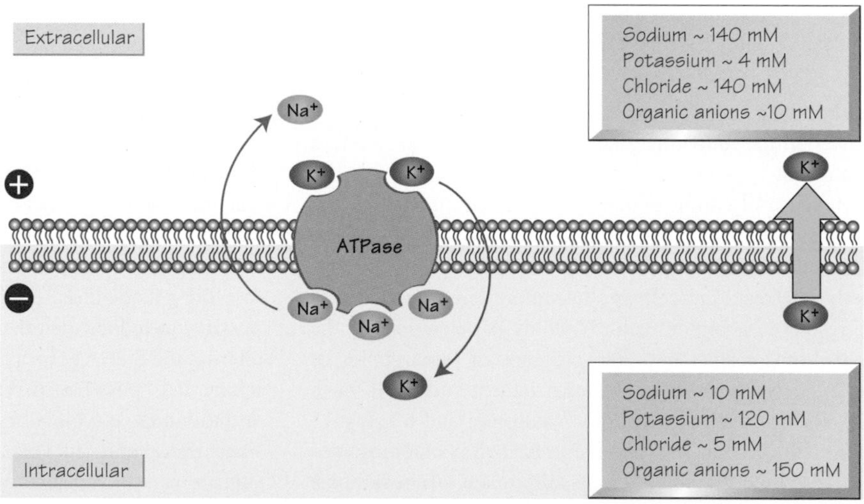

Extracellular
Sodium ~ 140 mM
Potassium ~ 4 mM
Chloride ~ 140 mM
Organic anions ~10 mM
Na⁺
K⁺
ATPase
Intracellular
Sodium ~ 10 mM
Potassium ~ 120 mM
Chloride ~ 5 mM
Organic anions ~ 150 mM

Physiological processes (e.g. nervous conduction, the release of transmitters and hormones, muscle contractility) depend on cell excitability. Therefore, excitability and excitation of cells is tightly regulated.

Resting membrane potential (V_m)

Each cell in the body has an **electrical potential difference** which is determined by the distribution of ions across the cell membrane (Chapter 2). The potential difference across the membrane is the **membrane potential**. In the resting state the inside of the cell is negative on the intracellular side with respect to the outside, and this is the **resting membrane potential** (Figure 18.1). A typical value for a neurone is **−70 mV**, for skeletal muscle it is **−90 mV**. The resting membrane potential is determined by ionic balances across the cell membrane. The movement of ions is determined by both their electrical gradients and chemical gradients as driving forces; this is the **electrochemical potential gradient**. The ionic balance is governed by relative **membrane permeability**. For example, if we consider K^+ and organic anions, both have high intracellular concentrations and the chemical gradient favours their movement out of the cell. However, the membrane is more permeable to K^+ compared with the organic anions, and so the net efflux is K^+ unaccompanied by the anions. This results in the cell becoming more negative with respect to the outside. The balance of electrical and chemical work for K^+ is summarised by the **Nernst equation**:

$$E = \frac{RT}{F} \log_e \frac{[K]_o}{[K]_i}$$

where: E = membrane potential; $[K]_o$ = extracellular potassium; R = gas constant; $[K]_i$ = intracellular potassium; T = Absolute temperature; F = Faraday's constant.

At physiological temperatures the equation can be simplified to:

$$E = 61.5 \log_{10} \frac{[K]_o}{[K]_i}$$

When the electrical and chemical gradients are in balance there is no net flux of ions and E is the **Nernst potential** for the ion in question (e.g. for K^+ it is approximately −90 mV; for Na^+ it is approximately +65 mV).

As the membrane potential is governed by a number of ions, the equation can be modified to include each ion (the **Goldman field equation**), but the contribution of each is determined by **membrane permeability**:

$$E = \frac{RT}{F} \log_e \frac{P_k[K]_o + P_{Na}[Na]_o + P_{Cl}[Cl]_i}{P_K[K]_i + P_{Na}[Na]_i + P_{Cl}[Cl]_o}$$

where P_{ion} takes account of the ion's permeability.

In the resting state, the cell membrane is substantially more permeable to K^+, such that the membrane is typically 70- to 100-fold more permeable to K^+ compared with Na^+. The consequence of this is that the resting membrane potential of cells lies close to the equilibrium potential for K^+ (approx. −90 mV). Hence the major determinant of membrane potential is the extracellular K^+ concentration. By contrast, as the membrane is relatively impermeable to Na^+ in the resting state then changes in extracellular Na^+ concentration have little impact on the resting membrane potential.

The sodium pump (3Na⁺/2K⁺ ATPase)

This is a membrane transporter that uses ATP to pump $3Na^+$ ions out of the cell in exchange for $2K^+$ ions into the cell (Figure 18.2). While the sodium pump is **electrogenic**, its primary role is to maintain or replenish ionic balances, with Na^+ concentrations being high extracellularly/low intracellularly and K^+ concentrations being low extracellularly/high intracellularly. Hence the role of the pump is to maintain concentration gradients. The pump is in opposition to the electrical gradient for K^+ and since the membrane is relatively permeable to K^+ these ions pass out of the cell through K^+ channels to approach the Nernst potential for K^+. This leads to the setting up of the resting membrane potential. Only a small proportion of K^+ ions pass out to establish the resting membrane potential, with little impact on the concentration gradient.

While the membrane potential is small, the narrow width of the cell membrane (~10 nm) means that the electrical gradient is large (7 million volts per metre). This means that proteins within the cell are under an appreciable electrical force, and so changes in membrane potential lead to conformational changes in these proteins, which have significant regional charges. These conformational changes underpin activities such as the opening of voltage-operated ion channels.

Maintenance of the resting membrane potential is crucial to excitability. When a cell starts to depolarise (e.g. the propagation of an action potential, in response to activation of receptors, stimulation of mechanoreceptors) the change in potential may take the cell to threshold potential (Chapter 19). At this point the changes in the electrical field lead to conformation changes in **voltage-operated** (or gated) **ion channels** (VOCs). For example, at threshold in a neurone this leads to activation of voltage-operated Na^+ channels and the initiation of the action potential. Other examples of excitation may lead to the release of neurotransmitters and hormones. In pancreatic beta-cells, increases in ATP levels lead to closure of K^+ channels and this initiates depolarisation, which opens voltage-operated Ca^{2+} channels and the influx of Ca^{2+} leads to insulin secretion. This couples insulin secretion to states of raised ATP and glucose.

Hypokalaemia

A small reduction in extracellular K^+ below its normal range (3.5–5.3 mM) leads to the resting membrane potential becoming more negative with respect to the outside (**hyperpolarisation**). As a consequence the cell becomes less excitable, as it is more difficult for the cell to reach threshold potential and generate an action potential. A common cause of hypokalaemia is the use of diuretics (drugs that act on the kidney to promote fluid loss and are used in chronic heart failure and hypertension; Chapter 32). Diuretics reduce circulating volume, which activates the renin-angiotensin-aldosterone system (RAAS) (Chapters 32 and 38). The increased levels of aldosterone act on the distal convoluted tubules in the kidney to promote Na^+ reabsorption with the loss of K^+ from the body (Chapter 38).

Correction of hypokalaemia can be achieved by the use of K^+ supplements, K^+ rich foods (e.g. bananas) or K-sparing diuretics (e.g. spironolactone) that interfere with the actions of aldosteorone.

Hyperkalaemia

Increases in extracellular K^+ levels lead to cells becoming less negative with respect to the outside (**depolarisation**) and this results in cell excitation. For this reason, KCl should never be given by rapid intravenous injection as widespread cellular depolarisation is likely to prove fatal, often through abnormalities in cardiac rhythm. Hyperkalaemia is often associated with renal disease or the use of ACE inhibitors (Chapter 32), which block the RAAS and reduce K^+ loss (Chapter 38).

19 Nervous conduction

Michael D Randall

Figure 19.1 Schematic diagram showing the activation of closed voltage-operated Na⁺ channels due to depolarisation

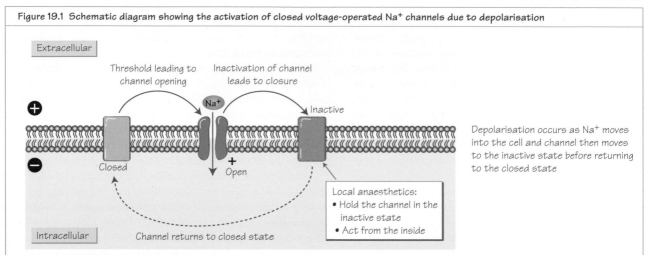

Depolarisation occurs as Na⁺ moves into the cell and channel then moves to the inactive state before returning to the closed state

Figure 19.2 A typical action potential

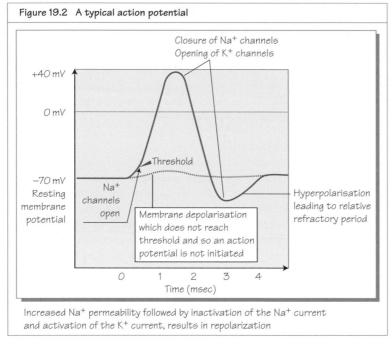

Increased Na⁺ permeability followed by inactivation of the Na⁺ current and activation of the K⁺ current, results in repolarization

Figure 19.3 Saltatory conduction

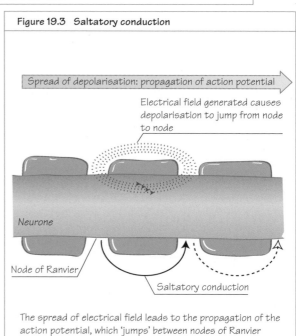

The spread of electrical field leads to the propagation of the action potential, which 'jumps' between nodes of Ranvier

Extracellular [K$^+$] essentially determines resting **membrane potential (V$_m$)** and ensures that excitation occurs at an appropriate time (Chapter 18). Excitation forms the basis of nervous conduction and also ensures the coupling of physiological responses (e.g. muscle contraction). Na$^+$ ions play a central role in the initiation and propagation of excitation (Figure 19.1).

Neurones typically have a **V$_m$ = −70 mV**, and following excitation (e.g. activation of receptors, the spread of nervous impulses) there is local **depolarisation** (i.e. the intracellular potential difference becomes less negative) and the membrane reaches **threshold**. At threshold, **voltage-operated Na$^+$ channels** ('fast' sodium channels) undergo a conformation change and the channel opens. The increase in Na$^+$ permeability causes an influx of Na$^+$ ions down their **electrochemical gradient** and, as determined by the **Nernst equation**, the movement of ions attempts to take the membrane towards the equilibrium potential for Na$^+$ (+65 mV).

Ion channels

Excitability is governed by ion channels. These are proteins that span the membrane and are permeable to specific ions. Their activity may be sensitive to voltage (voltage-operated) and their opening and closure are determined by the electrical environment. Other channel types are receptor-operated, in which events such as mechanical changes (e.g. stretch in **muscle spindle fibres**) cause the channel to open, leading to depolarisation (the **receptor generator potential**), which may lead to the initiation of action potentials.

The action potential

From **threshold** (approx. −50 mV) both the chemical and electrical gradients favour Na$^+$ influx (Figure 19.2). As the membrane depolarises to a potential of 0 mV, the electrical gradient dissipates and is no longer apparent at 0 mV. At this point it is the chemical gradient that continues to drive Na$^+$ influx such that the membrane potential becomes positive. As the membrane depolarises from 0 mV the electrical gradient starts to oppose force generated by the chemical gradient. The interplay of the chemical and electrical driving forces mean that there is depolarisation until (an **overshoot**) a peak membrane potential of approx. +40 mV is reached.

As the Na$^+$ channels open this leads to the next step, which is channel closure. At the same time, the depolarisation due to the Na$^+$ channels, leads to the activation of voltage-sensitive K$^+$ channels. The closure of Na$^+$ and activation of K$^+$ channels limits the depolarisation. More importantly, the opening of K$^+$ channels leads to K$^+$ efflux and this leads to the membrane to repolarise, i.e. initiates the return of membrane potential to the resting membrane potential and may overshoot to a **hyperpolarised** (more negative) and less excitable state.

Refractory period

The action potential is followed by a period (a few milliseconds) in which the cell cannot be excited. It has two components.

• **Absolute refractory period**: during which the cell cannot be excited, even at high stimuli. This is because the Na$^+$ channel has three kinetic states: **Close – Open – Inactivated**. Once the channel has opened it enters the inactive state before returning to the closed state. While in the inactive state the channel is closed and it cannot be activated. The period of time the channel is in the inactive state is the absolute refractory period.

• **Relative refractory period**: once the Na$^+$ channel returns to the closed state, the hyperpolarisation due to the K$^+$ efflux results in reduced excitability, with the Na$^+$ channels further from threshold and less likely to open. However, with increased stimulus (e.g. greater activation of mechanoreceptors and summation of receptor generator potentials) an action potential can be initiated, hence this refractory period is 'relative'.

The refractory period means that there is a maximum frequency of nervous impulses (~300 per second) and so nervous information is **frequency encoded** (the number of impulses correlates with the size of the stimulus).

Nervous conduction

The action potential is responsible for the transmission of electrical information. For this to occur, the action potential must spread or be propagated along the neurone. This is achieved by local depolarisation causing an adjacent region of the membrane to reach threshold, which causes the voltage operated Na$^+$ channels to open, leading to depolarisation and the genesis of an action potential along the nerve.

Saltatory conduction

To achieve rapid nervous conduction consistent with a fast-reacting nervous system, large nerves have a sheet of myelin to insulate the nerve (Figure 19.3). At intervals of 1–2 mm the myelin is absent and these areas are the **nodes of Ranvier**. This means that the wave of depolarisation 'jumps' from node to node and this leads to rapid conduction of electrical activity, referred to as '**saltatory conduction**'.

Speed of conduction

Larger diameter neurones are myelinated and have high conduction velocities. For example, Aα motor neurones have a diameter of 12–20 μm and conduction velocity of 70–120 m/s, whereas smaller nerves are unmyelinated and condition rates are slower, e.g. C pain fibres are unmyelinated with a diameter of ~1 μm and conduction velocities of 0.5–2.3 m/s.

Local anaesthetics

These are drugs (e.g. lidocaine) that block the transmission of pain by inhibiting action potential propagation. Local anaesthetics block action potential conduction in sensory nerves. They block voltage-operated Na$^+$ channels by binding to the channel in the 'Inactive' state. The channel is then held in the inactive state, and this prevents further activation and the propagation of action potentials. Many local anaesthetics show **use-dependence**, which means that as the frequency of action potentials increase, the level of blockade increases.

For local anaesthetics to act they must penetrate the cell membrane to act on the channel from the inside and this only occurs when the drug is in the uncharged form. Local anaesthetics are often weak bases and so show pH-dependence. As they are weak bases they are protonated (charged) at lower pHs and only at higher pH does the uncharged form predominate and it is in this form that the drug can penetrate the cell membrane and act on the channel from the intracellular side.

Cardiac action potentials (Chapter 30)

The classic neuronal action potential is not the only form of an action potential. Cardiac activity also involves the propagation of electrical activity. In the ventricles, the Na$^+$-channel-led depolarisation also activates voltage-operated Ca^{2+} channels, resulting in Ca^{2+} influx and cardiac contraction. The opening of the Ca^{2+} channels is prolonged, resulting in a plateau of the action potential.

20 Synaptic transmission

Michael D Randall

Figure 20.1 An idealised synapse showing the release of neurotransmitter leading to either excitation or inhibition

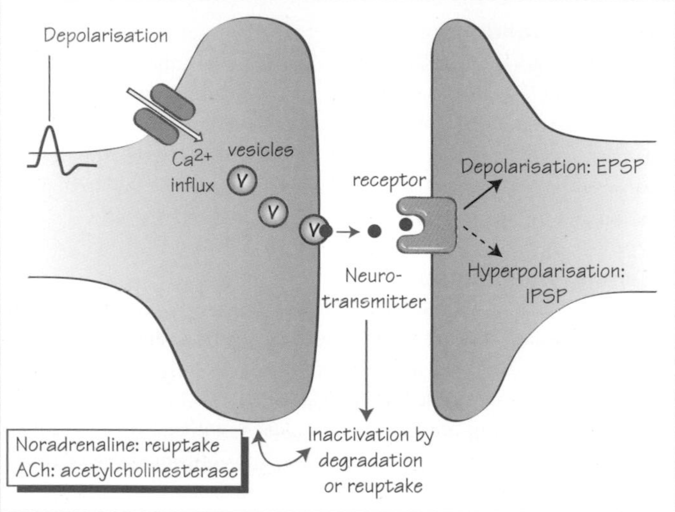

Depolarisation
Ca2+ influx
vesicles
receptor
Neuro-transmitter
Depolarisation: EPSP
Hyperpolarisation: IPSP
Inactivation by degradation or reuptake

Noradrenaline: reuptake
ACh: acetylcholinesterase

Figure 20.2 Schematic diagram of temporal and spatial summation

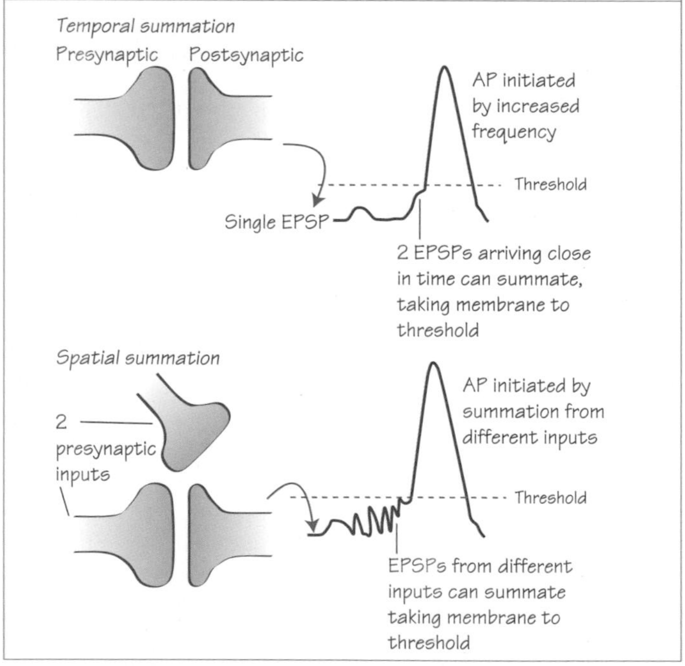

Temporal summation
Presynaptic   Postsynaptic

AP initiated by increased frequency
Single EPSP
Threshold
2 EPSPs arriving close in time can summate, taking membrane to threshold

Spatial summation

2 presynaptic inputs

AP initiated by summation from different inputs
Threshold
EPSPs from different inputs can summate taking membrane to threshold

---

Figure 20.3 A schematic diagram of the concept of presynaptic inhibition and autoinhibition

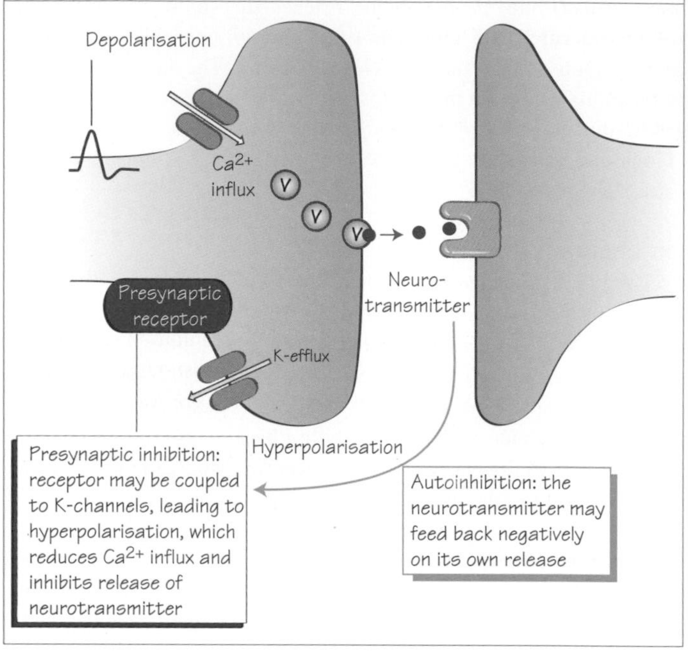

Depolarisation
Ca2+ influx
Presynaptic receptor
K-efflux
Neuro-transmitter
Hyperpolarisation

Presynaptic inhibition: receptor may be coupled to K-channels, leading to hyperpolarisation, which reduces Ca2+ influx and inhibits release of neurotransmitter

Autoinhibition: the neurotransmitter may feed back negatively on its own release

---

Figure 20.4 Spinal synapses as part of a reflex pathway, showing both excitation and inhibition

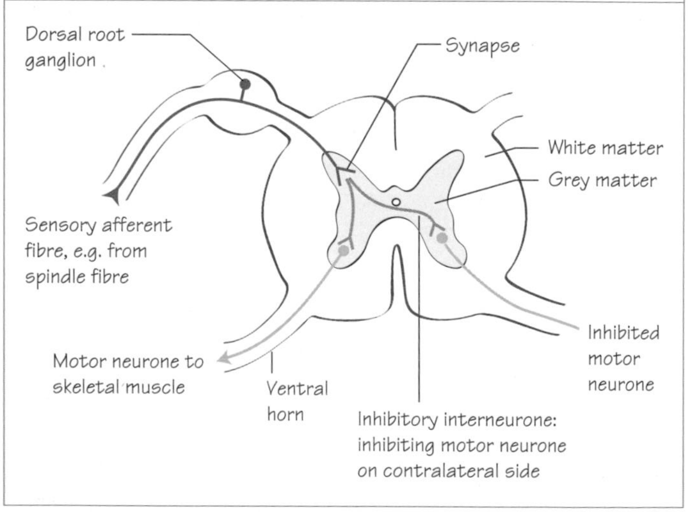

Dorsal root ganglion
Synapse
White matter
Grey matter
Sensory afferent fibre, e.g. from spindle fibre
Motor neurone to skeletal muscle
Ventral horn
Inhibitory interneurone: inhibiting motor neurone on contralateral side
Inhibited motor neurone

Nervous activity involves the spread of electrical charge via the generation and propagation of action potentials. Communication between neurones is predominantly via chemical transmission at synapses, in which an impulse in one fibre leads to the release of neurotransmitter, which acts on an adjacent neurone. In the autonomic nervous system a **presynaptic fibre** may synapse with a single **postsynaptic fibre**, which then releases neurotransmitters to control the target tissue. Synaptic transmission ensures that nervous conduction is **orthodromic**, i.e. unidirectional. In the central nervous system (CNS) a neurone may make up to 10 000 synapses with other neurones, reflecting the complexity and integration of connections with the CNS.

General principles

The arrival of the action potential at the presynaptic terminal leads to depolarisation, which activates voltage-sensitive Ca^{2+} channels resulting in Ca^{2+} influx. The rise in intracellular Ca^{2+} then leads to **exocytosis** of neurotransmitter vesicles and the release of neurotransmitter into the **synaptic cleft**. The neurotransmitter then binds to receptors on the postsynaptic terminal, leading to activation or inhibition of the neurone. The activation often involves depolarisation, leading to an **EPSP (excitatory postsynaptic potential)**, and inhibition often leads to hyperpolarisation with an **IPSP (inhibitory postsynaptic potential)**. The neurotransmitter is then degraded or taken up by transport mechanisms (Figure 20.1).

Temporal and spatial summation of impulses

The post-synaptic events, whether excitatory or inhibitory, may be additive. For example, if two excitatory impulses are close in time (i.e. temporally close) then the EPSPs in the post-synaptic cell may combine, leading to greater depolarisation and so increasing the probability of the cell reaching threshold and initiating an action potential. This leads to an enhancement of excitation, termed **temporal summation** (Figure 20.2).

For a post-synaptic neurone that has multiple presynaptic inputs, then the EPSPs (or IPSPs) derived from different connections can summate (or act in opposition) and so determine whether the cell reaches threshold and sets up an action potential. This is termed **spatial summation** (Figure 20.2).

The consequence of these properties of summation mean that information may be reinforced by high-frequency stimulation and that there is integration information from the different inputs.

Presynaptic inhibition

Synaptic transmission may be modulated by **presynaptic inhibition** (Figure 20.3). Under these circumstances a neurotransmitter (e.g. endogenous opioids such as the enkaphalins) or drug (e.g. opioids such as morphine) acts on presynaptic receptors, leading to hyperpolarisation, and this opposes the release of neurotransmitters. An example of this is when opioids act at μ-opioid receptors, leading to an inhibition of adenylyl cyclase, leading to a reduction in cAMP and the activation of a K-conductance. This results in hyperpolarisation, which stabilises the cell membrane and opposes synaptic transmission. This can explain the ability of opioids to inhibit pain transmission via sensory nerves and to cause constipation via inhibition of parasympathetic nerves responsible for lower gastrointestinal motility. There may also be **autoinhibition**. For example, at noradrenergic synapses the released noradrenaline may stimulate the target post-synaptic adrenoceptors but also act on presynaptic α_2-adrenoceptors, which reduce further transmitter release. This leads to negative feedback.

Cholinergic transmission

Acetylcholine (ACh) is involved at all autonomic ganglia and activates nicotinic receptors to activate postsynaptic fibres. It is also released by postganglionic parasympathetic fibres to activate muscarinic receptors on the target organ/tissue. ACh is also the neurotransmitter at neuromuscular junctions to stimulate nicotinic receptors on skeletal muscle. Once released, ACh is metabolised by **acetylcholinesterase (AChE)**, leading to inactivation and the reuptake of choline into the presynaptic terminal.

Noradrenergic transmission

Noradrenaline is the neurotransmitter that is released by sympathetic nerves and acts on the target tissues/organs. It activates alpha (α_1 and α_2)-adrenoceptors and beta (β_1 and β_2)-adrenoceptors. The activity of noradrenaline is terminated by **neuronal and non-neuronal uptake** via specific transporters. Following reuptake noradrenaline is metabolised by **monoamine oxidases**.

The neuronal reuptake of noradrenaline is a site of drug action and is inhibited by tricyclic antidepressants (e.g. amitripyline), which increase the levels of noradrenaline in the synaptic cleft. Some older antidepressants also act via inhibition of the monoamine oxidases.

Ionotropic neurotransmission

Ionotropic transmission is when the postsynaptic receptor is coupled to ion channels (ligand-gated), leading to a rapid depolarisation (excitation) or hyperpolarisation (inhibition). It occurs when a rapid 'on-off' response is required.

Metabotropic neurotransmission

Metabotropic transmission is when the postsynaptic receptor activation leads to a biochemical response in the target tissue, e.g. β-adrenoceptors activating adenylyl cyclase, leading to an increase in cAMP. In the heart, β_1-adrenoceptors increase cAMP, leading to an increase force and rate of contraction; in the airways, β_2-adrenoceptors increase intracellular cAMP, leading to relaxation of bronchial smooth muscle.

Inhibitory neurotransmission

Inhibition of nerve activity in the nervous system is key to nervous control. In the spinal cord, glycine, and in the brain, GABA, are examples of inhibitory transmissions. Both cause cellular hyperpolarisation by setting up IPSPs through inotropic receptors. In the spine, this dampens reflexes by having inhibitory modulation. In the brain, GABA is a key inhibitory transmitter that acts at $GABA_A$ receptors, in which the receptor complex is associated with a chloride channel, which in opening allows chloride influx and hyperpolarisation. The **benzodiazepines** (e.g. diazepam) enhance the actions of GABA at the $GABA_A$ receptors, leading to enhanced inhibition, resulting in sedation and anticonvulsive effects.

Spinal reflexes (Figure 20.4)

Synaptic transmission underpins spinal reflexes. The simple monosynaptic pathway involves sensory information (e.g. from spindle fibres, pain receptors) arriving at the dorsal root and activating a motorneurone via an excitatory synapse. This can lead to a simple reflex arc, e.g. the patella tendon reflex. The communication is more complex in that the sensory nerve can activate an inhibitory interneurone, which then inhibits for example a motor neurone on the contralateral side, resulting in inhibition of an opposing muscle.

21 Autonomic nervous system

Michael D Randall

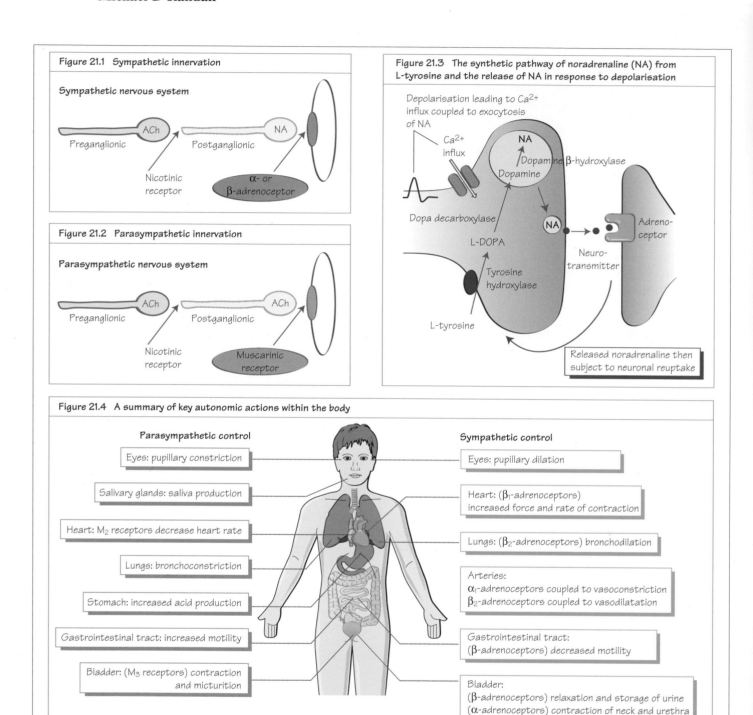

Figure 21.1 Sympathetic innervation

Sympathetic nervous system

Preganglionic — ACh — Postganglionic — NA

Nicotinic receptor

α- or β-adrenoceptor

Figure 21.2 Parasympathetic innervation

Parasympathetic nervous system

Preganglionic — ACh — Postganglionic — ACh

Nicotinic receptor

Muscarinic receptor

Figure 21.3 The synthetic pathway of noradrenaline (NA) from L-tyrosine and the release of NA in response to depolarisation

Depolarisation leading to Ca2+ influx coupled to exocytosis of NA

Ca2+ influx

NA

Dopamine β-hydroxylase

Dopamine

Dopa decarboxylase

L-DOPA

NA

Neurotransmitter

Adreno-ceptor

Tyrosine hydroxylase

L-tyrosine

Released noradrenaline then subject to neuronal reuptake

Figure 21.4 A summary of key autonomic actions within the body

Parasympathetic control

- Eyes: pupillary constriction
- Salivary glands: saliva production
- Heart: M₂ receptors decrease heart rate
- Lungs: bronchoconstriction
- Stomach: increased acid production
- Gastrointestinal tract: increased motility
- Bladder: (M₃ receptors) contraction and micturition

Sympathetic control

- Eyes: pupillary dilation
- Heart: (β₁-adrenoceptors) increased force and rate of contraction
- Lungs: (β₂-adrenoceptors) bronchodilation
- Arteries: α₁-adrenoceptors coupled to vasoconstriction β₂-adrenoceptors coupled to vasodilatation
- Gastrointestinal tract: (β-adrenoceptors) decreased motility
- Bladder: (β-adrenoceptors) relaxation and storage of urine (α-adrenoceptors) contraction of neck and urethra

The autonomic nervous system regulates involuntary actions such as breathing, the regulation of cardiac contractions, blood pressure control, gastrointestinal secretions and motility, control of pupil diameter, sweating, bladder control and sexual function.

The autonomic nervous system is divided into the **sympathetic** and **parasympathetic** systems (Figures 21.1 and 21.2). Both systems involve preganglionic and postganglionic fibres. In both cases, **acetylcholine** (ACh) is the neurotransmitter at the ganglionic synapse, where it stimulates ligand-gated **nicotinic receptors**, leading to the activation of the postganglionic fibres. These in turn lead to the activation of target receptors on the innervated tissue.

 Medical Sciences at a Glance, First Edition. Edited by Michael D Randall. © 2014 John Wiley & Sons, Ltd. Published 2014 by John Wiley & Sons, Ltd.

Parasympathetic control

In the parasympathetic nervous system, the ganglion is generally located close to, or in, the innervated organ and generally leads to more localised control. The postganglionic neurotransmitter is Ach, which acts at muscarinic receptors.

Muscarinic receptors are **G-protein-coupled receptors (GPCRs)** in which the subtypes M_1, M_3 and M_5 are coupled via $G_{q/11}$ to Ca^{2+} mobilisation; and M_2 and M_4 are G_i-linked to inhibition of formation of the second messenger cAMP (Chapter 7).

Sympathetic control

Anatomically this tends to provide more 'global' control, with the autonomic ganglia or synapses being located more centrally and closer to the spinal cord. The postganglionic neurotransmitter is **noradrenaline** (Figure 21.3), which acts at α- or β-**adrenoceptors**, depending on the tissue. An exception are the sweat glands, which are functionally sympathetic but have ACh as the neurotransmitter, which stimulates muscarinic (M) receptors.

An extension of the sympathetic nervous system is the **adrenal medulla**, which is essentially a sympathetic postganglionic fibre where ACh acts at nicotinic receptors to stimulate the release of **adrenaline** (and some noradrenaline) into the circulation. Adrenaline then exerts sympathetic actions (e.g. increase in heart rate and bronchodilation). This forms part of the 'fright, flight or fight' response.

Adrenoceptors

α_1-**adrenoceptors** are coupled via G-proteins ($G_{q/11}$) to activation of phospholipase C, which liberates inositol trisphophate (IP_3) and diacyl glycerol (DAG), leading to increases in intracellular Ca^{2+}.

α_2-**adrenoceptors** are negatively coupled via G_i to adenylyl cyclase, leading to reductions in cAMP.

β_1- **and** β_2-**adrenoceptors** are also GPCRs in which G_s is coupled to the activation of adenylyl cyclase and elevations in cAMP.

Autonomic regulation (Figure 21.4)

Cardiac control (Chapter 30)

Sympathetic: noradrenaline acts at β_1-adrenoceptors to increase the force (**inotropy**) and rate of cardiac contractions, (**positive chronotropy**).

Parasympathetic: ACh acts at M_2 receptors to reduce the heart rate (**negative chronotropy**).

Pharmacology: β-adrenoceptor antagonists (**beta-blockers**) are used to block cardiac β_1-adrenoceptors in the treatment of angina (e.g. atenolol) and heart failure (e.g. bisoprolol) (Chapter 35).

Vascular control (Chapter 31)

Sympathetic: noradrenaline acts at α_1- and α_2-adrenoceptors on vascular smooth muscle on arteries to cause **vasoconstriction**, and β_2-adrenoceptors (in skeletal muscle) to cause **vasodilatation**.

• α_1-adrenoceptor antagonists (e.g. prazosin) are used as antihypertensives but their use is limited by widespread side effects through interference of sympathetic control.

• *Adrenaline* is used to increase cardiac output and cause bronchodilation in anaphylactic shock.

• *Sympathomimetic agents:* these agents mimic the sympathetic nervous system and are widely used as **decongestants**. These actions can be direct (due to receptor agonism, e.g. phenylephrine) or indirect (by displacing and releasing noradrenaline, e.g. pseudoephedrine). They cause local vasoconstriction, reducing blood flow and mucus.

Central control of the cardiovascular system

In the cardiovascular control centres of the central nervous system noradrenaline activates α_2-adrenoceptors to decrease sympathetic outflow and increase vagal output.

Respiratory control (Chapter 26)

Sympathetic: circulating adrenaline acts at β_2-adrenoceptors to cause bronchodilation.

Parasympathetic: ACh acts at M_3 receptors to cause bronchoconstriction and increase mucus secretion.

• β_2-adrenoceptor agonists (e.g. salbutamol) are **bronchodilators** and are used as 'relievers' in asthma. Longer-acting β_2-agonists (e.g. salmeterol) are used for longer-term control as 'preventers' in asthma and chronic obstructive pulmonary disease (COPD).

• Muscarinic receptor antagonists (e.g. ipratropium) block parasympathetic bronchoconstriction and are used as bronchodilators in COPD.

• Beta-blockers (even β_1-selective) are contraindicated in asthma as they can block bronchial β_2-adrenoceptors, causing severe bronchospasm.

Gastrointestinal control (Chapters 42 and 43)

Salivary glands: parasympathetic control via ACh acting at M_3 receptors stimulates the production of saliva and increases blood flow. Sympathetic stimulation leads to the production of viscous saliva.

Gastric acid secretion: ACh acts at M_1 and M_3 receptors on parietal cells to stimulate gastric acid production.

Gastrointestinal motility: Muscarinic receptors are coupled to increased motility. Muscarinic receptor antagonists reduce motility and lead to constipation. They are sometimes used as antispasmodic agents.

Bladder control (Chapter 40)

Parasympathetic: ACh acts at M_3 receptors, which are coupled to contraction of the detrusor muscle, and at M receptors at the trigone and sphincter muscles leading to relaxation. These actions lead to bladder voiding.

Sympathetic: noradrenaline acts at β_2- and β_3-adrenoceptors to relax the detrusor muscle and at α_1-adrenoceptors at the trigone and sphincter muscles, leading to contraction.

Pharmacology: muscarinic receptor antagonists (e.g. oxybutynin) are used to relax the bladder and reduce the symptoms of overactive bladder. α_1-adrenoceptor antagonists (e.g. tamsulosin) are used to relax prostatic smooth muscle and so reduce prostatic obstruction.

Visual system

Sympathetic: α-adrenoceptors are coupled to pupilary dilation.

Parasympathetic: M_3 receptors are coupled to pupilary constriction.

Pharmacology: muscarinic receptor antagonists (e.g. tropicamide) are used as eye drops to dilate the pupils in ophthalmic examinations. Muscarinic agonists (e.g. pilocarpine) are used to constrict the pupils (miosis), which reduces pressure in closed-angle glaucoma.

Co-transmission

In addition to the 'classical' mediators of autonomic transmission, other mediators may also act in concert to form co-transmission. These are termed 'NANC' transmitters, as they are non-adrenergic and non-cholinergic. Important examples of co-transmitters include the purine ATP and neuropeptide Y (sympathetic), and vasoactive intestinal polypeptide and nitric oxide (parasympathetic), and these may be released in addition to the classical transmitter. Their release may enhance the actions of the 'classical' transmitter or be released differentially under certain circumstances (e.g. at different frequencies of stimulation).

Michael D Randall

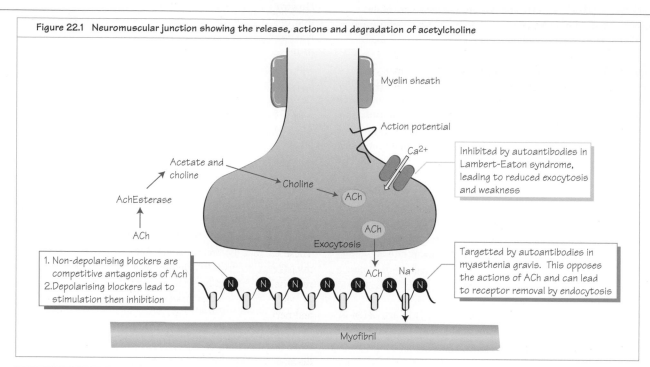

Figure 22.1 Neuromuscular junction showing the release, actions and degradation of acetylcholine

Myelin sheath

Action potential

Ca^{2+}

Acetate and choline

AchEsterase

ACh

Choline

ACh

Exocytosis

Inhibited by autoantibodies in Lambert-Eaton syndrome, leading to reduced exocytosis and weakness

1. Non-depolarising blockers are competitive antagonists of Ach
2. Depolarising blockers lead to stimulation then inhibition

ACh Na^+

Targetted by autoantibodies in myasthenia gravis. This opposes the actions of ACh and can lead to receptor removal by endocytosis

Myofibril

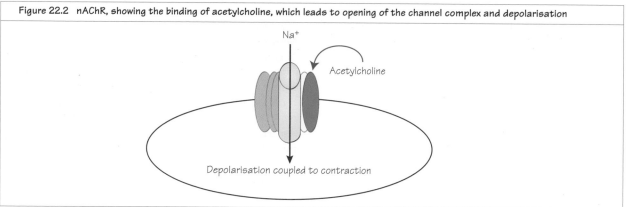

Figure 22.2   nAChR, showing the binding of acetylcholine, which leads to opening of the channel complex and depolarisation

Na^+

Acetylcholine

Depolarisation coupled to contraction

Neuromuscular junction (NMJ)

The neuromuscular junction (NMJ) is a specialised synapse between motor neurones and skeletal muscle, which enables nervous control of skeletal muscle contraction. At the NMJ, the neurone and skeletal membrane are brought into close contact by folding and the outside of the neurone is held in place by a **Schwann cell**. Anatomically, a collection of neuromuscular junctions form a **motor end plate**.

At the NMJ action potentials in the motor neurone cause depolarisation of the presynaptic terminal (**bouton**), which leads to the opening of voltage-operated (gated) Ca^{2+} channels and the influx of Ca^{2+} ions. The influx of Ca^{2+} ions then stimulates the **exocytosis** of synaptic vesicles containing the neurotransmitter **acetylcholine (ACh)** (Figure 22.1).

When released, ACh diffuses across the synaptic cleft (typically 50 nm) and stimulates postsynaptic **ionotropic nicotinic receptors**. The **nicotinic acetylcholine receptor** (nAChR) is an ion-channel complex of five transmembraneous subunits (α_2, β, δ, γ) and opens on activation by ACh. The open ion-channel complex is permeable to both Na^+ (influx) and K^+ (efflux), and following activation there is transient cellular depolarisation, which leads to a **miniature end plate potential (mEPP)** of typically 0.4 mV. The vesicles of ACh are of a relatively consistent size and so the transmission is quantal, with packages of excitation leading to steps in excitation. The mEPPs generated at the NMJ summate to form **excitatory post-synaptic potentials** (EPPs) and once threshold is reached lead to actions potential via voltage-operated Na^+ channels (sensitive to tetrodotoxin), which are propagated across the skeletal muscle by spreading depolarisation. The depolarisation of the skeletal muscle is coupled (via the T-tubular system) to Ca^{2+} release from the intracellular sarcoplasmic reticulum stores and the increase in intracellular Ca^{2+} leads to contraction of the skeletal muscle (Figures 22.1 and 22.2).

The actions of ACh (and therefore the signal for contraction) are terminated by **acetylcholinesterase (AChE)**, which breaks down ACh into acetate and choline. The choline is then recycled by reuptake by the presynaptic terminal. The reuptake mechanism can be blocked by hemicholinium.

Neuromuscular blockers

Neuromuscular transmission is targeted therapeutically by neuromuscular blockers, which are used in surgery to prevent muscle contraction, e.g. to prevent abdominal muscle contractions during abdominal surgery. Neuromuscular blockers are divided into two main classes.

Non-depolarising blockers (e.g. tubocurarine, pancuronium)

These drugs were developed from the neurotoxin curare, which was used in South American poisoned arrows.

These are competitive receptor antagonists of ACh at the nAChR. The onset of blockade leads to paralysis, as they block the actions of ACh. The blockade is dose-dependent and may be overcome by inhib-itors of AChE, which lead to increased levels of ACh to compete with the blocker.

Depolarising blockers (e.g. suxamethonium)

These are actually agonists at the nAChR and the onset of action is initially accompanied by stimulation, which leads to muscle twitches. However, the activation of the nAChR leads to prolonged depolarisation of the skeletal muscle and inactivation of the voltage-operated Na^+ channels that propagate the action potentials. It is the inactivation of these Na^+ channels that leads to failure of neuromuscular control and paralysis. In contrast to non-depolarising blockade, the inhibition by depolarising agents cannot be reversed by inhibition of AChE.

Toxins and the neuromuscular transmission

The exocytosis of vesicles can be blocked by **botulinum toxin**, which prevents fusion of the vesicles with the cell membrane, and this inhibition of release leads to paralysis.

The nAChR is sensitive to blockade by **α-bungarotoxin**. This is a snake-derived venon that binds irreversibly to the nAChR and is used extensively on neurophysiology to investigate the regulation of NMJs.

Inhibitors of acetylcholinesterase (AChE)

These prevent the breakdown of ACh and are used therapeutically in myasthenia gravis (MG). Inhibition also occurs with organophosphorus insecticides and nerve toxins, which lead to perpetual activation of neuromuscular transmission. Hence they are used in insecticides and nerve gases to disrupt neuromuscular control, leading to death.

AChE inhibitors are also used therapeutically to enhance the actions of ACh in the brain to improve cognitive function in Alzheimer's disease (Chapter 57).

Pathophysiology
Myasthenia gravis

This is a rare disease that affects neuromuscular transmission. It is associated with muscle weakness and an inability for prolonged muscle contraction due to impaired neuromuscular transmission. MG is caused by autoantibodies which bind to and block the nAChRs, so preventing the actions of ACh and muscle contraction. In some cases, the antibodies lead to endocytosis of the receptors and their removal from the membrane. To overcome the impaired actions of ACh inhibitors of AChE (e.g. neostigmine) are used to prevent the breakdown of ACh and so enhance its actions.

Lambert-Eaton myasthenic syndrome

This is characterised by the production of antibodies against the presynaptic Ca^{2+} channels involved in stimulating exocytosis of ACh vesicles. In this condition there is reduced ACh release, leading to weakness. However, the inhibitory effects of the antibodies can be overcome by increased Ca^{2+} influx and so the weakness can improve on exercise.

Structure of the respiratory system

Siobhan Loughna and Deborah Merrick

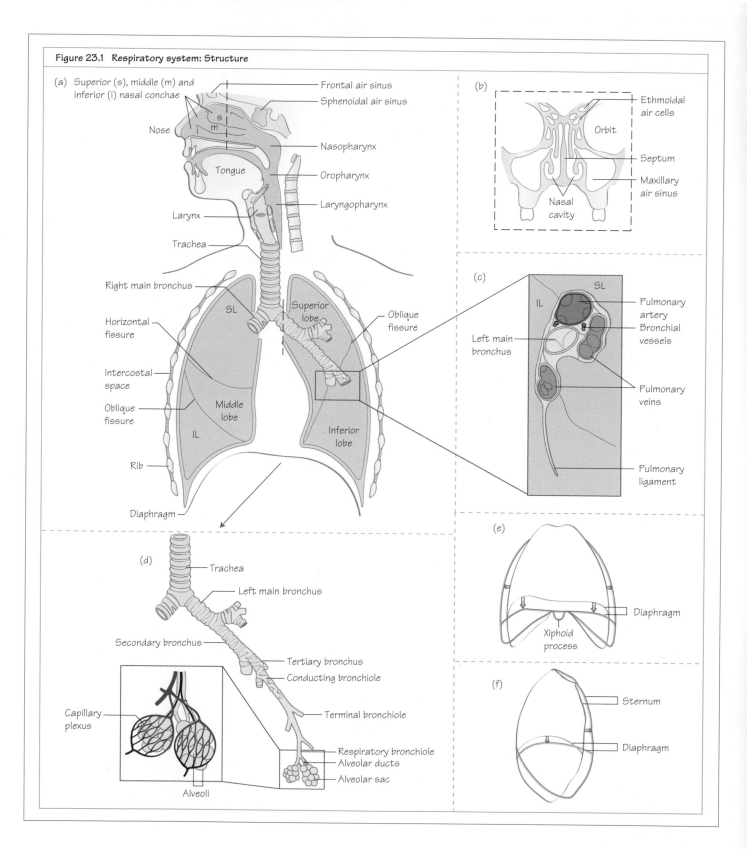

Figure 23.1 Respiratory system: Structure

(a) Superior (s), middle (m) and inferior (i) nasal conchae

- Frontal air sinus
- Sphenoidal air sinus
- Nasopharynx
- Oropharynx
- Laryngopharynx

Nose

Tongue

Larynx

Trachea

Right main bronchus

Horizontal fissure

Intercostal space

Oblique fissure

Rib

Diaphragm

SL

Superior lobe

Oblique fissure

Middle lobe

IL

Inferior lobe

(b)
- Ethmoidal air cells
- Orbit
- Septum
- Maxillary air sinus
- Nasal cavity

(c)
SL

IL

Left main bronchus

- Pulmonary artery
- Bronchial vessels
- Pulmonary veins
- Pulmonary ligament

(d)
- Trachea
- Left main bronchus
- Secondary bronchus
- Tertiary bronchus
- Conducting bronchiole
- Terminal bronchiole
- Respiratory bronchiole
- Alveolar ducts
- Alveolar sac

Capillary plexus

Alveoli

(e)
- Diaphragm
- Xiphoid process

(f)
- Sternum
- Diaphragm

The respiratory tract extends from the lips and nostrils to the alveoli of the lungs (Figure 23.1). It comprises a network of conducting and respiratory airways allowing air to pass into (inspiration) and out of (expiration) the lungs for gas exchange. The respiratory tract can be divided into upper and lower respiratory tracts for descriptive purposes.

Upper respiratory tract
Nasal cavities
These extend from the nostrils anteriorly to the posterior nasal apertures (choanae) posteriorly, and are divided into right and left halves by the nasal septum. Except for the vestibule of the nose, mucosa lines the nasal cavity. Air passing over the mucosa is warmed, filtered and moistened in preparation for efficient gas exchange, before passing further into the respiratory tract. The mucosa lining the majority of the respiratory tract is composed of **pseudostratified ciliated columnar epithelium** (respiratory epithelium). In certain areas within the nasal cavity the mucosa is modified for the specialised function of olfaction (olfactory epithelium). The nasal conchae, which increase the surface area, further divide each nasal cavity into four spaces: spheno-ethmoidal recess, superior nasal meatus, middle nasal meatus and inferior nasal meatus (Figure 23.1). The **paranasal sinuses** are air-filled cavities found within the frontal, maxilla, sphenoid and ethmoid bones (Figures 23.1 and 23.2). They communicate with the nasal cavities via small apertures.

Oral cavity
This extends from the lips anteriorly to the oropharynx posteriorly. It is divided into the oral vestibule and oral cavity proper. The oral vestibule is the slit-like space between the lips cheeks, teeth and gingivae. The oral cavity proper is the space posterior and medial to upper and lower dental arches; it contains the teeth and tongue.

Pharynx and larynx
This is the superior expansion of the alimentary system and is involved in the conduction of air to the larynx, trachea and lungs. It is a fibromuscular passage divided into three regions (Figure 23.1): **nasopharynx** (posterior to the nasal cavity), **oropharynx** (posterior to the oral cavity) and the **laryngopharynx** (posterior to the larynx). The **larynx** connects the oropharynx to the trachea. It has various important functions, including routing air into the lower respiratory tract, maintaining a patent respiratory tract and voice production.

Lower respiratory tract
Trachea and bronchial tree
The trachea is a fibrocartilaginous tube that extends from the larynx inferiorly and is characterised by C-shaped rings of hyaline cartilage contained within its walls. At vertebral level T4/5, the trachea bifurcates into two primary bronchi, with one passing to each lung. Within the lung, each bronchi divides repeatedly to form the bronchial tree (Figure 23.4). Each main bronchus divides into secondary bronchi (three on the right, two on the left – one to each lobe), which in turn divide into tertiary bronchi. The branching continues through terminal and respiratory bronchioles to alveolar ducts, alveolar sacs and the basic unit of gas exchange, the alveolus. The bronchioles are lined by ciliated simple columnar epithelium, transitioning to simple cuboidal epithelium in smaller peripheral branches. The alveoli are composed of type I pneumocytes (lining cells) and type II pneumocytes (surfactant producing cells).

Lungs
The lungs are divided by horizontal and oblique fissures into lobes, three on the right and two on the left (Figure 23.1). The root of the lung is formed by structures that enter and leave the lung (Figure 23.3). These include the main bronchus, a pulmonary artery supplying blood to the lung and two pulmonary veins draining blood from the lung. The bronchial vessels supply structures at the root of the lung, supporting tissues of the lung and viscera pleura. Innervation of the lungs is via the pulmonary plexuses containing parasympathetic and sympathetic fibres. **Parasympathetic innervation** (vagus nerves) causes bronchoconstriction, vasodilatation (pulmonary vessels) and secretomotor. **Sympathetic innvervation** is limited to mainly **circulating adrenaline**, which causes bronchodilation and inhibits secretions.

Pleura: a serous pleural sac that is composed of two membranes.
• Visceral pleura: covers the lungs and is adherent to its surface.
• Parietal pleura: lines the pulmonary cavities and is divided according to the region it lines: cervical, costal, diaphragmatic, mediastinal (Figure 23.1; right lung).

The mediastinal parietal pleura is continuous with the visceral pleura at the root of the lung. Serous pleural fluid is contained between the pleura membranes, allowing the two layers to glide over each other smoothly during respiration.

Thoracic wall
This is composed of bones, cartilages, muscles, vessels, nerves, fascia and skin. It provides protection for the thoracic organs and plays a role in respiration.

Thoracic cage: consists of 12 ribs and costal cartilages, 12 thoracic vertebrae and associated intervertebral discs, and the sternum. The ribs are described as true (1–7), false (8–10), or floating (11 and 12).

Intercostal muscles: comprise three muscle layers (external, internal and innermost) located within the intercostal spaces, between the ribs. These muscles receive innervation from the intercostal nerves (T1–T11) which run within the intercostal spaces. The intercostal muscles act as accessory muscles of respiration.

Diaphragm
The main muscle of respiration which forms the convex floor of the thoracic cavity. The diaphragm receives all motor innervation and some of its sensory innervation from the phrenic nerves (C3, 4, 5). The periphery of the diaphragm receives sensory innervation from the intercostal (T5–T11) and subcostal (T12) nerves.

Movements of the thoracic wall and diaphragm: change intrathoracic diameters and volumes during respiration, resulting in changes in intrathoracic pressure (Figures 23.5 and 23.6). During inspiration the vertical dimension of the central part of the thoracic cavity increases as the diaphragm descends. As the diaphragm relaxes, during expiration, the vertical dimension returns to a neutral position. The transverse dimension of the thoracic cavity also increases slightly during inspiration due to the intercostal muscles raising the lateral aspect of the ribs. The intercostal muscles also alter the anteroposterior dimension of the thorax by elevating the anterior ends of the ribs and sternum.

Lymphatic drainage of thoracic wall and respiratory tract
Lymph returns to the venous system via either the right lymphatic duct (draining right side of the thorax, head and neck and the right upper limb) or the thoracic duct (rest of body). Both lymphatic ducts drain into the junction of the subclavian and internal jugular veins (right and left venous angles respectively).

Steven Burr

Figure 24.1 Factors affecting the distributions of inhaled gases

(a) As chest expands airways widen, resistance to airflow decreases and inflation is easier, limits exhalation not inhalation

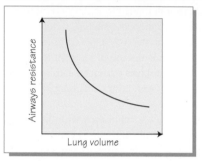

(b) As chest expands mechanical limits restrict volume, elastic forces increase and deflation is easier, limits inhalation not exhalation

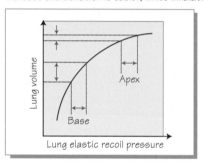

Same change in pressure yields a greater change in volume at bases than apical. Hence resting breathing is normally diaphragmatic

Figure 24.2 Alveolar gas exchange

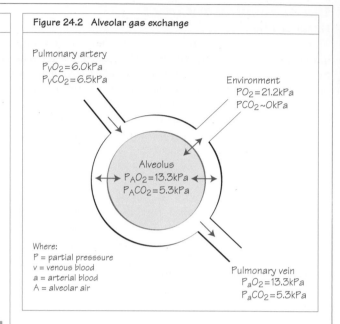

Pulmonary artery
$P_vO_2 = 6.0\,kPa$
$P_vCO_2 = 6.5\,kPa$

Environment
$PO_2 = 21.2\,kPa$
$PCO_2 \sim 0\,kPa$

Alveolus
$P_AO_2 = 13.3\,kPa$
$P_ACO_2 = 5.3\,kPa$

Pulmonary vein
$P_aO_2 = 13.3\,kPa$
$P_aCO_2 = 5.3\,kPa$

Where:
P = partial pressure
v = venous blood
a = arterial blood
A = alveolar air

Figure 24.3 Correlations between ventilation and perfusion

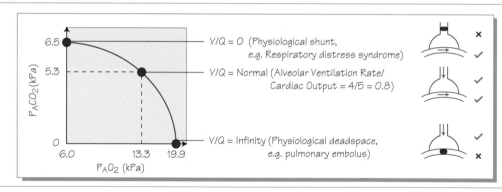

$V/Q = 0$ (Physiological shunt, e.g. Respiratory distress syndrome)

$V/Q = $ Normal (Alveolar Ventilation Rate/ Cardiac Output = 4/5 = 0.8)

$V/Q = $ Infinity (Physiological deadspace, e.g. pulmonary embolus)

The respiratory system serves to ensure that all tissues receive the O_2 they need and can dispose of the CO_2 they produce. Lungs exchange gases with atmosphere via the nasal cavity, which filters, warms and humidifies the air in preparation for efficient gas exchange. Blood carries gases to and from tissues, and has the intrinsic capacity to pick up O_2 and lose CO_2 if exposed to the right gaseous environment, and the lungs expose the blood to this type of environment.

Breathing

At rest we breathe at a respiratory rate of, on average, 12 breathes per minute, each with a volume of 0.5 L (with strenuous exercise this can rise to 120 L/min). The active inhalation phase lasts 2 s and the passive exhalation phase lasts 3 s. This normal respiration rate, depth and rhythm is called **eupnoea**. Breathing is therefore **tidal**, the last air to be inhaled is the first air to be exhaled. One-third of the air inhaled remains in the conducting airways at the end of inhalation and cannot take part in gas exchange. This relative proportion of **'dead space'** decreases with deeper breaths as the conducting airways contribute the same absolute volume. Thus deeper breaths are more efficient in moving air in and out of alveoli for gas exchange, but require more muscular effort. Two other critical internal factors that affect the distribution of inhaled gas and hence the efficiency of breathing, are airway resistance and lung compliance (Figure 24.1).

Airway resistance and conductance

Airway resistance is the opposition to airflow in the respiratory tree. Conductance (the reciprocal of resistance) is the change in flow for a unitary change in pressure, and usually limits exhalation. Airway resistance and conduction depend on friction and cross-sectional area. The major source of non-elastic resistance to air flow is friction in the respiratory passageways. **Resistance** in the respiratory tree is determined mostly by the diameters of the conducting tubules (i.e. trachea, bronchi, bronchioles, etc.). Gas flow stops at the terminal bronchioles, where airways have small diameters, but this is not a problem, as here diffusion is the main force driving gas movements. Therefore, the greatest resistance to gas flow occurs in the medium-sized bronchi and bronchioles. Although individual cross-sectional areas decrease with deeper penetration into the respiratory tree, total cross-sectional area increases. This means that there has to be very extensive damage to the small airways for ventilation to be affected.

Factors increasing airways resistance include: decreasing total lung volume; and increasing bronchomotor tone, age, mucus secretion and disease. Posture (through the effect of gravity) also affects airway resistance, as the height relative to heart affects blood vessel diameter and pressure on airways, while the abdominal contents either push up or pull down on the diaphragm altering lung volume by up to 1 L. Smooth muscle in the walls of the bronchioles has sensitive neural parasympathetic reflexes in response to inhaled irritants to prevent their deeper penetration (overreaction leads to asthma and can contribute to anaphylaxis).

Lung compliance and elastance

Compliance (the reciprocal of elastance, which is the ability to return to original shape after stretching) is the change in volume for a unitary change in pressure, and usually limits inhalation. As lung volume increases with expansion, then elasticity increases and compliance decreases (i.e. the more the lung inflates the harder it is to expand it further). Thus stiff lungs (e.g. with fibrosis) have low compliance and high elastic recoil (i.e. they are difficult to stretch and tend to return to resting position).

Surfactant decreases surface tension to maximise the compliance of lungs for inhalation. As surfactant becomes spread thinner during inflation it is less effective. So as alveoli become larger their surface tension decreases less, making it easier for small alveoli to expand and be recruited than it is for large alveoli.

It can be shown that for the same change in pressure, there is a greater change in lung volume at the lung base than at the apex (Figure 24.1b), because there is a greater range of mechanical movement at the diaphragm. Thus the lung acts as a more compliant structure at the lung base and it is easier to ventilate the lung base than the lung apex. We breathe from our lung bases at rest because of this reason.

With increasing age, tissue compliance increases (the lung is more compliant to air flow in, but does not collapse fully to push air out as elasticity has decreased), airways collapse more and thoracic compliance decreases (musculoskeletal elements become weaker and stiffer). The balance between lung tissue and thoracic compliance leads to peak ventilatory function in the third decade of life.

Diffusion and gas exchange

The lungs are a system for getting blood to one side and gas to the other side of alveolar membranes, so that gas exchange can occur between air and blood across the alveolar membrane (Figure 24.2). We inhale 21% O_2 and 0.03–0.04% CO_2, while exhaling 14% O_2 and 5% CO_2. Diffusion depends on large gradients for O_2 (19.9 kPa $P_AO_2 > 6.0$ kPa P_VO_2) and CO_2 (~0 kPa $P_ACO_2 < 6.5$ kPa P_VCO_2). Thus O_2 will diffuse into blood and CO_2 out of blood to achieve a P_aO_2 of 13.3 kPa and P_aCO_2 of 5.3 kPa. Diffusion also depends on a large combined alveolar surface area (70 m^2) and low diffusion resistance. Diffusion resistance depends on barrier thinness (0.5 μm, equal to one-tenth the width of an erythrocyte) and gas permeability (requiring low molecular weight and high solubility). O_2 exchange is complete within half a second of a blood cell arriving in a capillary. Erythrocytes spend about 1 s in a capillary, and so gas diffusion does not normally limit respiratory function.

Ventilation-perfusion coupling

To maximise the efficiency of gas exchange at the blood–gas interface, the amount of gas reaching the alveoli (ventilation) must be coupled to the flow of blood in pulmonary capillaries (perfusion). This is **ventilation-perfusion matching (V/Q)**, and it depends on local autoregulation of blood flow by altering vasomotor tone in response to P_AO_2 levels, and by altering bronchomotor tone in response to P_ACO_2 levels. Low O_2 causes vasoconstriction, while high O_2 causes vasodilatation. This is the opposite of what happens in the systemic circulation (e.g. low O_2 in a cerebral capillary would cause vasodilatation). High CO_2 dilates bronchioles, while low CO_2 constricts bronchioles. Thus gas is redirected to areas of the lung with adequate perfusion, while blood is similarly shunted to areas of the lung with adequate ventilation (Figure 24.3).

25 Gas transport

Steven Burr

Figure 25.1 Haemoglobin molecule

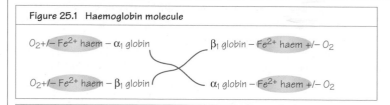

O2+/– Fe2+ haem – α1 globin
β1 globin – Fe2+ haem +/– O2
O2+/– Fe2+ haem – β1 globin
α1 globin – Fe2+ haem +/– O2

Figure 25.2 Oxyhaemoglobin dissociation curve

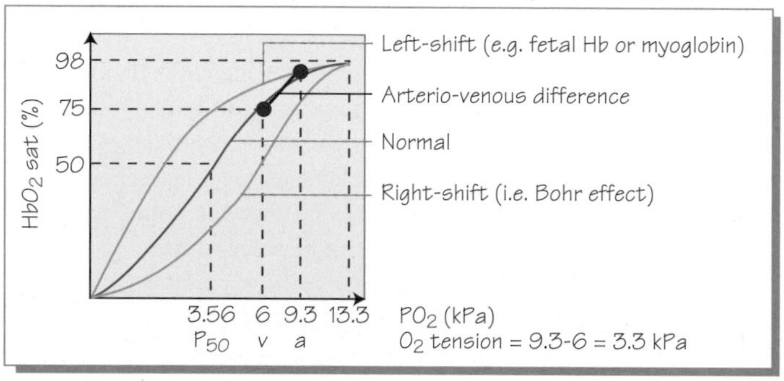

HbO2 sat (%)
98
75
50
Left-shift (e.g. fetal Hb or myoglobin)
Arterio-venous difference
Normal
Right-shift (i.e. Bohr effect)
3.56 6 9.3 13.3
P50 v a
PO2 (kPa)
O2 tension = 9.3-6 = 3.3 kPa

Figure 25.3 CO_2 transport

H+ + HCO3–
Carbaminos - plasma proteins
H2CO3
+ H2O
Dissolved
CO2
CO2
CO2
Red blood cell
Plasma
CO2+H2O
Carbaminos – Hb
Carbonic anhydrase
H-Hb
H2CO3
H+ + HCO3–
Cl– HCO3–
Capillary wall
Tissue fluid
Cell wall
0.5μm diffusion barrier

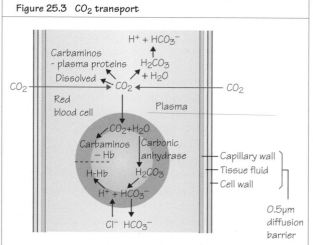

3 forms (CO_2, HCO_3^-, and carbaminos) in 2 compartments (plasma and cell). Arrows represent direction of events in metabolically active tissues (and are all reversed in the lungs)

Figure 25.4 CO_2 content of blood

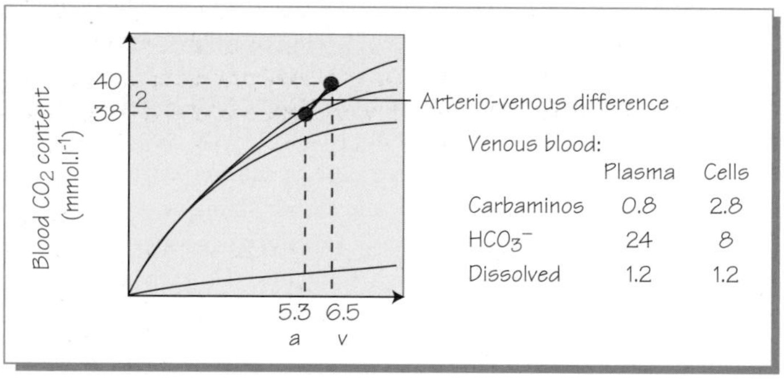

Blood CO2 content (mmol.l-1)
40
38
2
Arterio-venous difference
5.3 6.5
a v
Venous blood:
Plasma Cells
Carbaminos 0.8 2.8
HCO3– 24 8
Dissolved 1.2 1.2

Every minute at rest the human body consumes about 200 mL of oxygen (O_2) and produces about 200 mL of carbon dioxide (CO_2).

Oxygen

Forms of oxygen carriage and haemoglobin binding

O_2 is poorly soluble and so only 1.5% is transported dissolved in plasma. The remaining 98.5% is bound to **haemoglobin** (Hb) inside erythrocytes. Each erythrocyte contains 250–640 million Hb molecules (and there are 4.5–5.1 million erythrocytes per 1 mm^3 of blood). Hb is a protein composed of four polypeptide chain subunits. Each subunit is bound to an iron-containing porphyrin haem group. Because **ferrous** (Fe^{2+}) ions serve as O_2 binding sites, each Hb can rapidly and reversibly bind four O_2 molecules (Figure 25.1). A Hb molecule bound with O_2 is called **oxyhaemoglobin** (HbO_2), whereas a Hb molecule that has released its O_2 is called **deoxyhaemoglobin**. As O_2 binds it changes the optical absorption spectrum of the Hb and hence the colour of blood from cyan to red. Thus with an increase in the relative proportion of deoxyhaemoglobin to oxyhaemoglobin, a bluish discolouration of the skin and mucous membranes can be observed, which is referred to as **cyanosis**.

When the first O_2 molecule binds the first iron molecule, the Hb changes shape, and the affinity for the other three O_2 molecules progressively increases. Similarly, when the first O_2 is unloaded, the affinity for O_2 is decreased and it becomes progressively easier for the other three O_2 molecules to dissociate from the Hb. Hb is fully saturated when all four haem groups are bound to O_2. If fewer than all four haem groups are bound, the Hb is said to be partially saturated. Binding of the second is easier than the first, binding of the third is easier than the second, and binding of the fourth is easier than the third. The fourth O_2 molecule to bind has 300 times the affinity of the first. Thus, the affinity of Hb for O_2 changes depending on how much O_2 is bound to the Hb. The more saturated Hb is, then the easier it is to bind more O_2, and the harder it is to unbind O_2 from that Hb. So, binding gets more efficient as each O_2 binds, and release gets easier as each O_2 is released.

Oxyhaemoglobin dissociation curve

The association between O_2 and Hb is represented by a sigmoid-shaped (S-shaped) curve (Figure 25.2), because changes in affinity of Hb depend on O_2 saturation. The curve has a steep slope between 1 and 6 kPa PO_2 and a plateau between 9.3 and 13.3 kPa PO_2. The upper linear portion of the curve reflects where both O_2 loading in the lungs (from venous to arterial) and unloading in the tissues (from arterial to venous) occurs. Hb saturation (%; 'O_2 sats') depends on PO_2, not normally on Hb content. Near 100% Hb saturation implies healthy gas exchange, but could still occur with anaemia (reduced Hb content). O_2 content depends on both PO_2 and Hb content. So, low Hb content can cause tissue hypoxia, even if both PO_2 and Hb saturation are normal.

O_2 tension refers to the PO_2 difference between two sites, determining the direction and flow of O_2. Changes in O_2 tension do not correspond to equal changes in Hb saturation. As blood moves from arteries through tissues to veins there is a large decrease in PO_2 (13.3 to 6 kPa), associated with a much smaller decrease in Hb saturation (98% to 75%). PO_2 falls by more than 50%, whereas O_2 sats fall by less than 25%. This occurs because it is hardest to unload the first O_2 molecule and thus initially PO_2 falls without much decrease in O_2 sats. Hb is almost completely saturated at any PO_2 above 9.3 kPa, enabling normal O_2 delivery to tissues. When PO_2 decreases to below 9.3 kPa, Hb more readily gives up O_2. So, when blood arrives at tissues with low PO_2 it readily unloads O_2. A significant amount of O_2 is still available in venous blood and can be unloaded from blood to tissues if required (e.g. during vigorous exercise). Since Hb in arterial blood is 98% saturated, heavy breathing during exercise increases PO_2 above the normal 13.3 kPa, but causes almost no change in % saturation. Thus more Hb or increased cardiac output is needed to increase the transport of O_2.

Bohr effect

The Bohr effect is the decrease in affinity of Hb for O_2 (i.e. a 'right shift' in the dissociation curve; Figure 25.2). This occurs due to increased PCO_2 [H^+] or temperature in metabolically active tissues (or 2,3-diphosphoglycerate, which increases slowly in response to chronic hypoxia) when there is a need to unload O_2.

Carbon dioxide

There is almost three times as much CO_2 in *arterial* blood than there is O_2 (450–500 mL CO_2/L vs 200 mL O_2/L). CO_2 diffuses quicker across the lungs than O_2, and so exhalation of CO_2 is not limited by gas exchange. CO_2 is retained because it is not just a waste product of metabolism, it is critical for controlling the acidity of the body (see Chapter 27) and consequently for the control of ventilation (see Chapter 26). If O_2 consumption increases, then the removal rate of CO_2 from venous blood in the lungs needs to increase (e.g. via increasing ventilation or cardiac output) to keep arterial CO_2 constant.

Transformation and forms of carbon dioxide carriage

Dissolved CO_2 reacts with water in erythrocytes more efficiently than in plasma due to the presence of carbonic anhydrase. Within erythrocytes H^+ binds to Hb, so more CO_2 reacts and more bicarbonate is formed. Bicarbonate diffuses out of the erythrocyte in exchange for inward movement of chloride (known as the chloride shift), reaching equilibrium at 24 mmol/L of HCO_3^- in plasma. The third form of transport (after dissolved and as bicarbonate) is bound to protein (either Hb in erythrocytes or albumin in plasma) as carbamino compounds (Figure 25.3).

Carbon dioxide dissociation curve

Blood does not become saturated with CO_2 over the physiological range (Figure 25.4), unlike the oxyhaemoglobin dissociation curve, which does become saturated. Seventy per cent of CO_2 is transported as bicarbonate. There are more of all three forms (dissolved CO_2, HCO_3^- and carbaminos, in both plasma and erythrocytes) in venous blood, because PCO_2 is higher. However, the arteriovenous difference in CO_2 carriage needed for gas exchange is small. From P_aCO_2 of 5.3 kPa to P_vCO_2 of 6.5 kPa corresponds to a difference in blood CO_2 content of only 2 mmol/L.

Haldane effect

The Haldane effect is the increase in affinity of Hb for CO_2. This occurs due to the deoxygenation of Hb. CO_2 binds to the globin part of Hb, unlike O_2, which binds to the haem part of Hb. In metabolically active tissues, O_2 is unloaded, increasing affinity for CO_2, so CO_2 is loaded. In the lungs, O_2 is loaded, decreasing affinity for CO_2, so CO_2 is unloaded.

Steven Burr

Figure 26.1 Neural control of breathing

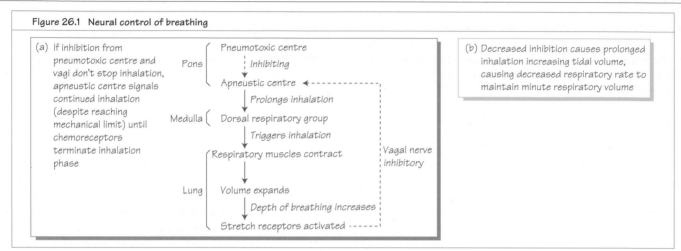

(a) If inhibition from pneumotoxic centre and vagi don't stop inhalation, apneustic centre signals continued inhalation (despite reaching mechanical limit) until chemoreceptors terminate inhalation phase

Pons — Pneumotoxic centre
↓ Inhibiting
Apneustic centre
↓ Prolongs inhalation
Medulla — Dorsal respiratory group
↓ Triggers inhalation
Respiratory muscles contract
↓
Lung — Volume expands
↓ Depth of breathing increases
Stretch receptors activated

Vagal nerve inhibitory

(b) Decreased inhibition causes prolonged inhalation increasing tidal volume, causing decreased respiratory rate to maintain minute respiratory volume

Figure 26.2 Integration of neural and chemical control

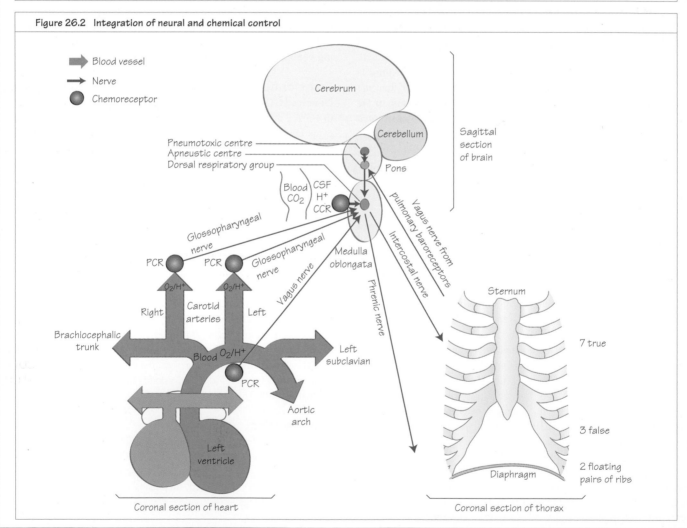

Neural generation of ventilatory pattern

We breathe automatically, and yet we can make instantaneous adjustments just by thinking about it. **Respiratory centres** in the **brainstem** maintain an optimum minute respiratory volume to meet the needs of metabolism, by controlling the relative contributions of both respiratory rate and tidal volume. The basic ventilatory rate and rhythm is produced by the **dorsal respiratory group** in the **medulla oblongata** by triggering the start of each inhalation (Figure 26.1). The duration of inhalation is prolonged by input from the **apneustic centre** in the **pons**, which itself receives inhibitory signals from both the **pneumotaxic centre** in the pons and vagal feedback from **lung baroreceptors** (which increases in response to progressive stretching). The lung baroreceptor (Hering-Breuer) reflex protects lungs from overinflation and is also implicated in fibrosis (where overstretching of unfibrosed areas prematurely curtails inhalation, decreasing tidal volume and increasing respiratory rate).

Chemical regulation of ventilatory pattern

The amount of O_2 consumed and CO_2 produced by the body varies depending on metabolic demand, and detection of chemical changes drives ventilation to match requirements. There are two types of chemoreceptor, which synapse with the respiratory centres in the brainstem to increase ventilation (Figure 26.2). **Central chemoreceptors** (CCRs) found on the ventrolateral surface of the medulla oblongata respond to increases in $[H^+]$ (and indirectly PCO_2) in cerebrospinal fluid (CSF). **Peripheral chemoreceptors** (PCRs) found within the aortic arch and carotid arteries respond when O_2 falls below 8 kPa in arterial blood (functioning despite severe hypoxia, because of their extremely high blood supply in proportion to their size). PCRs respond quickly to large changes (as they are in main arteries), but CCRs dominate under normal conditions to determine fine control (being more sensitive, as CSF has less protein to buffer pH compared with blood). Thus rising CO_2 normally drives ventilation. While CCRs adapt on gradual exposure to sustained **hypocapnia** or **hypercapnia**, PCRs do not adapt, and produce a respiratory drive as long as P_aO_2 remains low (e.g. providing a fixed threshold for breath-holding). CCRs and PCRs work together synergistically, but their relative importance can change depending on the conditions.

If respiratory centres cannot respond quickly enough to changing P_aCO_2 and P_aO_2 (e.g. following stroke, head injuries, brain tumours, or when sleeping at high altitudes), then Cheyne-Stokes respiration occurs (a cycle of breaths becoming shallower and less frequent, followed by an overcompensatory hyperventilation).

Acclimatisation to altitude and hypocapnia

Ascent above 2500 m leads to type I respiratory failure (hypoxia without hypercapnia). With increasing altitude, gravity is less, gases expand and the air becomes less dense. The volume fraction of O_2 remains the same, but because the total pressure decreases the P_AO_2 also decreases.

With sudden exposure, acute hypoxia is detected by peripheral chemoreceptors, which try to increase breathing, but as ventilation increases, P_aCO_2 falls and CSF becomes alkaline. Breathing more leads to death from alkalosis, but failing to breathe more leads to death from hypoxia. Peripheral receptors detect hypoxia but are overridden by central receptors detecting hypocapnia, and the hypoxic drive to increase ventilation is suppressed.

With gradual exposure, mountaineers can climb to 8850 m without O_2, due to acclimatisation. Mild hypoxia stimulates ventilation enough to raise CSF pH slightly. Choroid plexus cells respond by exporting HCO_3^- from CSF to blood. CSF pH is corrected (even though P_aCO_2 remains low), hypoxic drive is expressed and ventilation can increase further. Over a period of hours, breathing becomes controlled around a new lower P_aCO_2. Over a period of days, the alkalinity of the blood is corrected as the exported bicarbonate is excreted by kidneys.

Hypoxic drive dependence with hypercapnia

Pulmonary pathology can lead to type II respiratory failure (**hypoxia with hypercapnia**). With mild hypercapnia, $[HCO_3^-]$ is matched to PCO_2 in CSF, but not in blood (which has a larger volume and is renal dependent). Choroid plexus cells respond by importing HCO_3^- from blood to CSF. Chronically, CSF pH is corrected and ventilation is normal (and inadequate), even though P_aCO_2 remains high (i.e. CO_2 trapping). Thus a gradually increasing P_aCO_2 is associated with inadequate drive for ventilation, which in turn becomes progressively more dependent on the hypoxic drive from PCRs. This is problematic when associated with the need to offset hypoxia by breathing supplemental O_2. Correcting low P_aO_2 removes the drive to breathe and results in a need for artificial ventilation. Hence O_2 therapy is administered at the lowest tolerable level and monitored closely.

27 Acid-base physiology

Steven Burr

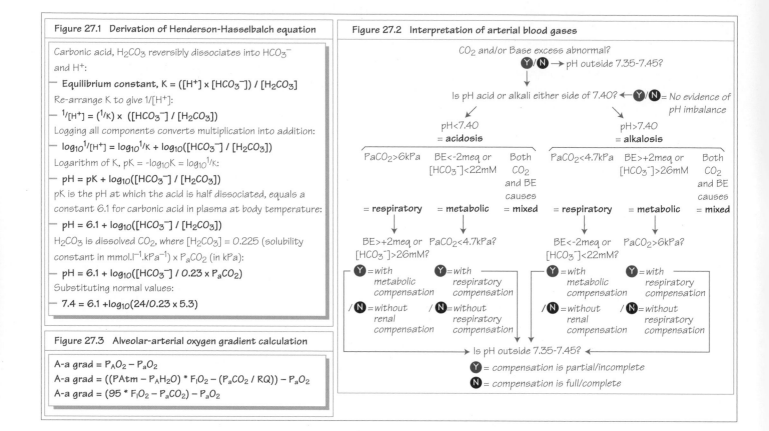

Figure 27.1 Derivation of Henderson-Hasselbalch equation

Carbonic acid, H_2CO_3 reversibly dissociates into HCO_3^- and H^+:

— Equilibrium constant, $K = ([H^+] \times [HCO_3^-]) / [H_2CO_3]$

Re-arrange K to give $1/[H^+]$:

— $1/[H^+] = (1/K) \times ([HCO_3^-] / [H_2CO_3])$

Logging all components converts multiplication into addition:

— $\log_{10} 1/[H^+] = \log_{10} 1/K + \log_{10}([HCO_3^-] / [H_2CO_3])$

Logarithm of K, $pK = -\log_{10}K = \log_{10} 1/K$:

— $pH = pK + \log_{10}([HCO_3^-] / [H_2CO_3])$

pK is the pH at which the acid is half dissociated, equals a constant 6.1 for carbonic acid in plasma at body temperature:

— $pH = 6.1 + \log_{10}([HCO_3^-] / [H_2CO_3])$

H_2CO_3 is dissolved CO_2, where $[H_2CO_3] = 0.225$ (solubility constant in $mmol.l^{-1}.kPa^{-1}$) $\times P_aCO_2$ (in kPa):

— $pH = 6.1 + \log_{10}([HCO_3^-] / 0.23 \times P_aCO_2)$

Substituting normal values:

— $7.4 = 6.1 + \log_{10}(24/0.23 \times 5.3)$

Figure 27.3 Alveolar-arterial oxygen gradient calculation

A-a grad $= P_AO_2 - P_aO_2$

A-a grad $= ((PAtm - P_AH_2O) * F_IO_2 - (P_aCO_2 / RQ)) - P_aO_2$

A-a grad $= (95 * F_IO_2 - P_aCO_2) - P_aO_2$

Figure 27.2 Interpretation of arterial blood gases

pH

The potential of hydrogen (pH) is a measure of the hydrogen ion concentration ($[H^+]$) in solution. It is conventionally expressed as $pH = \log_{10} 1/[H+] = -\log_{10} [H^+]$. The greatest range in $[H^+]$ is found in the gastrointestinal tract, where there are secretions in response to digestive requirements. There, gastric secretions can be as low as 1.1 and pancreatic secretions as high as 8.8. However, if blood becomes too acid or too alkaline there are serious consequences. If plasma pH falls below 6.8, enzymes are lethally denatured. If plasma pH rises above 7.6, free calcium concentration falls enough to produce fatal tetany. Therefore $[H^+]$ is kept within narrow bounds in blood. Mean normal extracellular $[H^+]$ is 40 nmol/L, equivalent to a pH of 7.4. The normal extracellular range is 35.5–44.7 nmol/L, which is equivalent to a pH range of 7.45–7.35 (as higher $[H^+]$ is more acidic and has a lower pH). Extracellular pH is kept close to 7.4, to maintain a gradient for $[H^+]$ removal from metabolically active tissues where the intracellular pH is normally 6.8–7.2.

Henderson-Hasselbalch equation

The dominant reaction governing extracellular $[H^+]$ and hence pH is: $CO_2 + H_2O = H_2CO_3 = HCO_3^- + H^+$ (Figure 27.1).

At a normal $PaCO_2$ of 5.3 kPa water in plasma dissolves 1.2 mmol/L. Dissolved CO_2 reacts with water forming H^+ and HCO_3. The reaction is reversible, with the amount reacting depending on [reactants] and [products]. If the amount of one constituent decreases, then the reaction is driven to produce more of that constituent in order to restore the equilibrium. At physiological equilibrium $[HCO_3] = 24$ mmol/L. and $[H^+] = 40$ nmol/L, so there is one million-fold less H^+ than HCO_3^- in blood. Thus changing how much CO_2 dissolves has a proportionally greater effect on H^+. Dissolved CO_2 depends directly on PCO_2. If PCO_2 rises, $[H^+]$ will rise; if PCO_2 falls, $[H^+]$ will fall. Thus, slow shallow breaths lead to less CO_2 exhaled, more CO_2 retained in blood, more free H^+ and consequently lower pH. Conversely, rapid deep breaths lead to more CO_2 exhaled, less CO_2 retained in blood, less free H^+ and consequently higher pH. Consequently, plasma pH depends primarily on the P_aCO_2 maintained by the lungs, and $[HCO_3^-]$, which is maintained by the kidneys. It is the relative not absolute values of these contributors that determine pH. A change in P_aCO_2 can be buffered by an equivalent relative change in $[HCO_3^-]$, and vice versa. The equation (Figure 27.1) enables calculation of the $[HCO_3^-]$ required to buffer an increase in P_aCO_2 and maintain a pH of 7.4. The required increase in $[HCO_3^-] = 10^{7.4-6.1+(\log 0.23 + \log PaCO2)}$ – existing $[HCO_3^-]$. For

Medical Sciences at a Glance, First Edition. Edited by Michael D Randall. © 2014 John Wiley & Sons, Ltd. Published 2014 by John Wiley & Sons, Ltd.

example, if P_aCO_2 increased from 5.3 kPa to 8 kPa, then $[HCO_3^-]$ has to increase by 12 (from 24 to 36) mmol/L to maintain pH at 7.4. In severe cases, the required increase is multiplied by the circulating volume (typically 5 L for an adult) and half this amount of sodium bicarbonate is administered either orally or intravenously before reassessing arterial blood gas status.

Acidosis, alkalosis and compensation

Acidosis and alkalosis refer to the process of becoming more acidic or alkali respectively. **Acidaemic** and **alkalemic** refer to the state of being more acid or alkali, while acidaemia and alkalemia specifically refer to the state of the blood. Changes in ventilation that cause acid-base imbalance are termed respiratory; all other non-ventilatory causes of acid-base imbalance are termed metabolic. Changes that act to restore normal acid-base balance are termed compensation. Causes of both imbalance and compensation can be respiratory, metabolic, or mixed/combined respiratory and metabolic (Figure 27.2). However, the lungs can adjust body pH much more rapidly than the kidneys. Altering ventilation can begin within seconds/minutes to compensate for acid-base imbalance, whereas altering kidney output takes hours/days to bring about effective renal compensation. Hence acute acid-base imbalances are likely to undergo complete respiratory compensation before renal compensation can take effect.

Respiratory alkali

Hyperventilation causes P_aCO_2 to fall (hypocapnia), for example to correct low P_aO_2 (hypoxia) on ascent to high altitude. So plasma pH rises = respiratory alkalosis. This can be compensated for (returning pH towards normal) by hypoventilation (if the cause of hyperventilation has ended), or by the kidneys increasing $[HCO_3^-]$ excretion.

Respiratory acid

Hypoventilation causes P_aCO_2 to rise (hypercapnia), for example when ventilation is impaired by disease. Plasma pH falls = respiratory acidosis. This can be compensated for by hyperventilation (if the cause of hypoventilation has ended), or by the kidneys increasing $[H^+]$ excretion.

Metabolic acid

If the tissues produce acid, for example with ketoacidosis (due to poorly controlled diabetes mellitus), this reacts with HCO_3^-. The fall in $[HCO_3^-]$ leads to a fall in pH = metabolic acidosis. This can be compensated for by increased ventilation to lower P_aCO_2, or by the kidneys increasing $[H^+]$ excretion.

Metabolic alkali

If plasma $[HCO_3^-]$ rises, for example vomiting causes loss of acid from the body (and hence a relative increase in plasma $[HCO_3^-]$), plasma pH rises = metabolic alkalosis. This can be compensated for by decreasing ventilation to raise P_aCO_2, or by the kidneys increasing $[HCO_3^-]$ excretion. Metabolic alkalosis can only be compensated for to a degree by hypoventilation because of the associated decrease in P_aO_2 leading to hypoxia.

Compensation

While renal metabolic compensation can occur at the same time as a non-renal metabolic cause of acid-base imbalance, respiratory compensation cannot occur at the same time as a respiratory cause of imbalance (i.e. hypoventilation and hyperventilation cannot occur together in time, although if the cause has stopped then compensation can follow).

Compensation may not occur, be partial, or complete. If neither P_aCO_2 nor $[HCO_3^-]$ have moved to compensate when one or the other would have been expected to change, then an apparently normal value can indicate an abnormality. Partial compensation occurs where there is evidence of P_aCO_2 or $[HCO_3^-]$ having moved to compensate, but the pH is not within the normal range. Complete compensation has occurred when the pH is within the normal range. Note that when deciding whether a case is either metabolic alkalosis with respiratory compensation or respiratory acidosis with metabolic compensation, assume that overcompensation does not occur (it would be inefficient for the body to expend resources in continuing to compensate beyond the midpoint pH of 7.40) unless there is evidence from the patient history to the contrary (e.g. imposing excessive or insufficient mechanical ventilation).

Arterial blood gases and alveolar-arterial gradient

Arterial blood gases are crucial for the management of all acute respiratory disorders and many chronic ones. Provided the patient has been at steady state for the preceding 20 minutes (i.e. breathing the same gas composition at the same rhythm), then a 0.5 mL blood sample is taken from their radial artery and analysed. Normal ranges are: pH = 7.40 (7.35–7.45); P_aO_2 = 10.6–13.3 kPa; P_aCO_2 = 4.7–6 kPa; and base excess (BE) =+2 to −2 meq/L (where BE is a derived value relative to a normal $[HCO_3^-]$ of 24 mmol/L). These values are a crucial indictor of prognosis as nobody dies with normal blood gases. Interpretation depends on identification of values that are clearly abnormal (severely so if O_2 is less than 8 kPa and/or CO_2 more than 7 kPa), and is supported by knowledge of the patient's history and whether there is any pre-existing disease (e.g. diabetes mellitus may contribute a metabolic acidosis).

Calculate the alveolar-arterial oxygen gradient (A-a grad, sometimes referred to as oxygen difference or A-a DO_2) to determine whether there is impaired gas transfer (indicating lung damage, as a large difference means poor gas exchange and a problem with the efficiency of ventilation-perfusion matching). A normal A-a grad (Figure 27.3) depends on atmospheric pressure (PAtm at sea level = 101.325 kPa), alveolar humidity (P_AH_2O is kept constant with normal respiratory tract physiology and hydration = 6.28 kPa), fractional concentration of oxygen in inspired gas (F_IO_2 for room air = 0.21093, but can differ if a patient is receiving supplemental oxygen) and aerobic metabolism (respiratory quotient = 1). The calculated A-a grad value is then classified as normal if it is less than a threshold determined by age (upper limits of normal A-a grad are: 2.5 kPa at 20 years; 3.2 kPa at 40 years; 3.7 kPa at 60 years; and 4.0 kPa at 80 years). For every 10% increase in F_IO_2, these normal A-a gradient thresholds increase by 0.66–0.93 kPa (a normal A-a gradient when breathing 100% oxygen = 8–9.3 kPa).

28 Respiratory pathophysiology

Steven Burr

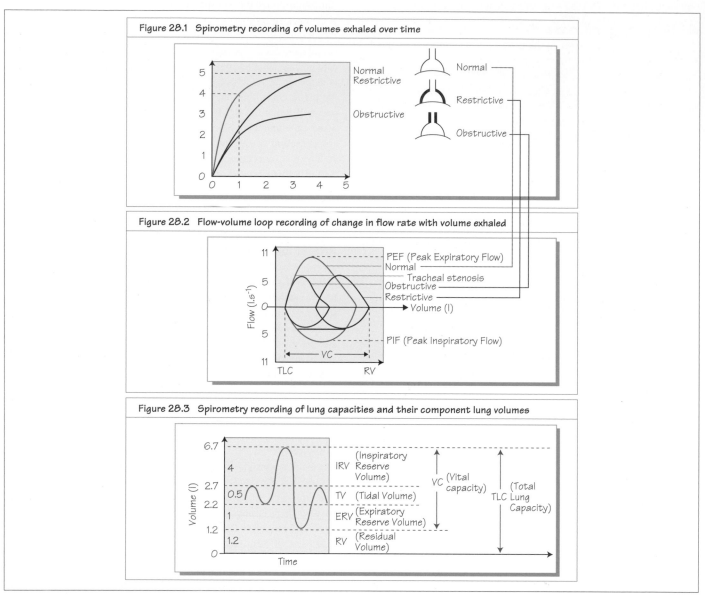

Figure 28.1 Spirometry recording of volumes exhaled over time

Figure 28.2 Flow-volume loop recording of change in flow rate with volume exhaled

Figure 28.3 Spirometry recording of lung capacities and their component lung volumes

The effect of disease on respiratory function is best demonstrated by changes in the measurements of air flow, lung volumes and gas transfer. Diagnosis, management and monitoring of respiratory problems rely on non-invasive measurements of the movement of air breathed in and out of the lungs, and the diffusion of gas between inspired air and the blood. Ventilation is assessed by both expiratory flow rate and lung volume measurements. Normal values will vary with gender, age, height, weight and ethnicity. Thus measured values are usually expressed as a percentage of average normal predicted values. Abnormal flow rates reflect changes in airway resistance indicating obstructive pathology; whereas abnormal lung volumes reflect changes in compliance indicating restrictive pathology.

Obstructive respiratory deficits

Increased airway resistance obstructs air flow and thus impairs exhalation. If airways are narrowed it is still possible to fill the lungs to capacity, but resistance will increase on exhalation, so air will come out more slowly. Possible pathological causes include **chronic obstructive pulmonary disease** (COPD), irreversible increases in airway resistance involving a combination of chronic bronchitis (recurrent inflammation with mucus secretion) and emphysema (permanent destructive enlargement of alveoli)), and **asthma** (reversible increases in airway resistance involving a combination of bronchoconstriction and inflammation).

Restrictive respiratory deficits

Decreased compliance restricts lung expansion and thus impairs inhalation. If lungs are difficult to fill to capacity because they are stiff, have weak muscles, or there is a problem with the chest wall, they will be less full before exhalation. Lung volume will be reduced, but air will come out at a normal rate. Possible physiological causes include obesity, pregnancy, or restrictive clothing. Possible pathological causes are parenchymal (e.g. pulmonary fibrosis, pulmonary oedema), chest wall (e.g. kyphoscoliosis, pneumothorax), or neuromuscular (e.g. myasthenia gravis). Mixed respiratory deficits are also possible (e.g. tumours or cystic fibrosis) or with a combination of obstructive and restrictive conditions (e.g. if both obese and asthmatic).

Spirometry

Spirometry records the volumes breathed in and out over time. Peak expiratory flow rate (PEFR) depends on the patient inhaling as deeply as possible and then exhaling as quickly as possible. Forced expiratory volume in the first second (FEV_1) and forced vital capacity (FVC) are measured by the same manoeuvre as PEFR, but the patient continues to try to breathe out until no more air can be exhaled (Figure 28.1). The FEV_1 is expressed as a percentage of FVC. PEFR is the simplest technique to perform, but it is less reliable for assessing conditions where airways are not affected uniformly. With variable airway damage, a very brief momentary high PEFR may still be achieved, whereas measuring over a whole second with FEV_1 would be a more reliable. With obstruction, FEV_1 will be less than 70% of predicted, but FVC will be more than 70% of normal. With restriction, FVC will be less than 70% of predicted, but FEV_1 will be more than 70% of FVC. A flow-volume loop is measured by the same manoeuvre as FEV_1 and FVC, but once no more air can be breathed out then the patient inhales as rapidly as possible until they can breathe no more air in (Figure 28.2). A flow-volume loop has the advantage of assessing inhalation as well as exhalation, along with producing shapes characteristic of certain conditions (Figure 28.2).

Lung volumes

The residual volume (and in turn total lung capacity and functional residual capacity) cannot be breathed out nor measured directly (Figure 28.3). Such unknown lung volumes can be measured indirectly by helium dilution. At a known point in the respiratory cycle (e.g. with only the residual volume remaining within the lungs) the patient starts breathing from (and to) a known volume (V1), which contains a known concentration of helium (C1). When the air between the unknown volume in the lungs and known volume containing helium have completely mixed, then the concentration of helium is re-measured (C2). Because helium is not normally present in air and is insoluble in blood, the helium will have redistributed equally only between the two volumes. The resulting dilution of the helium will be proportional to the increase in total volume. It is then possible to calculate the unknown volume that was in the lungs when the patient started breathing from V1. Thus the unknown lung volume = (C1/C2 − 1) × V1.

Effects of restrictive disease on lung volumes

A common effect of lung disease involving any kind of space-occupying lesion is that FRC, TLC and RV all decrease together. In contrast, weakness affecting both inspiratory and expiratory muscles causes FRC to remain unchanged. The lungs cannot be expanded fully, so the IRV and in turn TLC are decreased. Similarly, the lungs cannot be compressed fully, so the RV is increased by an amount equal to that by which the ERV is decreased (causing no overall change in FRC). The proportion of total lung capacity not involved in ventilation is often expressed as RV/TLC.

Effects of obstructive disease on lung volumes

The changes in lung volumes with COPD depend on the severity and relative contributions of chronic bronchitis and emphysema. FRC, TLC and RV all decrease slightly due to the reduction in airway volume associated with bronchoconstriction and mucus secretion caused by the chronic bronchitis. This has greatest effect on RV, because a larger proportion of RV is airways than for other lung volumes. However, if the emphysema is severe enough to collapse airways and trap air then RV will increase. In contrast, an upper tracheal stenosis or other localised obstruction (e.g. a tumour or foreign body obstruction) would not affect FRC, TLC, or RV.

Gas transfer

The efficiency of respiration can be limited by the diffusion of oxygen from alveolar air to pulmonary capillary blood. Gas transfer is measured using carbon monoxide (CO) as a surrogate for oxygen. The rate of transfer across the alveolar membrane can be calculated by fully exhaling then rapidly and maximally inhaling a single breath containing 0.3% CO, and holding that breath for 10 seconds before exhaling rapidly and maximally, and measuring the CO remaining in the exhaled air. Because P_VCO is negligible, and Hb is not saturated (because % CO is low), the rate of CO uptake, or permeability, is constant. A permeability factor (kCO) can be calculated from the decrease in alveolar fraction of CO over the time of the test (where: $kCO = log_e (F_ACO_0 / F_ACO_t) / t$).

Alveolar volume (V_A; not alveolar ventilation rate)
V_A in litres = TLC − total dead space volume.
Normally = 4–5 L.

Total lung carbon monoxide transfer (T_LCO)
T_LCO in L/ min.kPa^{-1} = $(kCO \times V_A) / (PAtm − PH_20)$.
Assume PAtm = 101.325 kPa, PH_20 = 6.28 kPa, and 1 mole of gas occupies 22.4 litres.
$\quad T_LCO$ in mmol.$min^{-1}.kPa^{-1}$ = $(T_LCO$ in l.$min^{-1}.kPa^{-1}$ / 22.4) × 1000.
Normally T_LCO = 6–10 mmol/min.kPa^{-1}.

Factors that would decrease ventilation-perfusion matching and hence decrease T_LCO include: decreased alveolar surface area (e.g. caused by emphysema); thickened alveolar-capillary membrane (e.g. diffusion distance increase caused by pulmonary oedema); decreased pulmonary capillary blood flow (e.g. pulmonary embolus/ischaemia; cf. exercise increases T_LCO because pulmonary capillary blood flow increases); and decreased Hb (e.g. anaemia). With anaemia, a correction factor can be applied to adjust T_LCO, in order to assess gas exchange independently of Hb.

Coefficient of carbon monoxide transfer (KCO; not kCO)
KCO = T_LCO / V_A,
i.e. Efficiency per lung unit = gas exchange capacity/number of contributing units. Normally KCO = 1.25–1.75 mmol/min.kPa^{-1}/L.

Effects of restrictive disease on gas transfer

With incomplete lung expansion V_A is very low by definition, and this is normally associated with an increased KCO and hence only a slightly decreased T_LCO. The increased KCO is due to smaller alveoli having an increased surface area to volume ratio, thus increasing diffusing capacity. NB A low V_A with an apparently normal KCO would actually reflect impaired transfer.

Effects of obstructive disease on gas transfer

With COPD, V_A is effectively reduced slightly because there is increased mucus lining airspaces and trapping of air, leading to its exclusion from ventilation. There are larger airspaces and reduced alveolar surface area (emphysema), and increased diffusion distance due to mucus (from bronchitis); so KCO decreases and because $T_LCO = V_A \times KCO$, T_LCO is very low. With asthma the pulmonary microcirculation is maintained and cardiac output increases, so KCO increases and T_LCO decreases slightly.

Siobhan Loughna and Deborah Merrick

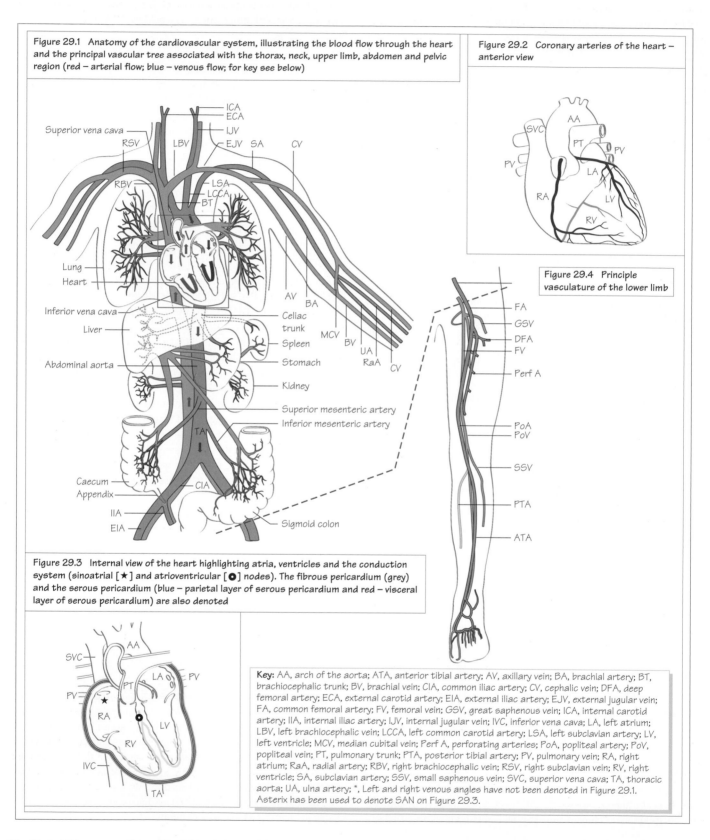

Figure 29.1 Anatomy of the cardiovascular system, illustrating the blood flow through the heart and the principal vascular tree associated with the thorax, neck, upper limb, abdomen and pelvic region (red – arterial flow; blue – venous flow; for key see below)

Figure 29.2 Coronary arteries of the heart – anterior view

Figure 29.4 Principle vasculature of the lower limb

Figure 29.3 Internal view of the heart highlighting atria, ventricles and the conduction system (sinoatrial [★] and atrioventricular [◉] nodes). The fibrous pericardium (grey) and the serous pericardium (blue – parietal layer of serous pericardium and red – visceral layer of serous pericardium) are also denoted

Key: AA, arch of the aorta; ATA, anterior tibial artery; AV, axillary vein; BA, brachial artery; BT, brachiocephalic trunk; BV, brachial vein; CIA, common iliac artery; CV, cephalic vein; DFA, deep femoral artery; ECA, external carotid artery; EIA, external iliac artery; EJV, external jugular vein; FA, common femoral artery; FV, femoral vein; GSV, great saphenous vein; ICA, internal carotid artery; IIA, internal iliac artery; IJV, internal jugular vein; IVC, inferior vena cava; LA, left atrium; LBV, left brachiocephalic vein; LCCA, left common carotid artery; LSA, left subclavian artery; LV, left ventricle; MCV, median cubital vein; Perf A, perforating arteries; PoA, popliteal artery; PoV, popliteal vein; PT, pulmonary trunk; PTA, posterior tibial artery; PV, pulmonary vein; RA, right atrium; RaA, radial artery; RBV, right brachiocephalic vein; RSV, right subclavian vein; RV, right ventricle; SA, subclavian artery; SSV, small saphenous vein; SVC, superior vena cava; TA, thoracic aorta; UA, ulna artery; *, Left and right venous angles have not been denoted in Figure 29.1. Asterix has been used to denote SAN on Figure 29.3.

The cardiovascular system comprises the heart and an extensive network of vessels, called the vascular tree (Figures 29.1, 29.2 and 29.3). The heart is a four-chambered pump that ensures an adequate supply of oxygenated blood is provided to all tissues of the body. The right side of the heart receives deoxygenated blood destined for the lungs (via the pulmonary circulation). The left side receives oxygenated blood from the lungs, which is pumped at high pressure to the rest of the body (**systemic circulation**).

The heart and pericardium

The heart: is a muscular organ located in the middle **mediastinum** (Figure 29.1). The muscular layer of the heart is the **myocardium**, and an epithelial layer called the **endocardium** is the internal lining. The myocardium is composed of bundles of cardiac muscle, some of which have specialised functions in initiating and coordinating the contraction of the heart musculature (sinoatrial [SA] and atrioventricular [AV] nodes, Figure 29.3). The heart has three surfaces (sternocostal, diaphragmatic and the base) with the apex of the heart located approximately 9 cm to the left of the midline at the fifth intercostal space. The heart is divided into four chambers by septa: left and right atria and left and right ventricles (Figure 29.3). The right side of the heart pumps blood into the pulmonary circuit and the left side into the systemic circuit (denoted by blue and red arrows respectively in Figure 29.1). The heart cycle commences with ventricular expansion and filling (**diastole**), and ends with ventricular shortening and emptying (**systole**). Deoxygenated blood from the body enters the right atrium via the **inferior and superior vena cavae** (**IVC** and **SVC**); this blood enters the right ventricle via the tricuspid valve. Ventricular contraction leads to the blood going to the lungs via the pulmonary trunk through the pulmonary valve. Upon oxygenation, blood then returns to the heart via the pulmonary veins to enter the left atrium; the blood enters the left ventricle via the mitral valve. Ventricular contraction pumps the oxygenated blood into the aorta, through the aortic valve, from where it is distributed around the body via the vascular tree. **Coronary arteries** provide the blood supply to the heart. The main coronary arteries are the right and left coronary arteries, which arise from the aorta just superior to the aortic valve (Figure 29.2). Deoxygenated blood is returned to the heart via the coronary veins, with most blood entering the right atrium of the heart via the coronary sinus. The heart receives sympathetic and parasympathetic innervation via the cardiac plexuses.

The pericardium: is divided into fibrous (outer) and serous (inner) parts to form a sac that encloses the heart (Figure 29.3). The fibrous portion of the pericardium is strong and relatively nondistensible, preventing excessive movement of the heart. It attaches to the diaphragm inferiorly, and superiorly blends into adventitia of great vessels. The fibrous pericardium is lined internally by the parietal layer of serous pericardium, whereas the visceral layer of serous pericardium covers the surface of the heart. There is a potential space between the two serous layers and a lubricant produced by these layers prevents friction of the heart.

The vascular tree

Arteries and veins: carry blood from and to the heart respectively. Their walls contain three layers: **tunica intima** (inner endothelial lining), **tunica media** (middle smooth muscle layer) and **tunica adventitia** (outer connective tissue layer). Arteries have a more prominent tunica media and can be classed as elastic, muscular, or arterioles. **Capillaries** arise from terminal arterioles; blood contained within them moves into venules and then into progressively larger veins as they approach the heart. Veins carry blood at lower pressure and often contain valves to prevent retrograde blood flow.

Blood supply of the thorax: the **aorta** is the main arterial trunk, which takes oxygenated blood from the heart and passes it to numerous branches to be distributed around the body. Its main divisions are the ascending aorta, arch of the aorta, thoracic (descending) aorta and abdominal aorta (Figure 29.1). The arch of the aorta has three main branches: the brachiocephalic (divides into the right subclavian and right common carotid), the left common carotid and the left subclavian arteries. With regard to the venous system, the subclavian vein comes from the upper limb and the jugular vein from the neck; both enter the brachiocephalic vein (right and left), which in turn enter the SVC (Figure 29.1). The **azygos system** drains much of the thorax, also entering the SVC. The IVC enters the thorax from the abdomen via an opening in the diaphragm and immediately enters the right atrium of the heart (Figure 29.3).

Blood supply of the head and neck: within the neck, the common **carotid arteries** branches to form the internal and external carotid arteries (left and right; Figure 29.1). These arteries and their branches supply the head and neck region. Venous blood is returned from the brain, superficial head and neck via the internal **jugular veins**. These veins (left and right) terminate by joining the corresponding subclavian vein to form the brachiocephalic vein (Figure 29.1). External jugular veins receive blood from the exterior of the cranium and deep parts of the face, to enter the subclavian vein.

Blood supply of the upper limbs: the subclavian arteries continue as the axillary arteries in the upper limbs, which in turn continue as the brachial arteries. The blood supply to the limb is predominately via the **brachial** and **axillary** arteries and their branches, such as the ulnar and radial arteries (Figure 29.1). The main veins (on the right and left) are the basilic and cephalic veins, which both empty into the axillary veins followed by the subclavian veins and finally brachiocephalic veins, which unite to form the SVC to return deoxygenated blood to the right atrium of the heart.

Blood supply of the abdomen, pelvis and perineum: the majority of the abdominal viscera are supplied by three anterior branches of the abdominal aorta: **celiac trunk, superior and inferior mesenteric arteries** (Figure 29.1). The liver receives blood from the hepatic artery (branch of celiac trunk) and the hepatic portal vein. The latter carries poorly oxygenated blood rich in nutrients from the gastrointestinal viscera (**portal circulation**). The abdominal aorta bifurcates into left and right common iliac arteries (Figure 29.1). These further divide into internal and external iliac arteries; branches of the former supply the majority of the pelvic viscera (exceptions include testes and ovaries) and perineum. Venous blood from the abdomen, pelvis and perineum returns to the heart via the IVC and the azygos system.

Blood supply of the lower limbs: the external iliac artery continues in each lower limb as the common **femoral artery**, providing the main blood supply (Figure 29.4). The common femoral artery divides into the superficial and deep femoral arteries. The superficial femoral artery continues as the **popliteal artery** as it passes posterior to the knee. The popliteal artery divides into the anterior and posterior **tibial arteries**, with the posterior branch giving rise to the fibular (peroneal) artery. The veins of the lower limbs are divided into a deep and superficial group. The deep group consists of the popliteal vein, which continues as the femoral vein in the thigh (Figure 29.4). The superficial group consist of the small saphenous vein (enters into the popliteal vein) and the great saphenous vein (enters the femoral vein).

30 Cardiac physiology

Michael D Randall

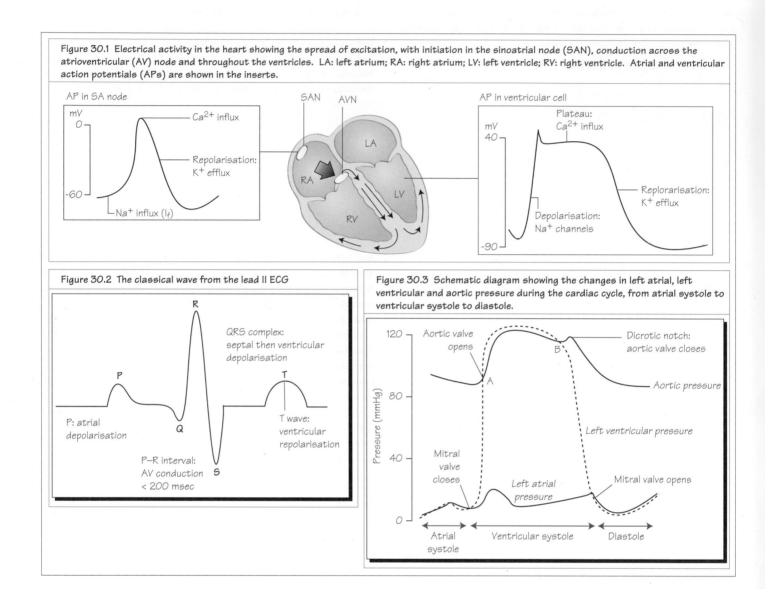

Figure 30.1 Electrical activity in the heart showing the spread of excitation, with initiation in the sinoatrial node (SAN), conduction across the atrioventricular (AV) node and throughout the ventricles. LA: left atrium; RA: right atrium; LV: left ventricle; RV: right ventricle. Atrial and ventricular action potentials (APs) are shown in the inserts.

Figure 30.2 The classical wave from the lead II ECG

Figure 30.3 Schematic diagram showing the changes in left atrial, left ventricular and aortic pressure during the cardiac cycle, from atrial systole to ventricular systole to diastole.

The purpose of the heart is for the **left ventricle** to pump blood around the systemic circulation to perfuse organs and tissues, and for the **right ventricle** to pump blood through the pulmonary circulation to enable gaseous exchange and delivery of oxygenated blood to the left atrium to prime the left ventricle. To achieve this the **cardiac cycle** is a highly coordinated process, which leads to rhythmic and synchronised contractions. **Ventricular systole** is the contractile period and **diastole** is when the heart is not contracting. **Coronary blood flow** supplies the cardiac muscle and only occurs during diastole.

Initiation of the heartbeat

The heartbeat is controlled by the propagation of action potentials leading to coordinated contraction of the cardiac muscle (Figure 30.1).

The heartbeat is initiated by the **sinoatrial node** (SAN), which is the **pacemaker**, as it has the highest intrinsic rate of depolarisation. The pacemaker is set by Na^+ influx via the I_f **current**. This leads to an initial depolarization (from $-60mV$) which takes the membrane to threshold ($-45mV$) and leads to the opening of voltage-operated Ca^{2+} channels, resulting in slow depolarization as there is no involvement of fast Na^+ channels. This is followed by repolarization as the Na^+ current switches off and K^+ channels open with K^+ efflux. The spread of depolarization from the SAN leads to atrial contraction.

To drive the ventricles, depolarisation is conducted across the **atrioventricular (AV) node** and the time required for this to occur leads to a delay (the **AV delay**). The depolarisation then spreads down the **Purkinje fibres** of the **bundle of His**. The Purkinje fibres are specialised conducting fibres that convey the spread of excitation to the ventricular muscle. The **excitation-contraction coupling** starts in the septum and spreads from the apex to the base of the ventricles. The spread of depolarisation is then followed by a wave of repolarisation.

The action potential in ventricular cells is prolonged compared with that in atrial cells and this ensures sufficient time for Ca^{2+} influx to couple to forceful contraction. The initial depolarisation is driven via **voltage-operated ('fast') Na^+ channels** and the plateau of depolarisation lasts typically 200 msec and is associated with Ca^{2+} influx via voltage-operated **L-type Ca^{2+} channels**, which leads to contraction of the ventricular mass. The spread of electrical activity between myocytes is mediated via **gap junctions** composed of connexins at the **intercalated discs** which join the cells.

The electrocardiogram (ECG)

The **ECG** is used to detect the electrical activity of the heart as conducted to the surface of the body via the body's salt solutions. It indicates electrical activity and is not a measure of mechanical events. The recording electrodes can be placed on the limbs and/or on the chest. The 'classical' ECG is referred to as lead II (recorded by an inferior lead, Figure 30.2) and is divided into the following.
• **P-waves**: atrial depolarisation. These are relatively small, reflecting the small mass of the atria.
• **P-R interval** (sometimes referred to as P-Q) (120–200 msec): a period due to conduction delay across the atrioventricular node.
• **QRS complex** an initial dip reflects the septal depolarisation and this is then followed by the spread of depolarisation from the apex to the base.
• **T wave**: ventricular repolarisation.
The ST length corresponds with ejection and the T-P interval corresponds with cardiac filling.

A positive deflection on the ECG reflects a wave of depolarisation towards (or a wave of repolarisation away from) the positive electrode. By comparing the relative magnitudes of ventricular QRS waveforms from different leads (e.g. I, II, III), vectoral analysis determines the 'cardiac axis' of depolarisation. This can be shifted to the right (e.g. pulmonary hypertension) or to the left (e.g. systemic hypertension).

Clinically, the ECG identifies disorders of rate, conduction (e.g. heart block where AV conduction is either slowed or completely blocked), rhythm (e.g. atrial flutter and fibrillation) and ischaemic heart disease (where the ST segment is elevated in myocardial infarction or depressed in ischaemia associated with angina).

Cardiac cycle (Figure 30.3)

The heart is designed to pump blood unidirectionally and to achieve this, intracardiac valves open and close during the cardiac cycle. During atrial systole atrial valves (**mitral** or **bicuspid** in the left atrium and **tricuspid** in the right) are open and allow blood into the ventricles, and as ventricular pressure increases the atrial valves shut. Normally 70% of blood flows directly from the atria to the ventricles and only 30% of flow is due to atrial contraction. Hence the atria act as primers to increase ventricular efficiency.

As the left ventricle fills, the aortic valve is shut as aortic pressure exceeds that in the ventricles. However, as pressure rises in the ventricles, due to contraction, the aortic valves open and blood is ejected

into the aorta. As there is **isovolumic relaxation** the aortic pressure then exceeds ventricular pressure and the aortic valve closes. An equivalent process occurs on the right side with the pulmonary valve opening into the pulmonary artery. Only when ventricular pressure is less than atrial pressure do the atrial valves open and the cycle is repeated.

Cardiac haemodynamics

The ventricular ejection of either the left or right ventricle is the **stroke volume**. In the healthy adult, the stroke volume is typically 70 mL and the volume ejected per minute is the **cardiac output**.

Cardiac output = Stroke volume × heart rate

At rest the stroke volume is ~70 mL and heart rate is typically 72 beat per minute and so cardiac output is of the order of 5 L per minute. This is increased according to demand (e.g. exercise) and can reach values of around 20–25 L in highly trained individuals.

Stroke volume is the volume ejected by each ventricle per cycle and is the difference between **end diastolic volume (EDV)** and **end systolic volume (ESV)**. The EDV is determined by the preload on the heart, which is governed by venous return (i.e. the volume of blood returning to the heart from the venous system and is related to venous tone, blood volume and posture). Stroke volume is affected by the contractility of cardiac muscle, which is governed by the **Frank-Starling relationship**. This states that the force of contraction is proportional the initial degree of fibre stretch. Mechanistically, as cardiac muscle is stretched there is an increase in calcium sensitivity of troponin C and so more contractile actin-myosin links are formed in the muscle, and the contractile response is enhanced. As a consequence, as the EDV increases then the force of contraction rises proportionately. This ensures that the stroke volumes of the right and left ventricles are matched.

The stroke volume is also affected by **afterload**, which is the force it has to work against. Afterload is determined by factors such as **peripheral resistance** and **aortic stiffness**. As afterload increases at a constant preload then stroke volume will decrease.

Autonomic control of the heart

Sympathetic: noradrenaline and circulating adrenaline act at β_1-**adrenoceptors**, which are coupled via adenylyl cyclase to an increase in intracellular cAMP. The increase in cAMP, via cAMP-dependent protein kinase, leads to increased Ca^{2+} entry and increased sensitivity of the contractile elements to Ca^{2+}. These changes lead to an increase in the force of contraction (**positive inotropic**). Sympathetic activity increases the Frank-Starling relationship such that an EDV gives an even greater increase in force of contraction. Sympathetic stimulation also increases the rate of pacemaker depolarisation and so increases heart rate (**positive chronotropic**).

Parasympathetic: acetylcholine from the vagus nerve acts on M_2 **muscarinic receptors**, which are negatively coupled to cAMP, and this leads to the activation of hyperpolarising K^+ currents to slow the pacemaker at the SAN and slow AV conduction. This slows the heart rate (**negative chronotropic**).

Cardiovascular physiology

Michael D Randall

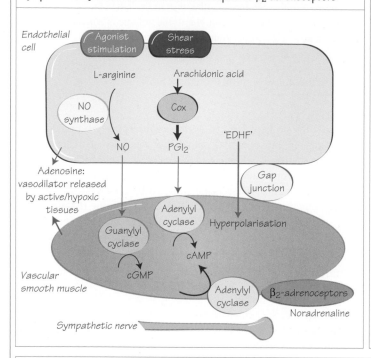

Figure 31.1 Mechanisms of vasodilatation involving endothelium-dependent mechanisms (NO, PGI$_2$, EDHF), the release of adenosine and sympathetically mediated vasodilatation coupled to β$_2$-adrenoceptors

Endothelial cell

Agonist stimulation   Shear stress

L-arginine   Arachidonic acid

NO synthase   Cox

NO   PGI$_2$ 'EDHF'

Adenosine: vasodilator released by active/hypoxic tissues

Gap junction

Guanylyl cyclase   Adenylyl cyclase   Hyperpolarisation

cGMP   cAMP

Vascular smooth muscle

Adenylyl cyclase   β$_2$-adrenoceptors

Noradrenaline

Sympathetic nerve

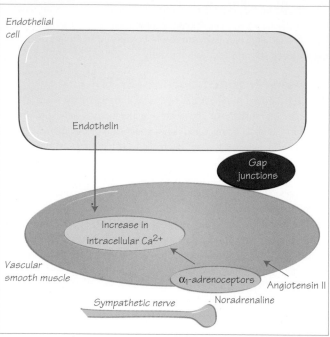

Figure 31.2 Mechanisms of vasoconstriction involving endothelins, and sympathetically mediated vasodilatation coupled to α$_1$-adrenoceptors. Circulating angiotensin II augments sympathetic vasoconstriction

Endothelial cell

Endothelin

Gap junctions

Increase in intracellular Ca^{2+}

Vascular smooth muscle

α$_1$-adrenoceptors   Angiotensin II

Sympathetic nerve   Noradrenaline

Figure 31.3 The vascular network with the exchange of fluid at the capillary network

Artery   Arterioles   Capillary bed   Venule   Vein

Colloidal osmotic pressure acts against movement of fluid

Fluid moves into tissues

Colloidal osmotic pressure promotes reabsorption

Hydrostatic pressure promotes movement of fluid into tissue

Reabsorption promoted by low venous pressure

| 100 mmHg | 35 mmHg | 27 mmHg | 15 mmHg | |
| Arterial pressure | Precapillary pressure | Capillary pressure | Venule pressure | The normal intravascular pressures are indicated |

The purpose of the cardiovascular system is to ensure perfusion of the tissues with blood, allowing for the delivery of nutrients and oxygen, and the removal of metabolites including CO_2. This is achieved by the **systemic circulation**, which delivers oxygenated blood via arteries and then arterioles (<50 μm in diameter) to the capillary network, where exchange occurs.

Regulation of vascular tone

Blood flow is driven by the increased pressure generated by the heart. Blood readily flows through low-resistance conduit arteries (e.g. the aorta then the superior mesenteric artery) to the tissues and organs. At this point the control of blood flow, and therefore tissue, perfusion is determined by **vascular resistance**. This impedes flow, meaning that blood follows the route of least resistance and is facilitated by vasodilatation and opposed by vasoconstriction.

Vascular resistance is determined by **Poiseuille's law**:

$$\text{Resistance} = \frac{(8 \times \text{viscosity} \times \text{length})}{(\pi r^4)}$$

Therefore vascular resistance is proportional to **1/radius⁴**, meaning that small decreases in radius lead to substantial increases in vascular resistance. Hence, small changes in vessel diameter, governed by vascular tone, have profound effects on blood flow and pressure.

Autonomic control of vascular tone

One of the key regulators of arterial diameter and resistance is the sympathetic nervous system. Sympathetic nerve fibres release noradrenaline, which activates α_1-adrenoceptors on the vascular smooth muscle, leading to an increase in intracellular Ca^{2+} via release from stores and Ca^{2+} influx via L-type calcium channels. This leads to vasoconstriction and increases vascular resistance. Sympathetic innervation and circulating adrenaline also stimulate β_2-adrenoceptors (coupled via adenylyl cyclase to cAMP), largely associated with arteries supplying skeletal muscle, leading to vasodilatation, which results in increased blood flow, for example during exercise (Figures 31.1 and 31.2).

Sympathetic control is also augmented by angiotensin II (AII) (Chapter 32) from the renin-angiotensin system. This system is activated by both indications of low blood pressure and sympathetic stimulation, and results in the release of renin by the juxtaglomerular (granular) cells of the kidney.

Endothelial autacoids and vascular control

The vascular endothelium is now recognised as a key regulator of vascular tone by the release of endothelium-derived autacoids (Figure 31.1). The archetypical endothelium-derived relaxant is the gas **nitric oxide (NO)**, which is derived from L-arginine via NO synthase. There is a tonic release of NO, which helps to modulate vascular resistance and control blood pressure. The release of NO also occurs in response to agonists and shear stress resulting from blood flow. This leads to flow-dependent dilatation to match blood flow to demand. NO acts on the vascular smooth muscle to stimulate guanylyl cyclase, which increases levels of cGMP, resulting in vasodilatation.

The endothelium also releases the prostanoid, **prostacyclin (PGI₂)**, and the so-called **endothelium-derived hyperpolarising factor (EDHF)**, which also causes vasodilatation. The activity of EDHF may, in part, be explained by the transfer of electrical current (hyperpolarisation) via gap junctions to the vascular smooth muscle.

The endothelium also releases peptides of the **endothelin** family, which are the most potent vasoconstrictors known.

Metabolic control

Metabolism may also regulate blood flow. Products of metabolism (e.g. **adenosine** from ATP) are released by very active tissues (e.g. cardiac muscle) to cause local vasodilatation and match blood flow to metabolic demand. When blood flow is transiently stopped to a tissue (e.g. a limb) the restoration of blood flow is at a greater rate, '**reactive hyperaemia**'. This response is due to the release of vasodilator mediators (e.g. prostanoids), metabolites (e.g. adenosine, K^+) and the activation of ATP-sensitive potassium channels.

Capillary exchange (Figure 31.3)

The movement of fluid at the capillary bed is tightly regulated. Arterial pressure provides **hydrostatic pressure**, which is the driving force for fluid (blood components but not red blood cells or large proteins) to move out of the circulation. This is the **precapillary pressure**. The

colloidal osmotic pressure, generated by the plasma proteins retained in the intravascular compartment, acts against fluid moving out.

Interstitial or tissue fluid is then reabsorbed into the venous circulation and the reabsorption of water is promoted by plasma protein colloidal osmotic pressure. The hydrostatic pressure in the venous circulation acts against reabsorption and so a low venous pressure promotes reabsorption.

The surface area of the capillary bed also plays a role and a large surface area facilitates exchange. For example, as skeletal muscle becomes active there is capillary recruitment to increase the surface area and so increase exchange.

This is summarised by Starling's equation:

$$\text{Fluid flow} \propto (P_c - P_i) - \sigma (\pi_p - \pi_i)$$

where P_c = capillary pressure and P_i = interstitial pressure, and so $(P_c - P_i)$ is the pressure gradient or hydrostatic force; π_p is the colloidal osmotic pressure in the plasma and π_i is the interstitial colloidal osmotic pressure such that $(\pi_p - \pi_i)$ is the colloidal osmotic gradient; σ is the reflection coefficient, which takes account of the difficulty of proteins to pass across the capillary wall.

The tissue pressure in the tissue is normally constant and so has little influence on fluid exchange. However, if it were to increase then it would alter the hydrostatic gradient and limit the movement of fluid into the extravascular compartment.

The reabsorption of fluid is usually less than that entering the interstitium and the lymphatic system plays a role is reabsorbing this excess fluid and also proteins that have escaped from the blood.

Oedema

This is the accumulation of fluid in the tissues and leads to swelling. This is a pathological event and may result from the following.

Low levels of protein (associated with liver disease as the liver is a key site of plasma protein synthesis, or malnutrition): the reduced colloidal osmotic pressure reduces the driving force for retention of fluid on the arterial side and reduces the driving force for reabsorption on the venous side. *Increased venous pressure* (associated with heart failure): the increase in venous pressure acts as hydrostatic force, which reduces the reabsorption of fluid in the venous side. In left-sided heart failure this leads to pulmonary oedema and in right-sided heart failure it leads to peripheral oedema. *Lymphatic obstruction*: this impedes return of fluid and proteins from the tissue via the lymphatic system to the veins. *Inflammation*: inflammatory mediators such as histamine can increase capillary permeability, leading to extravasation of fluid and oedema. *Arteriolar vasodilatation* (e.g. due to calcium channel inhibitors such as amlodipine): this leads to an increase in blood flow with an increase precapillary pressure and so increases the hydrostatic driving force for fluid to move out leading to oedema.

Venous return

The venous circulation is a low-pressure system whose role is to return blood to the heart ('venous return'). The movement of blood through the venous circulation is driven by the following.

Vascular tone: although veins are less muscular then arteries, venoconstriction promotes return to the heart and venodilatation reduces venous return. *Skeletal muscle pump*: in which leg muscles contract and squeeze blood from superficial veins to deep veins to the vena cava. Movement is facilitated by venous valves, which ensures unidirectional flow. *Breathing*: inspiration decreases intrathoracic pressure and provides a pressure gradient to promote venous return.

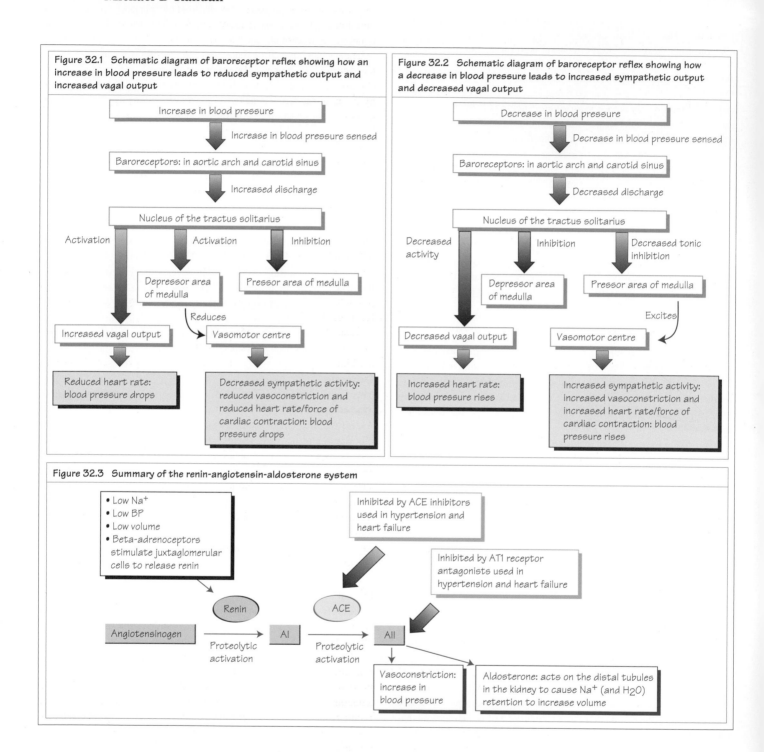

Figure 32.1 Schematic diagram of baroreceptor reflex showing how an increase in blood pressure leads to reduced sympathetic output and increased vagal output

Figure 32.2 Schematic diagram of baroreceptor reflex showing how a decrease in blood pressure leads to increased sympathetic output and decreased vagal output

Figure 32.3 Summary of the renin-angiotensin-aldosterone system

Blood pressure is a measure of the pressure in the systemic cardiovascular system and is reported as central arterial pressure (i.e. equivalent to that in a large artery at the height of the heart). The higher value is the **systolic blood pressure** as the left ventricle contracts and ejects, and the lower value is the **diastolic blood pressure** when the heart is not contracting. In a healthy adult, normal values are 120 mmHg (systolic) and 80 mmHg (diastolic), and mean arterial pressure is reported as:

Mean arterial pressure(MAP)

= diastolic pressure + 1/3 of the (pulse pressure)

where **pulse pressure** is the difference between systolic pressure and diastolic pressure.

MAP in a healthy adult is approximately 93 mmHg. The mean arterial pressure is the time-averaged pressure experienced by the systemic circulation.

Blood pressure is determined by **cardiac output** (CO) × **total peripheral resistance** (TPR) and is tightly controlled to ensure appropriate tissue perfusion. **Hypertension** is pathological and is a sustained increase in blood pressure at rest, such that diastolic blood pressure is ≥90 mmHg and systolic is ≥140 mmHg. In the healthy adult, blood pressure is tightly regulated by nervous and hormonal mechanisms.

Nervous control of blood pressure and baroreceptor control

Blood pressure is regulated in the short term by the autonomic nervous system, with sympathetic innervation of arterial smooth muscle leading to α_1-adrenoceptor-mediated vasoconstriction and an increase TPR (Chapter 31). To ensure maintenance of blood pressure, **baroreceptors** in the carotid sinus and aortic arch sense pressure, and as pressure increases there are increased impulses to the **nucleus of the solitary tract (nucleus tractus solitarius; NTS)** in the brain. Increases in pressure inhibit the 'pressor' area in the rostral ventrolateral medulla to reduce sympathetic output from the vasomotor centre. Increases in pressure also stimulate the 'depressor' area in the caudal ventrolateral medulla to inhibit sympathetic output from the vasomotor centre (Figure 32.1). This is accompanied by increased vagal output to lower blood pressure. Decreases in blood pressure lead to the 'pressor' centre dominating and decreased vagal output to restore blood pressure (Figure 32.2).

Postural control of blood pressure

Changes in posture lead to alterations in pressure due to the hydrostatic influence on the blood. For example, when changing from lying down to standing up, the change in fluid distribution would tend to cause a reduction in central blood pressure. The reduction in central arterial pressure would tend to lead to less pressure in the cerebral circulation and could lead to 'light headedness'. However, the **baroreceptor reflex** aims to maintain a relatively constant blood pressure with any change in posture. An initial drop in blood pressure would initiate a baroreceptor reflex, resulting in increased sympathetic activity (with peripheral vasoconstriction) and decreased vagal activity to maintain a relatively constant blood pressure. **Autonomic dysfunction** or drug treatments that interfere with volume control (diuretics) or α_1-adrenoceptor-mediated vasoconstriction (α_1-adrenoceptor antagonists) can impair these responses and lead to **postural** or **ortho-static hypotension** (i.e. when systolic blood pressure drops >20 mmHg) when changing from lying or sitting down to standing.

Volume control of blood pressure

In the longer term it is blood volume that has the greater influence on blood pressure, and this is tightly regulated. Volume is linked to Na^+ balance, as water follows Na^+ by osmosis. Blood volume and Na^+ balance are tightly controlled by the kidneys and this is achieved by the **renin-angiotensin-aldosterone system** (RAAS) (Chapter 38) (Figure 32.3). Low levels of Na^+ and low blood pressures are sensed by the **macula densa cells** of the **juxtaglomerular apparatus** in the kidneys, which respond by releasing renin. This is also stimulated by β-adrenoceptor-mediated sympathetic stimulation. **Renin** is a proteolytic enzyme that activates by cleavage of the circulating hormone **angiotensinogen** to form the peptide **angiotensin I (AI)**. Following this, AI is activated by the **angiotensin converting enzyme** (ACE), which is largely located in the lungs, to form **angiotensin II (AII)**. AII acts at the angiotensin AT_1 receptor and is a potent vasoconstrictor and also augments sympathetically induced vasoconstriction to increase blood pressure. AII also stimulates the release of the steroid hormone **aldosterone** from the zona glomerulosa of the adrenal cortex. Aldosterone then acts on distal tubular cells of the kidney to increase the number of sodium channels and sodium pumps, and this promotes the reasbsorption of Na^+ (with a concomitant loss of K^+), followed by water.

Vasopressin or the **antidiuretic hormone** (ADH) also plays a role in volume control (Chapter 38). ADH acts on the collecting ducts of the kidney, leading to the activation of **aquaporins** (water channels) and this promotes water reabsorption and volume control.

Hypertension

As defined above, this is the sustained and pathological increase in blood pressure. **Essential hypertension** accounts for 90–95% of cases and its aetiology is multifactorial, with no single identifiable cause. **Secondary hypertension** (5–10%) is when the increase in blood pressure is associated with another pathology, e.g. renal artery stenosis (associated with increased activation of RAAS), Conn's syndrome (associated with increased release of aldosterone), phaeochromocytoma (tumour-secreting catecholamines), or fluid-retaining drugs (e.g. steroids and non-steroidal anti-inflammatory drugs, NSAIDs). Secondary hypertension is usually treated by managing the associated condition. Essential hypertension is managed by lifestyle measures (e.g. weight loss, decreased alcohol consumption, increased physical activity) and may be treated with antihypertensives. As blood pressure is the product of cardiac output and TPR, the principle is to reduce one of these determinants.

Widely used antihypertensives include:
- **angiotensin converting enzyme (ACE) inhibitors** (e.g. ramipril): these reduce the production of AII and so reduce TPR. AT_1 receptor antagonists (e.g. losartan) are also used and inhibit the actions of AII;
- **calcium channel blockers** (e.g. amlodipine): these inhibit voltage-operated Ca^{2+} channels in vascular smooth muscle to cause vasodilatation and so reduce TPR;
- **diuretics** (e.g. thiazide-like agents such as indapamide): act on the distal convoluted tubule cells of the kidney to inhibit NaCl reabsorption (and so water reabsorption). These lead to a reduction in circulating volume and reduction in blood pressure. They also cause vasodilatation.

33 Blood: 1

Michael D Randall

Figure 33.1 Summary of haemopoiesis

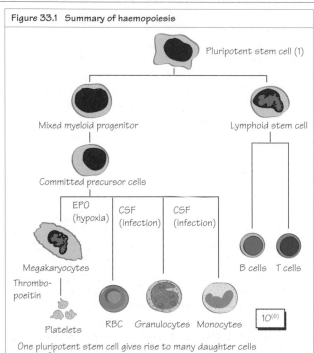

One pluripotent stem cell gives rise to many daughter cells (e.g. 10^6) via clonal expansion. The process is tightly regulated by factors such as thrombopoietin, erythropoietin (EPO) and colony-stimulating factors (CSFs)

Figure 33.2 Centrifuged blood sample to indicate its normal composition

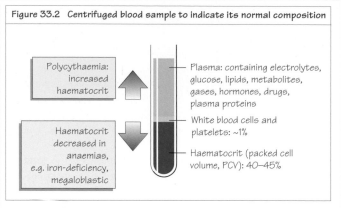

Table 33.1 Alterations in differential blood cell counts

Cell type	Increased	Decreased
Erythrocytes [Males 4.5–6.5 x 10^{12}/L] [Females 3.9–5.6 x10^{12}/L]	Polycythemia • Primary: stem cell defect leading to uncontrolled proliferation • Secondary: (Patho)physiological response to hypoxia associated with ascent to altitude, smoking and COPD	Anaemia • Microcytic associated with iron deficiency • Macrocytic associated with folate and/or vitamin B_{12} deficiency • Normocytic associated with chronic conditions, e.g. renal disease
Leucocytes [Total 4.0–11.0 x 10^9/L]	Leucocytosis	Leucopenia
Neutrophils [2.5–7.5 x 10^9/L]	Neutrophilia • Response to infections (bacterial/fungal) • Inflammation • Trauma	Neutropenia • Drug-induced as an adverse drug reaction. Patient may present with increased infections • Infection (viral, malaria)
Eosinophils [0.04–0.44 x 10^9/L]	Eosinophilia • Associated with allergy/atopy • Parasitic infections	
Monocytes [0.2–0.8 x 10^9/L]	Monocytosis • Associated with chronic infections, e.g. tuberculosis	
Lymphocytes [1.5–3.5 x 10^9/L]	Lymphocytosis • Response to infection (bacterial, viral) • Lymphoma – malignancy of lymphatic tissue leading to uncontrolled production	Lymphopenia • Inflammation – depletion of cells • Lymphoma – malignancy of lymphatic tissue impairing production • Steroids – anti-inflammatory actions reducing production
Platelets [150–400 x 10^9/L]	Thrombophilia • Increased risk of thrombosis	Thrombocytopenia • May be drug-induced as an adverse drug reaction • Idiopathic: no identifiable cause

The volume of blood in an adult is around 5 litres and is normally composed of **red blood cells** (RBCs: erythrocytes) for gas transport (Chapter 25), white blood cells (WBCs) (**neutrophils, eosinophils, basophils, monocytes** and **lymphocytes**) for defence/immunology and **platelets** (for clotting). The remainder is plasma, a solution of electrolytes, glucose, lipids, metabolites, gases, hormones, drugs and plasma proteins. **Serum** is coagulated plasma.

Control of blood production

Production of blood cells (**haemopoiesis**) is a tightly regulated process in which a **pluripotent stem cell** is committed to one cell line and undergoes many cell divisions, leading to **clonal expansion**. RBC production is stimulated by the polypeptide **erythropoietin** (EPO), which is released by renal peritubular cells in response to hypoxia. **Colony-stimulating factors** (**CSF**s), e.g. **G-CSF** (granulocyte CSF), act on the neutrophil cell line and are increased in infections to increase the WBC count (Figure 33.1).

Blood counts

The full blood count is the number of blood cells per volume of blood and is differentiated into RBCs, WBC types and platelets.

The amount of **haemoglobin** (Hb) in blood is expressed as (g) per 100 mL of blood and used to identify **anaemias**.

Haematocrit (packed cell volume, PCV) is the percentage of blood that is made up of RBCs. It is expressed as either a percentage (typically 40–45%) or as a fraction (0.40–0.45).

Mean corpuscular volume (MCV) is the volume (fl) of individual RBCs [normal range = 80–95 fl]. Increased MCV is described as **macrocytosis** and a decreased MCV as **microcytosis**.

Blood groups

These are determined by antigens (glycoproteins) expressed on RBC membranes and antibodies to other antigens may be in plasma. There are more than 400 groups, but **ABO** and **Rhesus** are the clinically important ones. **Group A** (A antigens and b-antibodies), **Group B** (B antigens and a-antibodies), **Group AB** (A and B antigens and no antibodies), and **Group O** (a and b antibodies).
• The **Rhesus D (RhD)** antigen confers the Rhesus status (positive). Patients are identified as being A, B, AB, or O, and are either Rh+ve or Rh−ve. This system is essential to ensure correct cross-matching of blood for transfusions, as exposure to an antigen from a different group leads to life-threatening **transfusion reactions**. This involves antibodies being raised against the foreign antigen, leading to a severe immune response with haemolysis of RBCs.

Blood from the **O Rh−ve** group is regarded as a **universal donor** as it lacks antigens and as such will not provoke an immune response. O−ve blood is therefore used in dire emergencies for transfusions until cross-matched blood is available.

Haemolytic disease of the newborn

Approximately 85% of the population are Rh+ve, consequently mothers who are Rh−ve are likely to carry to a Rh+ve fetus. In a first pregnancy this is unlikely to lead to complications, but at birth the transfer of fetal blood leads to the mother raising antibodies against the D-antigen. These antibodies would then attack a subsequent fetus that was Rh+ve, potentially leading to fetal death. To eliminate this risk the mother receives **anti-D immunisation** after the first birth to bind any D-antigens and so prevent the production of antibodies.

Anaemias

These are common clinical conditions with reduced Hb levels, leading to the symptoms of breathlessness, weakness, lethargy and tachycar-

dia. The patient may have pale conjunctiva, and anaemia is also associated with glossitis (painful red tongue) and angular cheilitis (fissures at corner of mouth).

Microcytic

Iron deficiency anaemia is the most common form of anaemia and develops once all of the body's iron stores have been depleted. This is usually secondary to negative iron balance through chronic blood loss due to **gastrointestinal bleeds** or **excessive menstrual bleeding**. The lack of iron results in impaired synthesis of Hb and RBCs, which are smaller than normal, i.e. **microcytic** (reduced MCV).

Normocytic

Anaemia associated with chronic conditions tends to be normocytic. An example of this is **renal anaemia**, in which patients with chronic kidney disease often develop normocytic anaemia due to reduced EPO production from the kidneys. It is managed with injections of EPO.

Macrocytic

The RBCs are macrocytic (increased MCV) and a common cause is **megaloblastic anaemia**. In this condition there is abnormal RBC maturation as a result of defective DNA synthesis, and the bone marrow contains **megaloblasts**. Megaloblastic anaemia is caused by deficiencies of either **vitamin B_{12} or folic acid**. Vitamin B_{12} is an essential cofactor for purine and pyrimidine synthesis (hence the defective DNA synthesis and impaired cell division). Folate is an essential substrate for thymidylate synthesis.

Pernicious anaemia is a version of megaloblastic anaemia in which the body raises antibodies against the **intrinsic factor** released from parietal cells in the stomach. The intrinsic factor normally binds to vitamin B_{12} and is essential for its absorption in the ileum. Therefore, in this condition there is impaired absorption of vitamin B_{12}, leading to deficiencies and megaloblastic anaemia, which is managed by injections of a vitamin B_{12} analogue.

Haemolytic anaemias

Haemolytic anaemias are characterised by increased RBC destruction. These can be acquired, for example through increased destruction associated with transfusion reactions or malaria. They can also be genetic and associated with abnormal forms of Hb that predispose to RBC destruction.
• **Sickle cell anaemia** involves a **single nucleotide polymorphism** in which there is a single amino acid substitution of glutamic acid with valine. This leads to abnormal Hb, which forms insoluble crystals at low O_2 tensions and the RBCs form fragile sickle shapes, which may block microcirculation.
• **Thalassaemias**: these are genetic conditions in which there is reduced rate of α or β globin units production. There are a range of variations, for example deletion of all four of the copies of the α-globin genes results in Hb with 4γ subunits being formed, which is incompatible with life and leads to death of the fetus. The loss of one or two of the α-globin genes is referred to as an α-thalassaemia trait and is not usually associated with anaemia (but MCV is usually low).

Aplastic anaemia

Aplastic anaemia is the lack of production of blood cells and platelets by the bone marrow. Mostly cases are acquired due to viral infection, radiation, or drugs causing damage to the bone marrow. This is a potentially fatal condition and is managed symptomatically by transfusions. Curative treatment is via bone marrow transplantation.

Michael D Randall

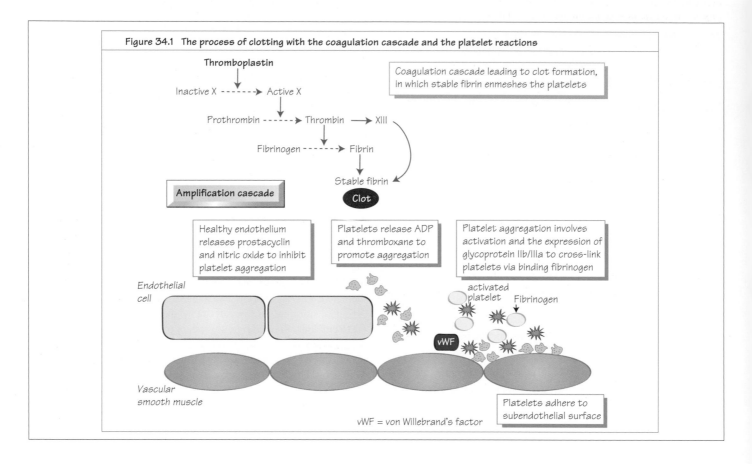

Figure 34.1 The process of clotting with the coagulation cascade and the platelet reactions

Thromboplastin

Inactive X - - - - - → Active X

Coagulation cascade leading to clot formation, in which stable fibrin enmeshes the platelets

Prothrombin - - - - - → Thrombin ——→ XIII

Fibrinogen - - - - - → Fibrin

Stable fibrin

Clot

Amplification cascade

Healthy endothelium releases prostacyclin and nitric oxide to inhibit platelet aggregation

Platelets release ADP and thromboxane to promote aggregation

Platelet aggregation involves activation and the expression of glycoprotein IIb/IIIa to cross-link platelets via binding fibrinogen

Endothelial cell

activated platelet   Fibrinogen

vWF

Vascular smooth muscle

Platelets adhere to subendothelial surface

vWF = von Willebrand's factor

Coagulation and thrombosis (Figure 34.1)

The process of haemostasis is the formation of clots at the site of damage to a blood vessel to prevent blood loss. It involves both coagulation (via plasma-borne proteins) and platelet aggregation.

Coagulation

Activation of the coagulation cascade results in the production of insoluble fibrin. This process involves many steps in which precursor coagulation factors are activated by activated factors. As such, the coagulation cascade is an **amplification cascade**, with each step resulting in a substantial activation of the next components. This means that a relatively small event can lead to large biological response. Many of the reactions involve **serine protease** activity cleaving the precursor factor, and the final product is stabilised fibrin, which enmeshes platelet aggregates.

The **initiation phase** (previously termed extrinsic pathway) involves the release of **thromboplastin** (tissue factor) from damaged tissues. Thromboplastin then complexes with activated factor VIIa in the plasma and this leads to the activation of factor X. Factor Xa then leads to the activation of prothrombin to thrombin, which hydrolyses fibrinogen to release fibrinopeptides A and B, which are polymerised to form fibrin. Thrombin also activates factor XIII to form XIIIa, which cross-links the fibrin.

Platelet adhesion and aggregation

In parallel with the coagulation cascade is the **platelet reaction**, in which platelets adhere to subendothelial surface on vessel damage and this is facilitated by binding to **von Willebrand's factor (vWF)**. **Platelet adhesion** then leads to the **release reaction**, in which platelets release **adenosine diphosphate** (ADP) and **thromboxane** (TXA_2) to promote platelet aggregation. ADP binds to receptors on platelets and this leads to the expression of **glycoprotein IIb/IIIa** in the platelet membranes and promotes cross-linking by binding vWF and fibrinogen. TXA_2 promotes aggregation by reducing intracellular levels of cAMP.

Thrombosis

Thrombosis is the unwanted formation of blood clots. On the venous side of the circulation thrombosis is largely associated with stasis of blood. For example, immobility may lead to the formation of **deep vein thrombosis** (DVTs) in the deep veins of the calf muscles in the legs. The thrombus may break off and enter the circulation where it can become lodged in the lungs. This is a life-threatening **pulmonary embolism** due to blockade of the pulmonary circulation.

Arterial thrombosis usually forms at atherosclerotic sites, in which the plaque may rupture, leading to platelet adhesion and aggregation. The resulting clot formation can lead to an arterial blockage. In the coronary circulation this leads to a **myocardial infarction** and in cerebral vessels formation of the blockage or an embolus results in a **thromboembolic stroke**.

Atrial fibrillation leads to impaired pumping of the blood from the left atrium and the stasis of blood predisposes towards thrombosis. Blood clots form and may then break off and enter the systemic circulation and become lodged in the cerebral circulation leading to a **transient ischaemic attack (TIA)**.

Anticoagulants

To prevent thrombosis the oral anticoagulant **warfarin** is used. Warfarin is a vitamin K antagonist and blocks the **vitamin K epoxide reductase** (VKOR), which is an enzyme in the liver responsible for the post-translational modification of coagulation factors. Warfarin therefore inhibits the synthesis of certain coagulation factors. Clinically, warfarin is a difficult drug to use and has many drug interactions. It requires extensive monitoring of its anticoagulant activity by measuring the **prothrombin time**, expressed as the **international normalised ratio** (**INR**).

Injectible anticoagulants are the **heparins**, which have immediate actions via activating antithrombin III in the plasma, which inhibits serine protease activities of some of the coagulation factors.

More recently **direct thrombin inhibitors** (e.g. dabigatran) have been introduced and do not require extensive monitoring.

Antiplatelet drugs

Low-dose (75 mg) **aspirin** is highly effective at reducing the risk of myocardial infarction and ischaemic stroke in at risk patients. Aspirin inhibits the cyclooxygenase enzyme responsible for producing prostacyclin in the endothelium (which inhibits platelet aggregation) and TX_2 in platelets. The actions of aspirin are irreversible, but since the endothelial cells have a nucleus they are, in time, able to produce new cyclooxygenases and so prostacyclin. However, platelets, which lack a nucleus, are incapable of producing more enzyme and therefore cannot produce TXA_2. Consequently aspirin shifts the balance to favour prostacyclin over TXA_2 and reduces the chances of platelet aggregation.

Clopidogrel is an ADP ($P2Y_{12}$) receptor antagonist and prevents ADP-induced expression of glycoprotein IIb/IIIa. Therefore, clopidogrel is also used to prevent platelet aggregation.

Problems with haemostasis

Haemophilias are genetic conditions in which affected patients have low or absent levels of Factor VIII (haemophilia A) or IX (haemophilia B) of the clotting cascade. This means that affected patients bleed profusely on minor trauma and require treatment with coagulation factor.

Von Willebrand's disease is an hereditary lack or defect in vWF and results in increased bruising and mucosal bleeding (e.g. nose bleeds).

Thrombocytopenia is a reduction in platelet count due to impaired production of platelets. It may be induced by the toxic or immunological effects of drugs on platelet production. It may also occur in the absence of an identifiable cause (idiopathic). The reduction in platelet count leads to easy bleeding and bruising.

Disseminated intravascular coagulation involves widespread and uncontrolled activation of the coagulant cascade throughout the vascular system. This may occur due to the presence of procoagulant material (e.g. amniotic fluid) in the circulation stimulating coagulation. The uncontrolled production of fibrin leads to the excessive consumption of coagulation factors and the patient is at risk of severe haemorrhage due to depletion of factors and platelets.

Leukaemias and lymphomas
Leukaemias

Leukaemias are haematological malignancies in which abnormal cells accumulate in the bone marrow and this may lead to bone marrow failure. The malignant transformation can result in the increased production of abnormal white blood cells, which increase the patient's susceptibility to infection. Associated bone marrow failure leads to anaemia and thrombocytopenia. There are number of different forms of leukaemia.

• **Acute leukaemias** usually have a short time course between discovery and death if they are untreated. There is failure of cell maturation, and useless cells accumulate in bone marrow and then spill over into the circulation. They are divided into **myeloid** or **lymphoblastic**, depending on which cell line is involved.

• **Chronic myeloid leukaemia** involves the replacement of normal bone marrow cells with cells with an abnormal chromosome (90% of patients have Philadelphia chromosome).

• **Chronic lymphocytic leukaemia** is the most common form and especially affects the elderly. It is characterised by abnormal lymphocytes in lymphoid tissue (including the bone).

Lymphomas

These are malignancies of the lymphatic tissue in which there is replacement of lymphoid tissue with abnormal cells. Depending on the histology, they are divided into either Hodgkin's disease or non-Hodgkin's lymphoma (high or low grade).

Management

Both leukaemias and lymphomas may be managed by anticancer chemotherapy (Chapter 65) and some leukaemias can be cured by bone marrow transplantation with stem cells following destruction of diseased bone marrow by high-dose chemotherapy and irradiation.

35 Cardiovascular pathophysiology

Michael D Randall

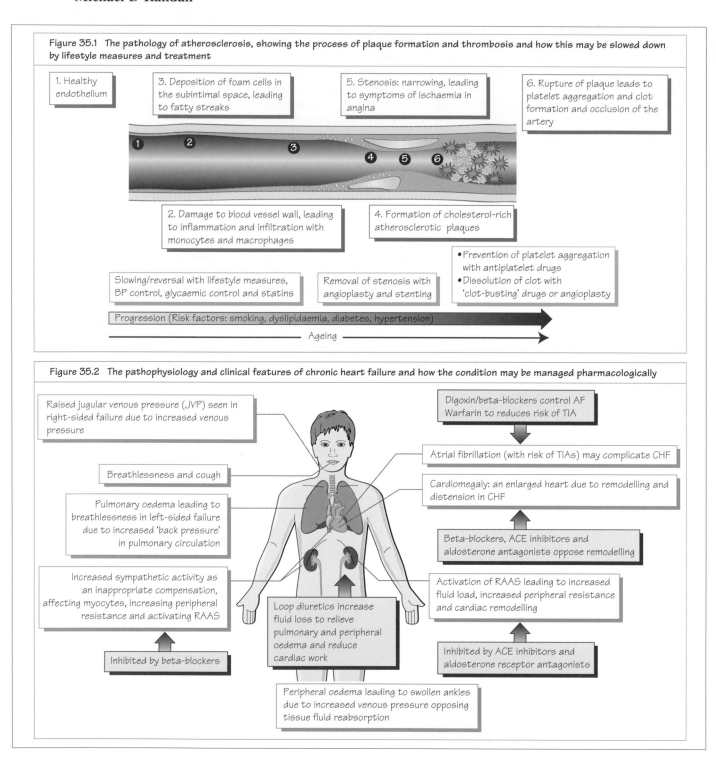

Figure 35.1 The pathology of atherosclerosis, showing the process of plaque formation and thrombosis and how this may be slowed down by lifestyle measures and treatment

1. Healthy endothelium

3. Deposition of foam cells in the subintimal space, leading to fatty streaks

5. Stenosis: narrowing, leading to symptoms of ischaemia in angina

6. Rupture of plaque leads to platelet aggregation and clot formation and occlusion of the artery

2. Damage to blood vessel wall, leading to inflammation and infiltration with monocytes and macrophages

4. Formation of cholesterol-rich atherosclerotic plaques

- Prevention of platelet aggregation with antiplatelet drugs
- Dissolution of clot with 'clot-busting' drugs or angioplasty

Slowing/reversal with lifestyle measures, BP control, glycaemic control and statins

Removal of stenosis with angioplasty and stenting

Progression (Risk factors: smoking, dyslipidaemia, diabetes, hypertension)

Ageing

Figure 35.2 The pathophysiology and clinical features of chronic heart failure and how the condition may be managed pharmacologically

Raised jugular venous pressure (JVP) seen in right-sided failure due to increased venous pressure

Digoxin/beta-blockers control AF Warfarin to reduces risk of TIA

Atrial fibrillation (with risk of TIAs) may complicate CHF

Breathlessness and cough

Cardiomegaly: an enlarged heart due to remodelling and distension in CHF

Pulmonary oedema leading to breathlessness in left-sided failure due to increased 'back pressure' in pulmonary circulation

Beta-blockers, ACE inhibitors and aldosterone antagonists oppose remodelling

Increased sympathetic activity as an inappropriate compensation, affecting myocytes, increasing peripheral resistance and activating RAAS

Activation of RAAS leading to increased fluid load, increased peripheral resistance and cardiac remodelling

Loop diuretics increase fluid loss to relieve pulmonary and peripheral oedema and reduce cardiac work

Inhibited by beta-blockers

Inhibited by ACE inhibitors and aldosterone receptor antagonists

Peripheral oedema leading to swollen ankles due to increased venous pressure opposing tissue fluid reabsorption

Cardiovascular disease is the biggest killer in the Western world. Ischaemic heart disease is the leading cause of death in the UK, with stroke (after cancer) accounting for the third-highest number of deaths. Cardiovascular disease is an inevitable consequence of the ageing process but is accelerated by the following risk factors (male gender, smoking, ethnicity: Indian subcontinent ethnicity is associated with an increased risk, diabetes: especially with poor glycaemic control, dyslipidaemia: high LDL cholesterol, low HDL cholesterol and high triglycerides; there may be a familial tendency, obesity, family history: close relative with premature cardiovascular disease).

Hypertension (Chapter 32)

This is a key cardiovascular disease and is a risk factor for developing ischaemic heart disease and chronic heart failure.

Ischaemic heart disease

Ischaemic heart disease (IHD) may manifest as either angina or myocardial infarction (MI) and is an important cause of chronic heart failure. In both cases, IHD is generally associated with **atherosclerosis** within the coronary arteries, leading to impaired blood flow or thromboembolic occlusion. In angina, the reductions in coronary blood flow mean that perfusion does not match demand, leading to ischaemia, which provokes the symptoms. **Stable angina** is characterised by chest pain (which may radiate down the left arm and to the jaw), which appears on exertion but is relieved by rest and/or the nitrate **glyceryl trinitrate** (**GTN**) given as a spray. Diagnosis may be based on symptoms and on ST-depression on the electrocardiogram (ECG) during an attack. Patients with stable angina receive beta-blockers (or rate-limiting calcium channel blockers), which reduce cardiac work and by increasing the time for diastole (when coronary flow occurs) increase coronary blood flow. GTN is used to relieve attacks and releases nitric oxide, which causes vasorelaxation, specifically venorelaxation, and this decreases venous return to the heart and so reduces cardiac work. Interventions include angioplasty with **stenting** (see below) or **coronary artery bypass grafting (CABG)**, in which a donor artery (e.g. internal mammary artery) is used to surgically restore the blood flow by bypassing the diseased artery.

Unstable angina is generally due to plaque rupture and the formation of a non-occlusive thromboembolism, or, vasospasm.

In **myocardial infarction** (**MI**) there is often **thromboembolic occlusion** of a coronary artery. The cessation of blood flow results in damage or infarction of the cardiac muscle starved of blood. MI may lead to acute left ventricular failure and/or arrhythmias, which are the leading cause of early mortality. The initial management of MI is now emergency angioplasty, in which a balloon is advanced into the coronary artery to open up the blockage and restore blood flow. This is followed by insertion of a **stent** (a metal cage) to prevent reformation of the narrowing (**restenosis**). Other treatments include the use of '**clot-busting' drugs** or **thrombolytic** agents that activate the plasma protein plasminogen to plasmin, which degrades fibrin that forms the clot, resulting in reperfusion. Following an MI, patients are often prescribed the combination of a **beta-blocker**, an **ACE inhibitor**, a **statin** and an **antiplatelet drug** (e.g. low-dose aspirin) for **secondary prevention**.

Ischaemic heart disease is often due to **atheroscelerosis** resulting from **atherogenesis** (Figure 35.1). The formation of changes to the intimal wall of the blood vessel begin in early adulthood with the formation of fatty streaks, and this process, over time, leads to the formation of cholesterol-rich atherosclerotic plaques which lead to partial occlusion of the artery (leading to angina) or they may rupture, leading to thrombus formation (leading to an MI in the coronary artery or stroke in the cerebral circulation). Atherogenesis is regarded as an inflammatory process and when injury occurs (as promoted by smoking, hypertension and possibly infection) activated monocytes and macrophages generate free radicals, which oxidise LDL cholesterol, which in turn damages its receptor and this leads to cholesterol being deposited at the point of the lesion. To slow down atherosclerosis the key approach is reduction of cardiovascular risk through lifestyle changes. Patients who have an elevated cardiovascular risk are prescribed statins.

Statins are cholesterol-lowering drugs that inhibit the endogenous production of cholesterol in the liver by inhibiting the enzyme hydroxyl-methylglutaryl coenzyme A reductase (**HMG-CoA reductase**), which catalyses the first committed step of cholesterol synthesis. This reduces cholesterol levels by reducing its synthesis and also leads to an upregulation of LDL cholesterol receptors, which promotes the uptake of cholesterol into liver cells. In addition to reducing cholesterol levels, statins may also stabilise cholesterol within the plaques, reducing the chances of a cardiovascular event.

Although total cholesterol should ideally be <5 mmol/L, statins are prescribed in relation to overall cardiovascular risk and are of benefit in patients with 'normal' cholesterol levels.

Chronic heart failure (Figure 34.2)

Hypertension and ischaemic heart disease are both key risk factors for the development of **chronic (or congestive) heart failure (CHF)**. Chronic refers to the long-term nature of this condition, in which the pumping ability of the heart is insufficient for the needs of the body. CHF involves a syndrome of neurohormonal adaptations that are inappropriate and exacerbate the condition.

• Activation of **renin-angiotensin-aldosterone system** (RAAS, Chapter 31): underperfusion of kidneys leads to increased activity of RAAS, resulting in AII-mediated vasoconstriction (with further underperfusion of the kidneys and further activation of RAAS) and aldosterone release, which increases Na^+ reabsorption and fluid retention (which increases cardiac workload and exacerbates CHF).

• Increased **sympathetic activity**: to attempt to increase cardiac work (but also results in activation of RAAS and vasoconstriction).

There is also a compensatory increase in the release of natriuretic peptides from the heart and levels of b-type natriuretic peptide (BNP) are used as markers of CHF.

In **left-sided cardiac failure** back pressure builds up in the pulmonary circulation, leading to pulmonary oedema and breathlessness. In **right-sided failure** there is increased venous pressure leading to peripheral oedema, typically swollen ankles.

CHF is diagnosed by reduced ejection fraction on an echocardiogram. It may also be identified by increased levels of BNP and pulmonary oedema observed on a chest X-ray.

CHF is managed by:

• **Loop diuretics** (e.g. furosemide): leading to substantial diuresis, reducing circulating volume and so cardiac work.

• **ACE inhibitors** (e.g. ramipril): to oppose to RAAS "overactivity" if it will.

• **Beta-blockers** (e.g. bisoprolol): low dose, cardioselective agents are used cautiously to oppose the toxic effects of excessive sympathetic stimulation of the heart.

• **Aldosterone receptor antagonists** (e.g. spironolactone): to oppose the toxic effects of aldosterone on the heart.

• **Digoxin:** inhibits the Na^+ pump (Chapter 18); intracellular Na^+ is then exchanged for calcium, resulting in an increase in force of contraction. Digoxin also increases vagal slowing of atrioventricular (AV) node conduction and is used in atrial fibrillation.

Cerebrovascular disease (Chapter 57)

Cerebrovascular disease (stroke) is either **thromboembolic** (about 90% of cases) or **haemorrhagic** (about 10% of cases). Thromboembolic or ischaemic stroke is often due to atherosclerosis in the cerebral circulation resulting in thrombosis, or due to clot formation associated with stasis of blood due to poor atrial ejection in **atrial fibrillation**. Anticoagulants (e.g. warfarin) or antiplatelet drugs are given for prophylaxis in atrial fibrillation.

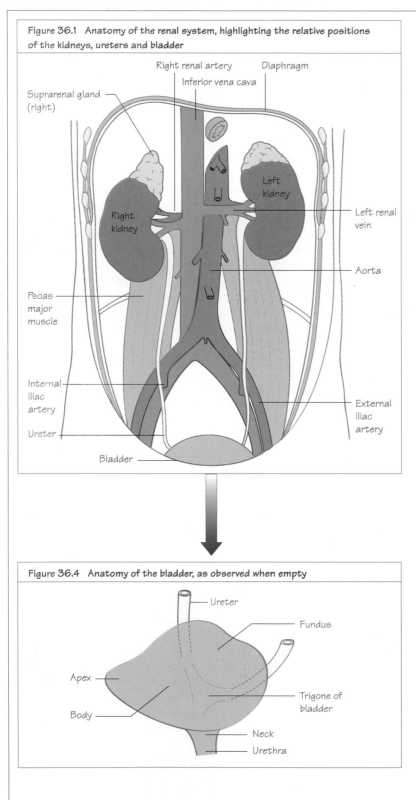

Figure 36.1 Anatomy of the renal system, highlighting the relative positions of the kidneys, ureters and bladder

Right renal artery
Diaphragm
Inferior vena cava
Suprarenal gland (right)
Left kidney
Right kidney
Left renal vein
Aorta
Psoas major muscle
Internal iliac artery
Ureter
External iliac artery
Bladder

Figure 36.4 Anatomy of the bladder, as observed when empty

Ureter
Fundus
Apex
Trigone of bladder
Body
Neck
Urethra

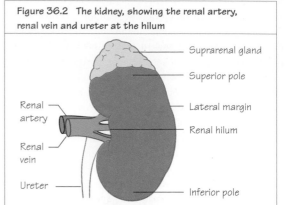

Figure 36.2 The kidney, showing the renal artery, renal vein and ureter at the hilum

Suprarenal gland
Superior pole
Renal artery
Lateral margin
Renal hilum
Renal vein
Ureter
Inferior pole

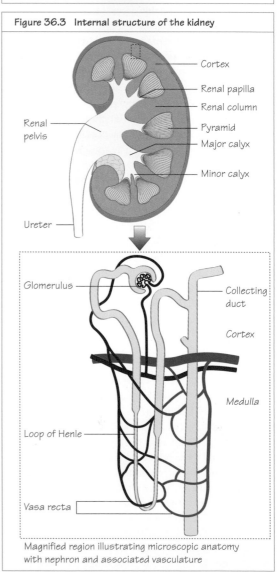

Figure 36.3 Internal structure of the kidney

Cortex
Renal papilla
Renal column
Pyramid
Major calyx
Renal pelvis
Minor calyx
Ureter

Glomerulus
Collecting duct
Cortex
Medulla
Loop of Henle
Vasa recta

Magnified region illustrating microscopic anatomy with nephron and associated vasculature

The renal system is involved in the removal of waste products, excess water and salts from the blood in the form of urine. It controls the level of water and electrolytes within the body and maintains the acid-base balance of blood. The renal system comprises the kidneys, ureters, bladder and urethra.

Kidneys and ureters
Kidneys
The kidneys are retroperitoneal organs located on the posterior abdominal wall at the level of T12-L3 vertebrae (Figure 36.1). Occupying a region either side of the vertebral column, the right kidney lies slightly lower than the left. The kidneys have some mobility, being able to move up to 2–3 cm during respiration and as a result of changes in body positioning (e.g. moving from erect to supine position). The kidneys have anterior and posterior surfaces, medial and lateral margins, and also superior and inferior poles (Figure 36.2). On the medial concave margin is a vertical slit called the renal hilum, which is the region where vessels, nerves and the renal pelvis enter/leave the kidney. The superomedial aspect of each kidney makes contact with the suprarenal (adrenal) gland. These two organs function independently, with a fascial septum separating them. The kidneys and suprarenal glands are surrounded by a protective layer of fat (perinephric fat), which in turn is enclosed by a layer of renal fascia. The kidneys receive their blood supply directly from the abdominal aorta, via the renal arteries (Figures 36.1 and 36.2). Close to the hilum, the right and left renal arteries divide into approximately five segmental arteries to supply the kidney. Venous blood drains through the renal veins to empty into the inferior vena cava (Figure 36.1). Lymphatic drainage of the kidney is to the lumbar lymph nodes. Innervation is from sympathetic, parasympathetic and visceral afferent fibres via the renal plexus.

Each kidney is composed of an **outer cortex** and an **inner medulla**. The medulla is composed of **renal pyramids** (approximately 10–18), which have an apex and base. The cortex extends to the base of the pyramid and between the pyramids, forming the renal columns (Figure 36.3). The cortex and medulla are composed of nephrons, which are the functional units of the kidney. Each **nephron** has a **glomerulus** (situated in the cortex) and a long tubule (**loop of Henle**) that extends into the medulla of the kidney, before uniting with a collecting tubule. Numerous blood vessels (**vasa recta**) are also found in the medulla (Figure 36.3).

Ureters
These are retroperitoneal muscular ducts (~25 cm in length) that carry urine from the kidneys to the bladder. The superior distended end of the ureter is called the renal pelvis, which is formed by the union of two to three major calices (Figure 36.3). A major calyx is formed by the union of two to three minor calices. Each minor calyx is indented by the renal papilla (apex of the renal pyramid), which has a perforated tip where large collecting ducts open to deliver urine into a major calyx. The ureters descend through the abdomen, running along the transverse processes of the lumbar vertebrae before crossing the pelvic brim by passing over the external iliac artery (Figure 36.1). The ureters descend along the lateral walls of the pelvis before entering the bladder. During their route from the kidney to the bladder the ureters are constricted at three sites: ureteropelvic junction, crossing external iliac artery (pelvic brim) and traversing the bladder wall (Figure 36.1). Arteries supplying the ureters are numerous, including branches from the renal arteries, abdominal aorta, testicular/ovarian arteries and branches of the internal iliac arteries. Veins draining the ureters accompany the arteries and are similarly named; lymphatic drainage is to the lumbar, common iliac, external iliac and internal iliac lymph nodes.

Bladder and urethra
Bladder (Chapter 40)
The bladder is a subperitoneal hollow muscular organ located in the pelvis. It functions to collect urine and then expel the waste fluid into the urethra during the process of micturition. When empty, the bladder has an apex, body, neck and fundus, lying posterior to the pubic bones (Figure 36.4). The bladder extends superiorly as it fills, reaching as high as the level of the umbilicus when full. The bladder wall is composed predominantly of the detrusor muscle. The **trigone muscle** of the bladder is a smooth triangular region of the mucosa between the ureteric orifices and the internal urethral orifice (Figure 36.4). Branches of the internal iliac arteries supply the bladder; namely, superior vesical arteries supply the anterosuperior aspects of the bladder, and inferior vesical arteries (male) or vaginal arteries (female) supply inferoposterior aspects. Veins draining the bladder correspond to the arteries they accompany, acting as tributaries to the internal iliac vein. Lymph from the bladder drains to the external iliac (superior surface of bladder), internal iliac (fundus) and sacral or common iliac (neck) lymph nodes. Parasympathetic fibres innervating the bladder arise from the sacral spinal cord levels, conveyed by the pelvic splanchnic nerves and inferior hypogastric plexuses. Sympathetic innervation is conveyed from T11-L2/L3 spinal cord levels to pelvic plexuses through the hypogastric plexuses and nerves. Sensory fibres (visceral afferents) transmitting sensations (e.g. pain from overdistention) follow the course of the parasympathetic (from inferior bladder) or sympathetic (from superior bladder) fibres.

Urethra
This is a muscular tube passing from the internal urethral orifice of the bladder to the external urethral orifice of the glans penis (male) or vestibule of the vagina (female). The urethra functions as an exit route for urine out of the body, varying in length in males (~20 cm) compared with females (~4 cm). Blood supply to the urethra is from the branches of the internal iliac arteries, including internal pudendal arteries and vaginal arteries (female) or prostatic branches of the inferior vesical and middle rectal arteries (male). Veins accompanying the arteries are named accordingly. Most lymph draining from the urethra enters the internal iliac nodes and to a lesser extent the inguinal lymph nodes.

37 Renal physiology: filtration and tubular function

Sue Chan

Figure 37.1 Kidney nephron

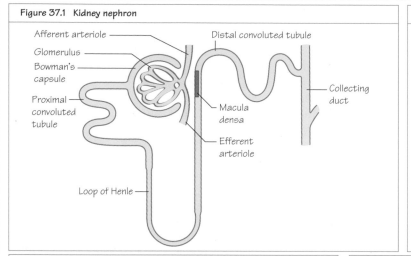

Figure 37.2 Starling forces and filtration

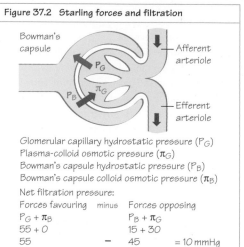

Glomerular capillary hydrostatic pressure (P_G)
Plasma-colloid osmotic pressure (π_G)
Bowman's capsule hydrostatic pressure (P_B)
Bowman's capsule colloid osmotic pressure (π_B)

Net filtration pressure:

Forces favouring	minus	Forces opposing	
$P_G + \pi_B$		$P_B + \pi_G$	
55 + 0		15 + 30	
55	−	45	= 10 mmHg

Figure 37.3 Proximal convoluted tubule (PCT)

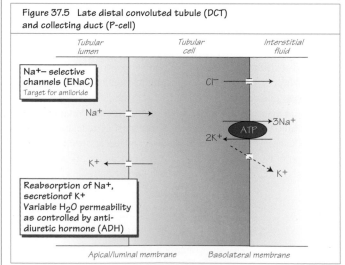

Figure 37.4 Early distal convoluted tubule (DCT)

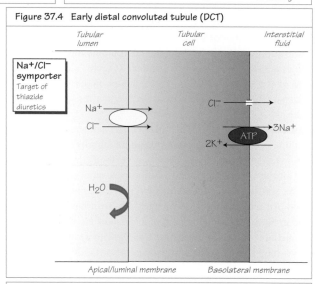

Figure 37.5 Late distal convoluted tubule (DCT) and collecting duct (P-cell)

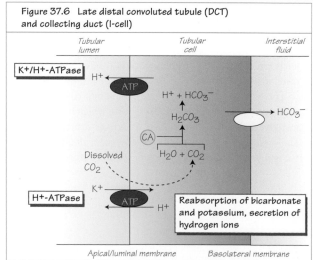

Figure 37.6 Late distal convoluted tubule (DCT) and collecting duct (I-cell)

Each nephron consists of a cup-shaped Bowman's capsule surrounding the glomerulus, which then passes to the proximal convoluted tubule, the loop of Henle, with the distal convoluted tubule draining into the collecting duct (Figure 37.1). There are two types of nephron: cortical (70–80%), with short loop of Henle and a network of peritubular capillaries supplying the tubular system; and juxtamedullary (20–30%), with long loop of Henle and specialised peritubular capillaries consisting of long vascular loops (vasa recta).

Filtration

The excretion of substances in urine is dependent on three processes: **filtration, reabsorption** and **secretion**. Urine formation begins with **filtration** of large amounts of fluid through the glomerular capillaries into the Bowman's space. Blood enters the network of glomerular capillaries via an afferent capillary, and leaves through an efferent arteriole, rather than a venule. Vasoconstriction of the afferent arteriole creates high hydrostatic pressure inside the glomerular capillaries to force the movement of water and solutes across the capillary wall. The glomerular capillary membrane is comprised of three layers (instead of the usual two): capillary endothelial cells form a layer with 70 nm pores or fenestrae; a basement membrane of negatively charged collagen and glycoproteins; then the epithelial visceral layer of the Bowman's capsule, known as **podocytes**, having long, foot-like projections that interdigitate to give filtration slits (slit pores, 25–65 nm). This **glomerular filter**, with each of the three layers having a negative charge, limits the filtration of a substance on both its molecular charge and size. The ultrafiltrate therefore consists of water, electrolytes, small molecules (<70 kDa) such as glucose, urea and amino acids, and is virtually protein-free.

Starling forces (Chapter 31) determine the movement of fluid between plasma and interstitium (tubule), summarised in Figure 37.2. **Renal blood flow** and **glomerular filtration rate** (**GFR**) are maintained at a relatively constant level, a process known as **autoregulation**. This involves two feedback mechanisms: an intrinsic **myogenic** property of blood vessels to resist stretching during increased arterial pressures; and the **tubuloglomerular feedback** involving the **macula densa**, a short segment of tubular cells (at the end of the ascending limb of the loop of Henle), which together with vascular **granular** cells (medial layer of the afferent arteriole adjacent to the vascular poles of the glomerulus) form the **juxtaglomerular apparatus**. The macula densa cells sense changes in tubular fluid NaCl concentration and volume/flow rate in volume delivery in the distal tubule, secreting vasoactive substances that control the vascular tone of blood vessels (such as adenosine, prostaglandins) and the control of renin release from the granular cells (see Chapter 39).

GFR can provide an estimate of the efficiency of renal filtration and hence renal function. In clinical medicine, creatinine (a metabolite of skeletal muscle creatine phosphate breakdown) is used to **estimate GFR** as it is almost completely cleared from the body by glomerular filtration.

The ultrafiltrate passes along the nephron tubule where its volume and content are altered by the processes of **reabsorption** (movement of filtered substance from tubular lumen to tubular capillaries) and **secretion** (movement of substances from vascular compartment to tubular fluid).

Proximal convoluted tubule (PCT)

Continuous with the Bowman's space, the proximal convoluted tubule lies entirely in the cortex. The first part of the tubule is highly convoluted with the second straighter part leading on to the loop of Henle.

Reabsorption

This is the predominant site of solute and water reabsorption: approximately 65% of filtered water, Na^+, K^+, Cl^- and other solutes, together with almost all of the glucose and amino acids in the ultrafiltrate. The tubular epithelial cells have a large apical membrane surface area due to the presence of many microvilli, together with a large number of mitochondria, to support the active transport process. Tubular reabsorption of all solutes is dependent, either directly or indirectly, on the **Na^+/K^+-ATPase pump**, present on the basolateral membrane (Figure 37.3). Active extrusion of Na^+ creates a low Na^+ concentration within the tubular cell, providing a concentration and electrical gradient for luminal Na^+ to move into the tubular cell, driving reabsorption of glucose and amino acids (co-transporters via secondary active transport) and the secretion of H^+ (Na^+/H^+ antiporter), with concomitant indirect reabsorption of filtered bicarbonate (via carbonic anhydrase) (Figure 37.3). Water is reabsorbed, driven by the tubular osmotic gradient established by solute reabsorption, by osmosis across 'leaky' tight junctions and via aquaporin water channels.

Secretion

The PCT is an important site for the secretion of organic acids and bases such as bile salts, oxalates and catecholamines. In addition to waste products of metabolism, the kidney also removes a large number of drugs and their metabolites (including thiazide-like diuretics, furosemide, penicillins, opioids) and toxins. Secretion is mainly an active process.

Loop of Henle

The loop of Henle extends into the medulla (descending thin limb), with the thick segment of the ascending limb responsible for the reabsorption of a further 25% of the filtered Na^+ load. The countercurrent multiplier system for the production of the hyperosmotic renal medulla, a key element in concentration of urine, is described in Chapter 38.

Distal convoluted tubule (DCT)

The early DCT reabsorbs Na^+, K^+ and Cl^- but is virtually impermeable to water and urea, thus diluting the tubular fluid (Figure 37.4). Sodium is reabsorbed together with chloride ions via the Na^+/Cl^- co-transporter, the Na^+ gradient for this Na^+ ion movement created by, once again, the basolateral Na^+/K^+-ATPase pump.

Late DCT and cortical collecting duct

These segments have similar functional characteristics, comprising of two distinct cell types with different transport properties.

Principal or P-cells

Sodium reabsorption and potassium secretion depends on the activity of the basolateral Na^+/K^+-ATPase pump. The hormone aldosterone can upregulate the expression of the Na^+/K^+-ATPase pump and the epithelial Na^+ channel, promoting increased sodium (and hence water) reabsorption together with increased potassium elimination (Figure 37.5). Additionally, vasopressin (or antidiuretic hormone) can cause increased transepithelial water transport.

Intercalated or I-cells

These cells are highly abundant with mitochondria, and are involved in active secretion of H^+ ions (via H^+-ATPase and K^+/H^+-ATPase) and reabsorption of bicarbonate and potassium ions (Figure 37.6). Thus, these cells play a key role in acid-base balance.

Renal physiology: loop of Henle

Sue Chan

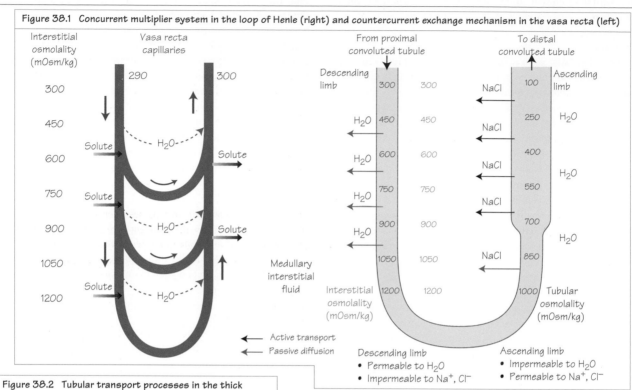

Figure 38.1 Concurrent multiplier system in the loop of Henle (right) and countercurrent exchange mechanism in the vasa recta (left)

Interstitial osmolality (mOsm/kg): 300, 450, 600, 750, 900, 1050, 1200

Vasa recta capillaries: 290 — 300

Solute, H₂O, Solute

From proximal convoluted tubule — To distal convoluted tubule

Descending limb: 300, 450, 600, 750, 900, 1050, 1200 (interstitial osmolality mOsm/kg)

Ascending limb: 100, 250, 400, 550, 700, 850, 1000 (tubular osmolality mOsm/kg)

NaCl, H₂O

Medullary interstitial fluid

← Active transport
← Passive diffusion

Descending limb
• Permeable to H₂O
• Impermeable to Na⁺, Cl⁻

Ascending limb
• Impermeable to H₂O
• Permeable to Na⁺, Cl⁻

Figure 38.2 Tubular transport processes in the thick ascending loop

Na⁺/K⁺/2Cl⁻ symporter
• Movement of Na⁺, K⁺ and 2Cl⁻ from apical membrane into cell as a result of Na⁺ gradient created by basolateral Na⁺/K⁺ ATPase pump
• Target for loop diuretics (such as furosemide)

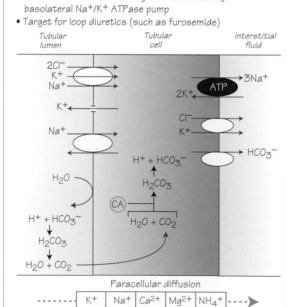

Tubular lumen — Tubular cell — Interstitial fluid

2Cl⁻, K⁺, Na⁺

3Na⁺, 2K⁺, ATP

K⁺

Cl⁻, K⁺

Na⁺

H⁺ + HCO₃⁻ → HCO₃⁻

H₂O

H₂CO₃ (CA) H₂O + CO₂

H⁺ + HCO₃⁻
↓
H₂CO₃
↓
H₂O + CO₂

Paracellular diffusion

-------- | K⁺ | Na⁺ | Ca²⁺ | Mg²⁺ | NH₄⁺ | ---->

Table 38.1 Permeability properties of nephron segments involved in urine concentration and dilution

Tubule segment	Permeability			Effects of ADH
	NaCl	Urea	Water	
Loop of Henle				
Thin descending limb	Very low ↑	Very low ↑	High	
Thin ascending limb	Very high	Moderate	Impermeable	
Thick ascending limb	Moderate	Very low ↑	Impermeable	NaCl reabsorption
Distal convoluted tubule	Moderate	Very low ↑	Variable	Water resorption late DCT
Collecting duct				
Cortical	Low ↑	Very low ↑	Variable	Water resorption
Medullary	Low ↑	Moderate	Variable	Water and urea resorption

The loop of Henle and the distal nephron are involved in the process of urine concentration. There are two key basic requirements: a **hyperosmotic renal medullary interstitium**, which provides the osmotic gradient for water reabsorption; and actions of **antidiuretic hormone (ADH)** (or vasopressin), which increase the water permeability in the late distal convoluted tubule and the collecting duct.

The loop of Henle consists of three functionally distinct segments: the **thin descending limb** and the **thin ascending limb** (only present in long loops of Henle of juxtamedullary nephrons) have thin epithelial membranes with poorly developed brush borders, few mitochondria and hence metabolic activity; the epithelial cells of the **ascending limb of Henle** have highly invaginated apical membranes and an abundance of mitochondria.

Tubular fluid entering the descending limb of the loop of Henle is isotonic with plasma/interstitial fluid (~290 mOsm/kg). The thin descending limb is highly permeable to water with very low permeability to solutes (such as NaCl and urea). Much of the water reabsorption in the loop of Henle (~20% of the filtered water) occurs along this segment. Thus, tubular fluid moving towards the tip of the loop becomes more solute concentrated (Figure 38.1). Meanwhile, the ascending segments are impermeable to water (an important feature in the process of concentration of urine). The thin segment has much lower solute reabsorptive capacity than that of the thick segment. As in the proximal convoluted tubule, the basolateral **Na$^+$/K$^+$-ATPase pump** maintains a low intracellular Na$^+$ concentration and this provides a favourable gradient for the reabsorption of tubular Na$^+$ ions, primarily via the apical **Na$^+$/K$^+$/2Cl$^-$ symporter**, with the apical K$^+$ channel enabling K$^+$ transported via Na$^+$/K$^+$/2Cl$^-$ transporter to be recycled back (Figure 38.2). This creates a slight positive charge in the tubular lumen, sufficient to force cations (such as Ca^{2+} and Mg^{2+}) to diffuse paracellularly into the interstitial fluid. There is also a Na$^+$-H$^+$ antiporter in apical membrane that enables Na$^+$ reabsorption and H$^+$ secretion (with HCO$_3^-$ reabsorption) (Figure 38.2). The tubular fluid in the ascending limb becomes more dilute (hypo-osmotic) as it flows towards the distal convoluted tubule due to this high solute reabsorption (Figure 38.1).

Countercurrent multiplication

This mechanism is dependent on both the form and the function of the loop of Henle: the two parallel limbs of the descending and ascending limbs with the flow of tubular fluid running in opposite directions (**countercurrent flow**) increases or 'multiplies' the osmotic gradient between tubular fluid and interstitial space.

The most important element in the development and maintenance of the high medullary osmolality is the active transport of Na$^+$ and co-transport of other ions from the thick ascending limb into the interstitium. The active pump mechanism allows a gradient of 200 mOsm/kg to be created across the tubular walls along the length of the tubule (Figure 38.1). As the **ascending limb** is impermeable to water, solute reabsorption occurs in the absence of accompanying water reabsorption, with high solute concentration in the renal medulla. As the **descending limb** is very permeable to water, the tubular fluid osmolality quickly becomes equal with that of the renal medullary interstitium, increasing as the tubular fluid flows towards the tip of the loop of Henle (Figure 38.1).

At the junction of the medulla with the cortex, the interstitium osmolality is ~300 mOsm/kg, virtually all of this is due to NaCl. The osmolality of the medullary interstitial fluid increases progressively to about 1200 mOsm/kg in the pelvic tip of the medulla, with NaCl and urea contributing equally to the hyperosmotic interstitium here. Approximately 50% of filtered urea is reabsorbed in the proximal convoluted tubule. However, the lack of permeability to urea in the thick ascending limb of the loop of Henle and the distal convoluted tubule results in the increased concentration of urea as it passes along the tubule, as water and other solutes are reabsorbed. The medullary collecting duct is relatively permeable to urea and so urea diffuses down its concentration gradient (via UT-A transporters) into the medulla, where some of urea passes back into the thin segments of the loop of Henle. Thus, the different permeability of segments (Table 38.1) of the nephron leads to the 'recycling' of urea.

The medullary capillaries, in particular the **vasa recta**, are highly permeable to solutes and water. The parallel configuration of the long vascular loops of the vasa recta means that although a large amount of fluid and solute exchange occurs across the capillary walls (between the plasma and the medullary interstitium), there is little net dilution of the concentration of the interstitial fluid at each level of the renal medulla (Figure 38.1). This **countercurrent exchange** process minimises dissipation of the built-up solute gradient by diffusion into the capillary system, preserving hyperosmolality of the renal medulla.

Distal nephron and actions of antidiuretic hormone, ADH

The water permeability of the late distal tubule and the collecting duct is dependent on the plasma concentration of antidiuretic hormone, ADH (Table 38.1). In the absence of ADH, the P-cells are almost impermeable to water and fail to reabsorb water while continuing to reabsorb solute, thus dilute urine is excreted. At high levels of ADH, water permeability is greatly enhanced, particularly in the cortical collecting duct, with a large amount of water reabsorbed into the renal cortex, where it is quickly taken away by peritubular capillaries. ADH also increases the transport of urea out of the medullary collecting duct, further increasing the renal medullary hyperosmolality, thus promoting the gradient for water reabsorption and the production of concentrated urine.

Sue Chan

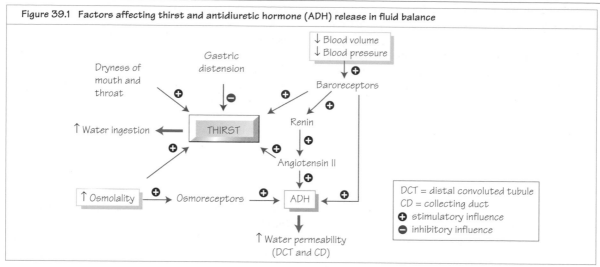

Figure 39.1   Factors affecting thirst and antidiuretic hormone (ADH) release in fluid balance

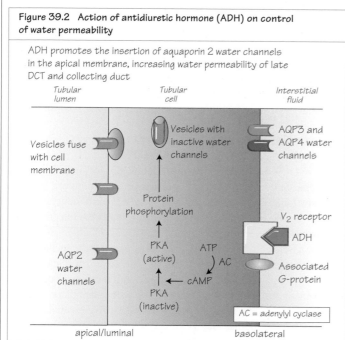

Figure 39.2   Action of antidiuretic hormone (ADH) on control of water permeability

ADH promotes the insertion of aquaporin 2 water channels in the apical membrane, increasing water permeability of late DCT and collecting duct

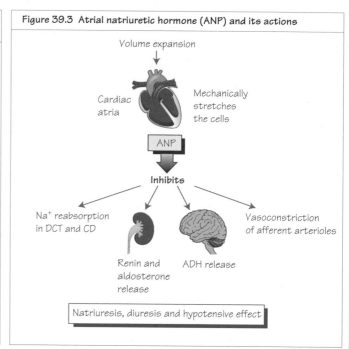

Figure 39.3   Atrial natriuretic hormone (ANP) and its actions

Water constitutes approximately 60% of the healthy human body, with the water in the intracellular and extracellular (interstitial fluid and blood plasma) compartments in osmotic equilibrium. Sodium and chloride ions are abundant in extracellular fluid, while in intracellular fluid, these ions are at low levels with a high concentration of potassium ions. The osmotic effect of these solutes acting across cell membranes determines the distribution of fluid between extracellular and intracellular compartments. Alterations to extracellular fluid osmolality can cause cell swelling or shrinking, which can lead to cell death. The kidney plays a key role in the close regulation of extracellular fluid osmolality via two primary mechanisms: the osmoreceptor-antidiuretic hormone (ADH, or vasopressin) system; and the thirst mechanism.

Antidiuretic hormone

The secretion of **antidiuretic hormone** (ADH, also known as vasopressin, Chapter 45) from the posterior pituitary is influenced by the osmolality of body fluids (osmotic), and the volume and pressure of the vascular system (Figure 39.1). **Osmotic control** of ADH secretion is highly sensitive, with a change of 1% being sufficient to alter ADH release. Shrinkage of **osmoreceptor cells** located in the anterior hypothalamus (close to supraoptic nuclei) in response to an increase in extracellular fluid osmolality (due to water deficit, for example) leads to nerve signals being sent to hypothalamic ADH-producing neuroendocrine cells (Chapter 45), culminating in the release of ADH from axon termini in the posterior pituitary. At the kidney, ADH interact with V_2 receptors on principal (P) cells, promoting the translocation of **aquaporin-2 water channels** to the apical membrane, which results in increased water reabsorption and excretion of a small volume of concentrated urine (Figure 39.2). The water conserved dilutes extracellular solutes, thereby correcting the initial hyperosmotic extracellular fluid. The opposite sequence of events occurs with hypo-osmotic extracellular fluid (such as with excess water ingestion).

Haemodynamic control of ADH release involves receptors in low pressure (left atrium and large pulmonary vessels) and high pressure (aortic arch and carotid sinus) regions of the circulation, which detect changes in blood volume and pressure, with afferent signals leading to appropriate control of ADH release to restore blood volume/pressure to normal (Figure 39.1). This is a much less sensitive mechanism than that of osmotic control; change of 5–10% reduction in blood volume is required for plasma ADH levels to change appreciably.

Fluid intake is regulated by the **thirst response**, the conscious desire to drink water. Neural centres involved in regulating water intake (thirst centre) located in the hypothalamus (in regions similar to those in control of ADH release) respond to a number of stimuli (Figure 39.1). It seems that the ADH and thirst systems work in concert to maintain water balance (Figure a), although with regard to body fluid osmolality, ADH secretion is secreted at a lower threshold than that for thirst. Thus, an increase in plasma osmolality evokes thirst with water ingestion and secretion of ADH with resultant conservation of water, while a fall in plasma osmolality leads to suppressed thirst and a lack of ADH release with enhanced renal water excretion.

Other hormones in renal excretion of salt and water

The **renin-angiotensin-aldosterone system** (Chapter 32) plays an important role in regulating sodium and water reabsorption. **Renin** is secreted by granular cells (juxtaglomerular apparatus, Chapter 37) in response to activation of sympathetic nervous system (via β_2-adrenoceptors), reduced renal perfusion pressure (afferent arteriole baroreceptors), or a fall in tubular fluid [NaCl] sensed by tubular macula densa cells – usually due to a decrease in glomerular filtration rate resulting in slower filtrate movement through the proximal tubule and thus more time for reabsorption, leading to a lower [NaCl] in the tubular fluid at the macula densa; tubuloglomerular feedback (Chapter 37). **Angiotensin II** stimulates release of aldosterone, arteriolar vasoconstriction (efferent more than afferent), ADH secretion and thirst, and enhances renal NaCl reabsorption. **Aldosterone** is secreted by

zona glomerulosa cells of the adrenal cortex (Chapter 48); it promotes Na^+ (and hence water) reabsorption, with K^+ elimination, by upregulation of the expression of Na^+/Cl^- co-transporter (early DCT), the epithelial Na^+ channel and basolateral Na^+/K^+-ATPase pump in principal (P) cells of the late DCT and collecting duct. Overall, activation of the renin-angiotensin-aldosterone system results in increased total peripheral resistance, thus increasing blood pressure and raising GFR, together with Na^+ and water reabsorption.

A number of natriuretic hormones contribute to volume regulation. **Atrial natriuretic peptide** (ANP) is released from cardiac atrial muscle fibres in response to atrial stretching as a result of increased blood volume. The combined actions of ANP lead to increased excretion of NaCl and water, which helps to compensate for the excess blood volume (Figure 39.3).

Disorders

- **Diabetes insipidus (DI)**: arises from lack of ADH production (central or pituitary DI), or ADH insensitivity in the kidney (nephrogenic DI). Excessive volume of dilute urine is produced (polyuria), due to lack of antidiuresis activity of ADH.
- **Syndrome of inappropriate antidiuretic hormone secretion (SIADH)**: may arise from many causes (central nervous system pathology, malignancy, drugs). Reduced water excretion (small volume of highly concentrated urine) with hyponatraemia (<135 mmol/L, due to dilution effect of water retention).
- **Hyperaldosteronism**: (primary, such as aldosterone-secreting adrenal adenoma [**Conn's syndrome**]; secondary, such as renin-producing tumour or reduced blood supply as in renal artery stenosis): presents with hypertension (water retention), hypernatraemia and hypokalaemia.
- **Hypoaldosteronism** (low aldosterone levels, with primary adrenal insufficiency as in Addison's disease or common form of congenital adrenal hyperplasia [Chapter 48]): leads to hyponatraemia and hyperkalaemia; patients may experience postural hypotension and muscle weakness.

Diuretics

- **Osmotic diuretics** (such a mannitol): freely filtered, increasing the osmolality of the tubular fluid, thus reducing water reabsorption. Used in management of cerebral oedema.
- **Loop diuretics** (such as furosemide): block the $Na^+/K^+/2Cl^-$ symporter of the thick ascending limb of loop of Henle, thus reducing the hyperosmolality of the renal medullary interstitium required for urine concentration. Also, reduction of NaCl entry into macula densa, with resultant increase in renin release from granular cells. Used in management of chronic heart failure (Chapter 35) and in renal failure (to improve diuresis).
- **Thiazide-like diuretics** (such as chlortalidone): inhibit Na^+/Cl^- co-transporter in early DCT. Ineffective in moderate renal impairment as renal secretion by the PCT weak acid transporter is required prior to acting on DCT.
- **Potassium-sparing diuretics** include aldosterone receptor antagonist spironolactone and sodium channel blockers such as amiloride. Weak diuretics may be used to offset hypokalaemia often seen with thiazide-like and loop diuretics.

Michael D Randall

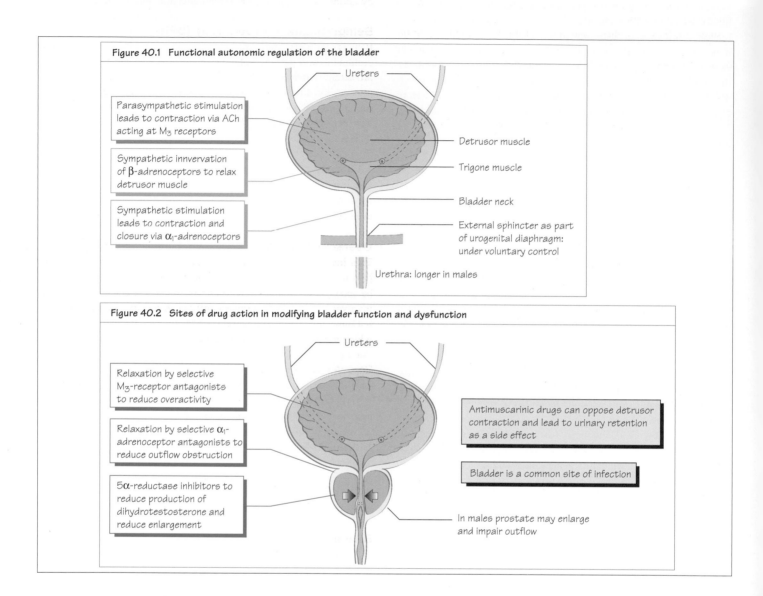

Figure 40.1 Functional autonomic regulation of the bladder

Ureters

Parasympathetic stimulation leads to contraction via ACh acting at M_3 receptors

Sympathetic innervation of β-adrenoceptors to relax detrusor muscle

Sympathetic stimulation leads to contraction and closure via α_1-adrenoceptors

Detrusor muscle

Trigone muscle

Bladder neck

External sphincter as part of urogenital diaphragm: under voluntary control

Urethra: longer in males

Figure 40.2 Sites of drug action in modifying bladder function and dysfunction

Ureters

Relaxation by selective M_3-receptor antagonists to reduce overactivity

Relaxation by selective α_1-adrenoceptor antagonists to reduce outflow obstruction

5α-reductase inhibitors to reduce production of dihydrotestosterone and reduce enlargement

Antimuscarinic drugs can oppose detrusor contraction and lead to urinary retention as a side effect

Bladder is a common site of infection

In males prostate may enlarge and impair outflow

The urinary bladder is a muscular organ in the pelvis that stores normally sterile urine prior to **micturition**. In the healthy adult, the volume of the bladder is typically 300–500 mL. The bladder receives urine (at approximately 1 mL/min) from the kidneys via two muscular **ureters** (Chapter 36) that enter the bladder low down near the neck. The ureters drain into the bladder via **vesico-ureteric junction**, which ensures that flow is unidirectional and that there is no reflux of urine from the bladder to the kidneys, which could lead to infection. The bladder then stores urine prior to its elimination through the external sphincter and then via the **urethra** (Chapter 36).

The bladder is made up of the following.

• **Detrusor muscle**: this is smooth muscle in the body of the bladder. When relaxed, it enables the bladder to hold urine and when it contracts there is an increase in internal pressure and so urine is voided.

• **Trigone muscle**: this is triangular smooth muscle at the base of the bladder at the urethral opening.

• **Urothelium**: the inner transitional epithelial layer of the bladder, which may release mediators (such as ATP) to regulate tone.

Autonomic control (Figure 40.1)

The key innervation of the detrusor muscle is **parasympathetic** via acetylcholine acting at muscarinic M_3 receptors, which leads to contraction and micturition. Sympathetic innervation results in noradrenaline acting at β_2- and β_3-adrenoceptors to relax the detrusor muscle, resulting in the bladder relaxing and storing urine. Noradrenaline also acts at α_1-adrenoceptors to contract the neck of the bladder and urethra to facilitate the storage of urine.

Somatic control

The external sphincter is made up of skeletal muscle associated with the **urogenital diaphragm** and is regulated via the somatic nervous system such that acetylcholine acts at nicotinic receptors to cause contraction of the urethra.

Micturition

Once the internal pressure reaches a certain level this stretches sensory fibres and initiates the **micturition reflex**, which is autonomic but regulated by the brain, which either facilitates or inhibits the reflex. The micturition reflex leads to bladder emptying via contraction of the detrusor muscle, leading to an increase in pressure and relaxation of the external sphincter.

Disorders of bladder function
Cystitis
Irritation of the bladder by chemicals or due to infection leads to the common symptoms of discomfort and an urge to pass urine. **Urinary**

tract infections (**UTI**) are relatively common, especially in females, who have a shorter urethra compared with males. UTIs may present with increased frequency of urination, often with a burning sensation. *Escherichia coli* is the commonest cause of UTIs and readily managed by antibiotic therapy (trimethoprim as a first choice agent).

Benign prostatic hypertrophy (BPH)
BPH is characterised by enlargement of the prostate gland around the urethra in males and is common over the age of 50 years. The enlarged prostate impairs urinary outflow and so leads to a frequent desire to pass urine with hesitancy, poor outflow and incomplete emptying. The stagnation of urine may also predispose towards infections. The obstruction of urinary outflow also poses a risk of renal failure.

Selective α_1-**adrenoceptor antagonists** (e.g. tamsulosin) are used to relax smooth muscle in the prostate and the neck of the bladder to aid urine flow. Prostatic enlargement is also testosterone-dependent and **inhibitors of 5α-reductase** (e.g. finasteride), the enzyme that converts testosterone to the more potent dihydrotestosterone, are also used (Figure 40.2).

Overactive bladder
This involves increased bladder contractility with increased urge to pass urine, leading to increased frequency, and there may or may not be incontinence or leakage. Common pharmacological management involves use of **selective muscarinic receptor antagonists** (e.g. oxybutynin) to inhibit involuntary contractions of the detrusor muscle which are responsible for the increased activity.

Stress incontinence
This is common in women and is caused by either sphincter weakness or urethral hypermobility. This is common following pregnancy and associated with weakness of the pelvic floor.

Stones
The urinary tract is susceptible to the formation of stones rich in calcium salts such as calcium oxalate. These can lead to obstruction and severe pain in the ureters. In the bladder, stone formation can become the focus of infection.

Side effects of drugs
Drugs that have antimuscarinic side effects (such as tricyclic antidepressants) are associated with urinary retention because they impair parasympathetically mediated voiding of the bladder.

Deborah Merrick

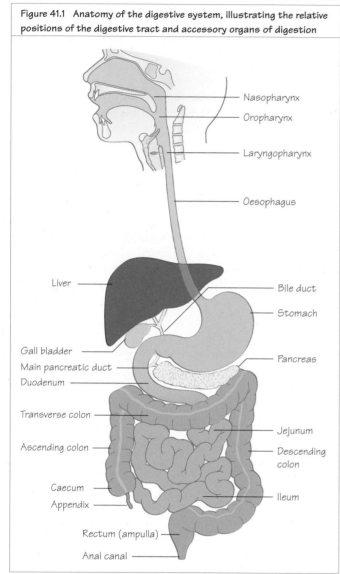

Figure 41.1 Anatomy of the digestive system, illustrating the relative positions of the digestive tract and accessory organs of digestion

Nasopharynx
Oropharynx
Laryngopharynx
Oesophagus
Liver
Bile duct
Stomach
Gall bladder
Main pancreatic duct
Pancreas
Duodenum
Transverse colon
Ascending colon
Jejunum
Descending colon
Caecum
Appendix
Ileum
Rectum (ampulla)
Anal canal

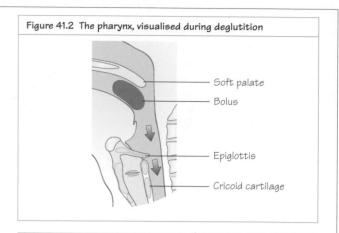

Figure 41.2 The pharynx, visualised during deglutition

Soft palate
Bolus
Epiglottis
Cricoid cartilage

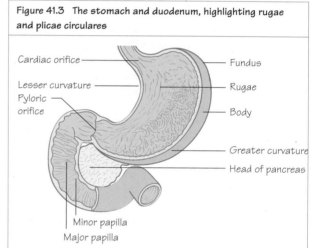

Figure 41.3 The stomach and duodenum, highlighting rugae and plicae circulares

Cardiac orifice
Fundus
Lesser curvature
Rugae
Pyloric orifice
Body
Greater curvature
Head of pancreas
Minor papilla
Major papilla

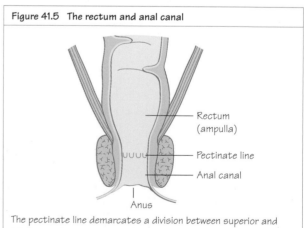

Figure 41.5 The rectum and anal canal

Rectum (ampulla)
Pectinate line
Anal canal
Anus

The pectinate line demarcates a division between superior and inferior anal canal. Superiorly – vasculature is from inferior mesenteric arteries/veins (portal) and lymphatic drainage is via internal iliac lymph nodes. Inferiorly – vessels are from internal iliac arteries/veins (caval) and lymph drains to superficial inguinal lymph nodes

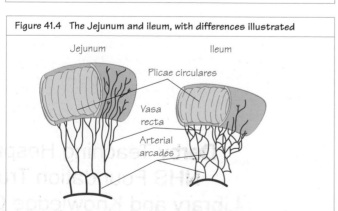

Figure 41.4 The Jejunum and ileum, with differences illustrated

Jejunum
Ileum
Plicae circulares
Vasa recta
Arterial arcades

The digestive system extends from the lips to the anus and consists of a series of organs and glands. The digestive tract is a tube-like passageway that conducts the food we eat, allowing absorption of vital nutrients along most of its length. Accessory organs (e.g. pancreas) secrete substances that aid digestion.

Digestive tract

Mucosa lines the hollow organs of the digestive tract. In the mouth, stomach and small intestines the mucosa contains glands that produce secretions to help digest food. Contraction of the smooth muscle within the walls of the digestive tract helps move food along its length.

Oral cavity: consists of the oral vestibule and the oral cavity proper. Food entering the oral cavity is chewed (mastication) and mixed with saliva to form a ball (bolus) of food. The tongue pushes the bolus upwards and backwards against the hard palate to enter the oropharynx (Figures 41.1 and 41.2).

Pharynx: a funnel-shaped muscular structure situated posterior to the nasal cavity (nasopharynx), oral cavity (oropharynx) and larynx (laryngopharynx). During the process of swallowing (deglutition), the nasopharynx becomes shut off from the oropharynx by elevation of the soft palate. The larynx and laryngopharynx are pulled upwards, while the epiglottis prevents food from entering the airways (Figure 41.2). Successive waves of contraction of the pharyngeal constrictor muscles move the bolus into the oesophagus.

Oesophagus: a muscular tube connecting the pharynx superiorly to the stomach inferiorly (~25 cm in length). It passes from the level of cricoid cartilage (opposite C6 vertebrae), running posterior to the trachea. It descends through the thorax, entering the abdomen by piercing the diaphragm at vertebral level T10. During its descent the oesophagus is compressed by three structures: the arch of aorta, left main bronchus and diaphragm.

Stomach: dilated portion of the digestive tract located in the upper abdomen. The stomach has two orifices (cardiac and pyloric), two curvatures (greater and lesser), a fundus, body, pyloric antrum and pylorus. The inner mucosal lining is thrown into multiple longitudinal folds (rugae) which become obliterated when the stomach becomes distended (Figure 41.3).

Small intestines: the major site of absorption within the digestive tract. Its longitudinal muscle forms a continuous layer around the gut. Its outer wall is smooth, whereas the internal mucous membrane is thrown into multiple folds called plicae circulares.
• *Duodenum*: ~25 cm in length, beginning at the pyloric sphincter and is C-shaped, curving around the head of the pancreas. Secretions from the accessory organs of digestion enter the duodenum at the major and minor papilla (Figure 41.3).
• *Jejunum and ileum*: ~6 m in length, the jejunum commences at the duodenojejunal flexure and the ileum terminates by joining the large intestines at the ileocaecal junction. There is no distinct dividing feature separating the jejunum and ileum, but some subtle differences are noted. For example, the jejunum has a wider diameter, thicker walls and contains increased number of plicae circulares (Figure 41.4).

Large intestines: function to absorb water and to store undigested food before excretion from the body as faeces (defecation). The longitudinal muscle of the large intestines is arranged in three bands called the teniae coli, and its walls, unlike the small intestines, are sacculated.
• *Caecum and appendix*: the caecum is a blind-ended pouch that joins the ileum and ascending colon. Attached to its posteromedial surface is the appendix.
• *Ascending colon*: extends from the caecum to the right lobe of the liver (hepatic flexure or right colic flexure), where it turns and becomes continuous with the transverse colon.
• *Transverse colon*: passes to the left colic flexure (splenic flexure), then turns and continues at the descending colon.
• *Descending colon*: descends from the left colic flexure to the pelvic brim where it becomes continuous with the sigmoid colon.
• *Sigmoid colon*: named according to its S-shaped appearance; continuous with the rectum at vertebral level S3.

Rectum and anal canal: the rectum passes inferiorly, following the curvature of the sacrum and coccyx. It dilates (rectal ampulla) before piercing the pelvic floor to become continuous with the anal canal. The short anal canal (~4 cm) passes posteroinferiorly to open at the anus. Halfway along its length is the pectinate line, which demarcates a distinct change in innervation and vascular supply of the anal canal (Figure 41.5). The lateral walls of the canal are kept in apposition by levator ani and the anal sphincters muscles until defecation.

Vasculature of the digestive tract

Arterial supply is predominantly from branches of the external carotid arteries (oral cavity and pharynx), inferior thyroid arteries and descending thoracic aorta (oesophagus), abdominal aorta (inferior oesophagus through to superior half of the anal canal) and internal iliac arteries (inferior anal canal). Veins draining the digestive tract correspond to the arteries they accompany. Likewise, deep lymphatic vessels also accompany the major blood vessels, traversing one or more lymph nodes before draining predominantly into the thoracic duct or right lymphatic duct.

Innervation of the digestive tract

This is by the autonomic nervous system (including enteric nervous system) as well as visceral afferents. In general, sympathetic innervation reduces blood flow (vasoconstrictor) and decreases secretions and motility (peristalsis) of the digestive tract. Parasympathetic stimulation increases motility and secretion. The enteric system, found within the tract walls, is principally composed of myenteric (Auerbach's) and submucosal (Meissner's) plexuses controlling movement and secretion.

Accessory organs of digestion

Pancreas: exocrine function produces pancreatic enzymatic juices to aid digestion. The pancreatic secretions pass into the main and accessory pancreatic ducts to enter the duodenum via the major and minor papilla respectively.

Liver and gall bladder: the liver produces bile, which is stored and concentrated in the gall bladder. Bile leaves the gall bladder via the cystic duct and then the bile duct to enter the duodenum at the major papilla (Figures 41.1 and 41.3).

42 Upper gastrointestinal physiology

Michael D Randall

Figure 42.1 The control of saliva production

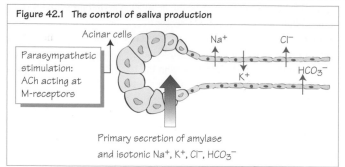

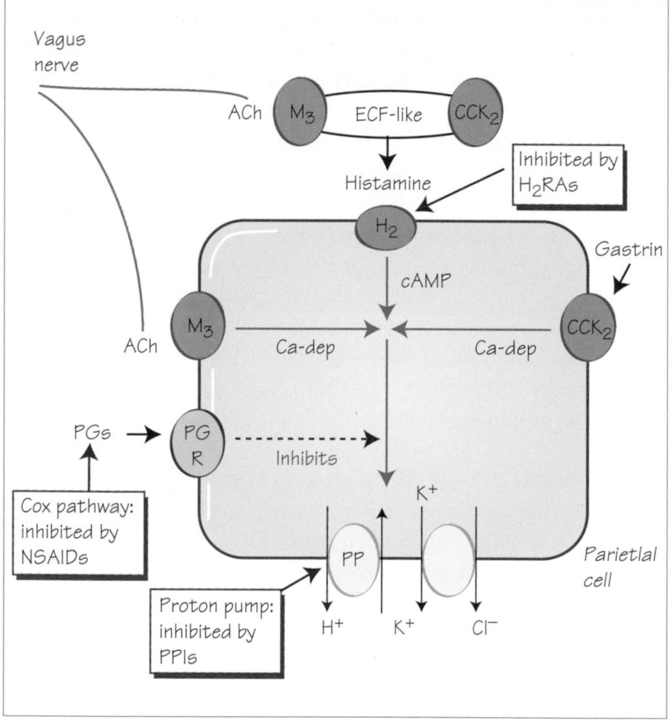

Acinar cells

Parasympathetic stimulation: ACh acting at M-receptors

Na$^+$ Cl$^-$ K$^+$ HCO$_3^-$

Primary secretion of amylase and isotonic Na$^+$, K$^+$, Cl$^-$, HCO$_3^-$

Figure 42.4 The regulation of acid release from a parietal cell

Vagus nerve

ACh M$_3$ ECF-like CCK$_2$

Inhibited by H$_2$RAs

Histamine

H$_2$

cAMP

Gastrin

M$_3$ Ca-dep Ca-dep CCK$_2$

ACh

PGs → PG R Inhibits

Cox pathway: inhibited by NSAIDs

K$^+$

PP

Parietlal cell

Proton pump: inhibited by PPIs

H$^+$ K$^+$ Cl$^-$

Figure 42.2 Cephalic and gastric phases of gastric acid secretion

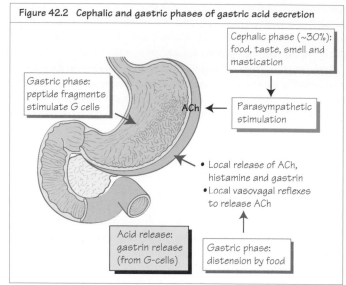

Cephalic phase (~30%): food, taste, smell and mastication

Gastric phase: peptide fragments stimulate G cells

ACh

Parasympathetic stimulation

- Local release of ACh, histamine and gastrin
- Local vasovagal reflexes to release ACh

Acid release: gastrin release (from G-cells)

Gastric phase: distension by food

Figure 42.3 Intestinal phase of gastric acid secretion

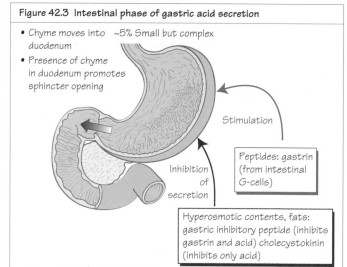

- Chyme moves into duodenum
- Presence of chyme in duodenum promotes sphincter opening

~5% Small but complex

Stimulation

Inhibition of secretion

Peptides: gastrin (from intestinal G-cells)

Hyperosmotic contents, fats: gastric inhibitory peptide (inhibits gastrin and acid) cholecystokinin (inhibits only acid)

Salivation

The process of digestion starts in the mouth with mastication, in which the physical breakdown of food is combined with saliva. Salivation occurs as saliva is produced by the parotid, submandibular and sublingual glands, and saliva lubricates the mouth, aids dental hygiene, adds fluid to the food and initiates the breakdown of starches by addition of amylase. **Acinar cells** secrete amylase and electrolytes with similar tonicity to plasma, and striated and excitatory ducts modify secretions. A healthy human produces about 1–1.5 L of saliva per day.

Control of salivation (Figure 42.1)

This process is under autonomic control with parasympathetic nerves releasing acetylcholine (ACh) to act at muscarinic receptors to increase the production of saliva and increase blood flow to promote fluid movement. Parasympathetic nerves also release vasoactive intestinal polypeptide (VIP), which causes vasodilatation to enhance saliva secretion. Parasympathetic control makes the saliva watery (hypotonic relative to plasma), while sympathetic control increases its viscosity. Drugs with antimuscarinic side effects may block the production of saliva as a side effect, leading to a dry mouth.

Gastric physiology

The food is then swallowed, which is largely a reflex action (controlled via the swallowing centre in the medulla and lower pons), and the bolus of food then passes down the oesophagus via peristalsis, through the lower oesophageal sphincter and into the stomach. Food is retained in the stomach for several hours, during which time the gastric mucosa releases acid (pH of the gastric contents is pH1–1.5) and proteolytic enzymes to initiate the breakdown of proteins. **Chief cells** of gastric mucosa release **pepsinogens** and the acid environment activates these to form **pepsins**. This is also an autocatalytic process as the newly formed pepsin activates further pepsinogens, which are endopeptidases and so act within peptide chain. The acidic environment is also the optimum pH for pepsin activity.

Gastric acid secretion (Figures 42.2, 42.3 and 42.4)

The production of gastric acid is a tightly regulated process. Parietal cells of the gastric mucosa contain H^+/K^+ ATPases (**proton pumps**) on their lumenal surfaces and these antiport H^+ out of the cell in exchange for K^+. Gastric acid secretion is under **cephalic control** (central control stimulated by the presence of food in the mouth and chewing), which involves direct parasympathetic vagal stimulation and indirect parasympathetic control via the release of histamine from enterochromaffin (ECF)-like cells. For direct control, ACh acts at muscarinic M_3 receptors, which couple via increasing intracellular calcium to activate the proton pump. **Histamine** released from the ECF-like cells acts on histamine H_2 receptors to increase cAMP, which also activates the proton pump via phosphorylation. The final stimulatory pathway is via the hormone gastrin. Gastrin is released by G-cells of the antrum and leads to the **gastric phase**. The release of gastrin is stimulated by the presence of the food in the stomach, passes via the bloodstream to act on the stomach and the **gastrin** acts at cholesytokinin CCK_2 receptors to stimulate histamine release from the ECF-like cells and also directly on parietal CCK_2 receptors to cause calcium-dependent proton pump activation. The final phase of control is the **intestinal phase**, in which protein digestion products stimulate the release of gastrin from G-cells.

Cytoprotection

The acidic and proteolytic secretions of the gastric mucosa are likely to cause erosion and so the local production of prostaglandins (PGE_2 and PGI_2) stimulates bicarbonate and mucus secretion by superficial epithelial cells. These prostaglandins also act on the parietal cells to inhibit the proton pump.

Roles of the stomach

Food is retained in the stomach for a number of hours and so the stomach acts as a storage site. Fatty foods tend to float to the top and solid foods are retained for longer periods of time. During this time the acidic environment sterilises the contents and activated pepsin digests protein, to give the end product chyme. Some absorption of small molecules occurs from the stomach.

Parietal cells also release an **intrinsic factor** (**IF**), a glycoprotein that binds to vitamin B_{12}, and this complex enables this vitamin to be absorbed in the small intestines. A lack of IF due to surgical loss of the stomach or autoimmune disease is associated with vitamin B_{12} deficiency and leads to megaloblastic anaemia (Chapter 33).

Dyspepsia

This is a common complaint that affects the upper gastrointestinal tract and encompasses:

- **gastro-oesophageal reflux disease**: acidic gastric contents reflux up and damage the oesophagus;
- **gastritis**: inflammation of the stomach;
- **peptic ulceration**: damage and erosion of the stomach or duodenum such that an ulcer forms; this may lead to bleeding.

Peptic ulceration

The principal cause of peptic ulceration is due to infection with *Helicobacter pylori*, which can lead inflammation and ulceration. About 70% of gastric ulcers and 90% of duodenal ulcers are associated with *H. pylori* infection. The second most important cause of ulceration is due to non-steroidal anti-inflammatory drugs (NSAIDs) which inhibit the production of cytoprotective prostanoids and so promote acid secretion and reduce gastric protection.

Pharmacology of dyspepsia

Symptoms of dyspepsia may be relieved by antacids such as magnesium hydroxide, which neutralise the acid. Suppression of acid release is a far more effective approach and involves either the use of **histamine H_2 receptor antagonists (H₂RAs)** (e.g. ranitidine), which block histamine-induced acid secretion, or **proton pump inhibitors (PPIs)** (e.g. omeprazole), which irreversibly block the proton pump (and therefore the final common pathway of acid secretion).

The most appropriate treatment for *H. pylori*-dependent ulceration is the use of 'triple therapy', with two antibiotics (from clarithromycin, amoxicillin and metronidazole) to eradicate the infection, and a PPI.

Michael D Randall

Figure 43.1 A schematic summary of the metabolism of disaccharides on the brush border and the facilitated transport of monosaccharides into the enterocytes and passing through the basolateral layer for absorption to the capillary network

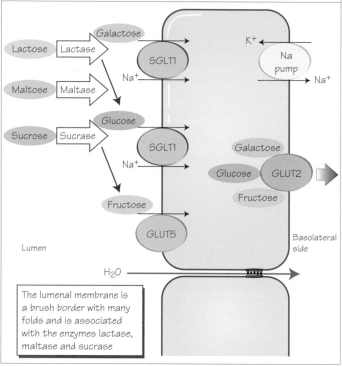

The lumenal membrane is a brush border with many folds and is associated with the enzymes lactase, maltase and sucrase

Figure 43.2 A schematic summary of the degradation of proteins and the absorption of small peptide and amino acids

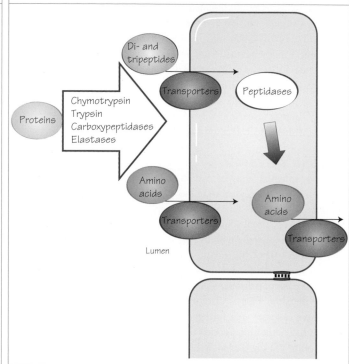

Figure 43.3 A schematic summary of the metabolism of lipids and their reconstitution in the enterocytes

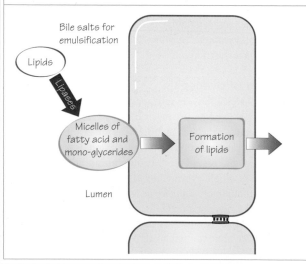

Figure 43.4 A schematic summary of the control of motility in the gastrointestinal tract

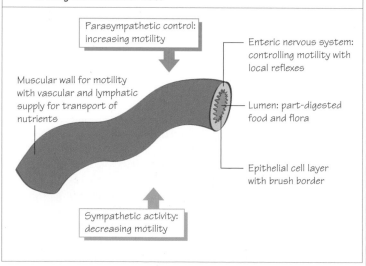

The principal role of the lower gastrointestinal tract is to provide a large volume for the processes of digestion and a large surface area for the absorption of nutrients.

Duodenum

As **chyme** passes from the stomach into the duodenum, it is acted on by pancreatic secretions that contain **lipases** to digest lipids, **pancre-**

atic amylases to break down carbohydrates, **nucleases** to break down nucleic acids and precursors to **proteolytic enzymes** (chymotrypsinogen, trypsinogen, procarboxypeptidases A and B and proelastases), which are activated by trypsin (to chymotrypsin, trypsin, carboxypeptidases A and B and elastases respectively) to break down a variety of proteins. This process of activation is to prevent autodigestion.

The **pancreatic secretions** are also rich in bicarbonate to neutralise the stomach acid and inhibit the activity of pepsins, and the pH in the small intestines is ~ 5.3. The pancreatic enzymes are made by the acinar cells of the exocrine pancreas feeding into epithelium-lined ducts. The secretion of enzymes is stimulated via **cholecystokinin** (CCK) in response to the presence of fats and protein in the duodenum. The epithelial cells in the secretory ducts release bicarbonate and this is promoted by the hormone **secretin**, released by the duodenal cells in response to acid entering the duodenum.

Hepatic products are also released from the gall bladder at this site, and they contain bile salts, which emulsify fat. The bile salts are efficiently recycled (90–95% are reabsorbed in the terminal ileum and this is referred to as **enterohepatic cycling** (Chapter 44)).

Jejunum and ileum
The duodenum leads into the jejunum and ileum, which provide a muscular wall for peristalsis and large surface area for absorption of nutrients. Structurally the lumenal side is made up of villi and the epithelial cells have a brush border of microvilli to increase the surface area.

Absorption of monosaccharides (Figure 43.1)
This occurs predominantly in the duodenum and jejunum. Carbohydrates are broken down to monosaccharides, and the brush borders contain **disaccharidases** to break down disaccharides (maltase breaks down maltose to glucose; sucrose breaks down sucrose to glucose and fructose; and lactase breaks down lactose to galactose and glucose). The monosaccharides are then **co-transported** into the epithelial cells (**enterocytes**) of the villi via a sodium co-transporter (e.g. **SGLT1**: the sodium-glucose transporter protein-1, which transports either glucose or galactose) driven by the concentration gradient for sodium created by the basolateral sodium pump. The monosaccharides then pass out of the basolateral membrane via the **GLUT2** transporter into the dense capillary network to complete absorption into the body.

Absorption of peptides and amino acids (Figure 43.2)
Di- and tri-peptides from protein degradation, including those formed by the brush border peptidases, are transported efficiently across the cell membranes. This is driven via the electrochemical difference for protons across the membrane, generated via Na^+:H^+ exchange. Inside the cell, peptides are then further broken down by peptidases to amino acids, which are then absorbed systemically.

Amino acids are transported, predominantly in the ileum, by specific amino acid transporters.

Absorption of lipids (Figure 43.3)
Emulsified fat is broken down by lipases to liberate free fatty acids and monoglycerides, which form micelles with hydrophobic cores and hydrophilic shells. These micelles promote the delivery of lipids to the microvilli membranes and the hydrophobic core can then pass into the epithelial cells. Once inside the cells, fats are formed and these are transported by the lymphatic system to enter the blood at the thoracic duct.

Absorption of electrolytes
The passage of Na^+ is driven by the sodium pump in the basolateral membrane, which keeps intracellular Na^+ low and generates a diffusion gradient from the lumen so that Na^+ enters via both transporters and channels.

Potassium is taken up in the small intestines but its movement in the colon depends on it electrochemical gradient from the lumen to the epithelial layer. Hence large volumes associated diarrhoea may promote secretion of potassium, leading to hypokalaemia.

Calcium balance is regulated via activated vitamin D (calcitriol), which increases the amount of a calcium-binding protein in the brush border. This occurs largely in the duodenum and jejunum.

Absorption of water
In health, some 99% of ingested (~2 L/day) and secreted (~7 L/day) water is reabsorbed in the gastrointestinal tract and this occurs predominantly in the small intestines. Epithelial cells are connected by tight junctions. These are more permeable to water in the duodenum and this decreases down the lower gastrointestinal tract. Therefore, in the upper areas, substantial amounts of water are reabsorbed by the paracellular route, and this is driven by osmotic gradients generated via electrolyte absorption, largely driven by the Na^+ pump.

Large intestines
The colon, which leads to the rectum and anus, forms the final section of the lower intestinal tract. The role of the colon is the final absorption of water and electrolytes to form more solid faeces.

Motility (Figure 43.4)
The lower gastrointestinal tract is made up of muscular tubes that are responsible for propelling the contents through the tract via peristalsis. This is a highly regulated process, as too rapid a transit limits the time for absorption of water and may lead to diarrhoea, while too slow a transit can lead to constipation. The gastrointestinal tract is under autonomic control, where, broadly speaking, parasympathetic stimulation enhances motility and sympathetic activation inhibits motility. The **enteric nervous system** (made up of submucosal and myenteric plexuses) is a well-developed arrangement of local neurones that coordinate local motor and secretory activity. The enteric nervous system can work in the absence of autonomic control and provides local reflex control in response to stimuli via sensory afferents from chemo and mechanoreceptors.

Pathophysiology
The lower gastrointestinal tract is affected by a number of pathologies. Viral and bacterial infections are common occurrences and can lead to secretory diarrhoea.

The primary treatment of diarrhoea is **oral rehydration therapy**, in which a solution of glucose and electrolytes is given. The uptake of glucose is coupled to Na^+ and this leads to the update of Na^+, which is followed osmotically by water, leading to rehydration.

In other conditions, motility may be affected, and reduced smooth muscle activity leads to constipation. Reduced smooth muscle activity can be a side effect of opioid drugs, which act at opioid receptors to cause presynaptic inhibition of parasympathetic activity (Chapter 20), and so constipation is a common side effect of opioids.

Inflammatory bowel diseases (ulcerative colitis and Crohn's disease) are autoimmune diseases that result in severe inflammation within the gastrointestinal system.

44 The liver

Michael D Randall

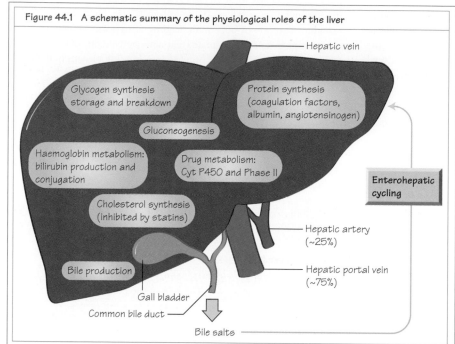

Figure 44.1 A schematic summary of the physiological roles of the liver

- Hepatic vein
- Glycogen synthesis storage and breakdown
- Protein synthesis (coagulation factors, albumin, angiotensinogen)
- Gluconeogenesis
- Haemoglobin metabolism: bilirubin production and conjugation
- Drug metabolism: Cyt P450 and Phase II
- Cholesterol synthesis (inhibited by statins)
- Enterohepatic cycling
- Hepatic artery (~25%)
- Hepatic portal vein (~75%)
- Bile production
- Gall bladder
- Common bile duct
- Bile salts

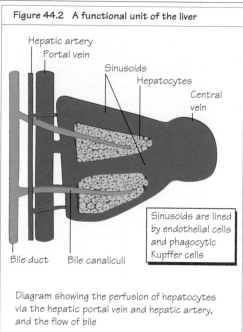

Figure 44.2 A functional unit of the liver

- Hepatic artery
- Portal vein
- Sinusoids
- Hepatocytes
- Central vein
- Bile duct
- Bile canaliculi

Sinusoids are lined by endothelial cells and phagocytic Kupffer cells

Diagram showing the perfusion of hepatocytes via the hepatic portal vein and hepatic artery, and the flow of bile

Table 44.1 Key liver function tests and their significance.
Typical normal ranges are given but these can vary between different assays and laboratories

Marker	Typical normal ranges	Clinical significance
Bilirubin	3–17 µmol/L	• Increased if there is increased red blood cell breakdown (haemolysis), intrahepatic dysfunction or cholestasis • Accumulation of bilirubin in the blood leads to jaundice (yellow colouration of the skin and sclera)
Aminotransferases, e.g. Alanine aminotransferase (ALT)	ALT: 5–45 iu/L	• These may leak out of damaged hepatocytes • Elevated levels are consistent with ongoing hepatocellular damage
Alkaline phosphatase (ALP)	40–120 iu/L	• Produced by a number of tissues including the liver, placenta and bone • ALP is excreted by the bile ducts which is impaired in cholestasis, leading to increased plasma levels
Gamma glutamyl transpeptidase (γGT)	<70 iu/L (males) <40 iu/L (females)	• Elevated levels may indicate alcohol abuse or induction of drug metabolism • Levels are also raised in cholestasis
Albumin	35–50 g/L	• Levels decrease as the synthetic activity of the liver is reduced in liver disease • Indicates impaired synthetic activity of liver
International normalised ratio	1–1.2	• Coagulation of the blood takes longer when the synthesis of coagulation factors is impaired in liver disease • Indicates impaired synthetic activity of liver

The liver is the central biochemical (and largest) organ, playing many roles to ensure homeostasis (Figure 44.1). In the adult, the liver weighs approximately 1.5 kg and receives approximately 25% of cardiac output. Seventy five per cent of liver blood flow is derived from the **hepatic portal vein**, which drains the gastrointestinal tract and so delivers nutrients to the liver, and toxins, which may be metabolised before entering the systemic circulation. The remaining blood flow is from the hepatic artery.

The liver is made up of thousands of functional units called lobules, which feed into a central vein. The hepatocytes are bathed in sinusoids, which receive blood from the hepatic portal vein and the hepatic arteries. The sinusoids are surrounded by an endothelium and also contain **phagocytic Kupffer cells**. The hepatocytes then form and feed into bile canaliculi, leading to bile ductules and then bile ducts, taking the bile to the gall bladder for storage (Figure 44.2).

Metabolic roles

The liver is a key store of energy in the form of glycogen and is active in both glycogen synthesis from glucose, and glyogenolysis to liberate glucose. The synthesis of glycogen is promoted by insulin, following the cellular uptake of glucose from the blood derived from the gastrointestinal tract. The liver also plays a role in **gluconeogenesis**, in which glucose is synthesised from non-carbohydrates such as certain amino acids, glycerol (from lipids), pyruvate and lactate (Chapter 12).

Synthesis of proteins

Many **plasma-borne proteins** are synthesised in the liver. These include coagulation factors (all except factor VIII), transport albumins (present in the plasma and contribute towards oncotic pressure), angiotensinogen (the precursor to the renin-angiotensin-aldosterone system [RAAS] pathway) and thrombopoietin (a peptide that regulates platelet production).

Lipid metabolism

Some 75% of cholesterol in the body is made endogenously by the liver and the remainder is from the diet. **Cholesterol** is synthesised from acetyl-CoA, which forms 3-hydroxy-3-methyl-glutaryl-CoA that is then acted on by enzyme **HMG CoA reductase** to form mevalonate and, ultimately, 27-carbon atom cholesterol. HMG CoA reductase is the first committed step in the pathway and is inhibited by cholesterol-lowering drugs (statins; Chapter 35).

The liver synthesises triglycerides from esterification of fatty acid acyl-Co-As with glycerol-3-phosphate.

Lipids are transported around the body by lipoproteins, and hepatocytes express low-density lipoprotein (LDL) receptors for the uptake of cholesterol derived from cellular degradation around the body. The liver also produces very-low-density lipoprotein (VLDL) for the transport of cholesterol and triglycerides and LDL cholesterol.

Haemoglobin and bilirubin

Red blood cells are broken down by the reticuloendothelial system of the liver, spleen and bone marrow. The iron is efficiently recycled and the porphyrin moiety of haem derived from haemoglobin is converted in the spleen and hepatocytes to bilirubin. Bilirubin is highly water insoluble and is conjugated in the liver to form water-soluble conjugates.

Bile

The liver produces 400–800 mL of bile per day and is made up of water, electrolytes, bile salts (derived from cholesterol), conjugated bilirubin, cholesterol, lecithin and some amino acids. It is stored in the gall bladder and excreted down the bile duct into the duodenum. The release of bile is principally stimulated by cholecystokinin as a consequence of food entering the duodenum. Bile is a detergent used to emulsify fats prior to digestion by lipases. Accordingly, bile will also promote the absorption of fat-soluble vitamins (A, D, E and K). Some 95% of bile salts are reabsorbed by **enterohepatic cycling**, in which constituents are reabsorbed in the ileum.

Drug metabolism

The liver plays a central role in drug metabolism and usually results in the production of an inactive compound that is more readily excreted (into the bile or via the kidneys), although in some cases drugs (in the form of **prodrugs**) are activated by hepatic metabolism. Drug metabolism is divided into **phase I** and **phase II**. Phase I generally involves oxidation (but may also involve reduction or hydrolysis) and this often involves hepatic oxidation via the **cytochrome P450** (CYP450) family. These reactions involve reduced NADP, molecular oxygen and CYP450 isoenzymes. Phase II involves a transferase reaction and conjugation (glucuronidation, methylation, sulphation, acetylation, glutathione conjugates, amino acid conjugates, mercapturic acid formation) to promote elimination. Phase I and phase II reactions usually happen sequentially.

Hormone metabolism

A number of steroid hormones (oestrogens, testosterone, aldosterone, cortisol), peptide hormones (insulin, growth hormone) and thyroxine are metabolised in the liver. In the cases of cortisol, oestrogens and testosterone, their metabolism involves conjugation to promote excretion.

Cholestasis

This is the inability of the liver to either produce or excrete bile. It may be due to intrahepatic problems, leading to the inability of the intrahepatic biliary ductules to produce bile, or may be extrahepatic due to blockage of the bile duct, e.g. due to gall stones.

Liver function tests (LFTs)

These are standard biochemical tests that measure a number of markers in the blood which may suggest altered liver biochemistry (Table 44.1). The battery of tests should be analysed to 'build up a picture' of possible pathologies and changes.

Liver disease

Liver disease may be acute (for example due to viral infection in hepatitis) or chronic (for example alcoholic liver disease). Liver failure has many pathophysiological effects, including the following.

• **Hyperbilirubinaemia**: with jaundice, nausea and itching as toxic effects of bilirubin.
• **Ascites**: fluid accumulation in the peritoneal cavity, partly associated with increased levels of aldosterone (due to impaired hepatic metabolism) leading to Na$^+$ and fluid retention. Acites is be managed by draining and/or diuretics (Chapter 39).
• **Increased bleeding**: due to impaired synthesis of coagulation factors.
• **Oesophageal varices**: increased portal pressure may lead to pathological dilation of veins in the oesophagus. These may rupture and lead to severe blood loss.
• **Encephalopathy:** impaired metabolism of nitrogenous toxins from gut flora may lead to altered neurotransmitter production in the brain, leading to changes in personality and behaviour.

45 Hypothalamus and pituitary

Sue Chan

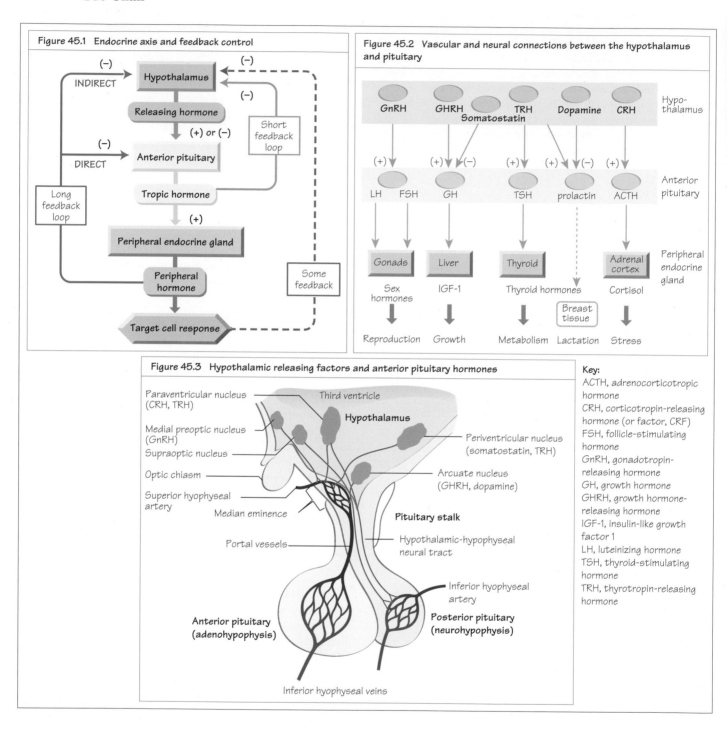

Figure 45.1 Endocrine axis and feedback control

Figure 45.2 Vascular and neural connections between the hypothalamus and pituitary

Figure 45.3 Hypothalamic releasing factors and anterior pituitary hormones

Key:
ACTH, adrenocorticotropic hormone
CRH, corticotropin-releasing hormone (or factor, CRF)
FSH, follicle-stimulating hormone
GnRH, gonadotropin-releasing hormone
GH, growth hormone
GHRH, growth hormone-releasing hormone
IGF-1, insulin-like growth factor 1
LH, luteinizing hormone
TSH, thyroid-stimulating hormone
TRH, thyrotropin-releasing hormone

The endocrine system is composed of several ductless glands that secrete chemical messengers known as **hormones** directly into the bloodstream. At target tissues, hormones interact with specific high-affinity receptors located on the plasma membrane, as in the case of protein (peptide) hormones or amines, or intracellularly (nuclear, cytosolic) as with thyroid and steroid hormones. Hormones exert their functions in four broad physiological areas: maintenance of internal environment, energy balance, growth and development, and reproduction.

Regulation of endocrine secretion

This involves feedback loop control systems that are tuned to set-points, which may be modified by circadian rhythm, seasonal cycles, age and other influences such as stress. Many hormones function as

Table 45.1 Secretory cells of the anterior pituitary

Cell type	% of endocrine population	Hormone	Structure
Acidophil cells somatotroph	~50	Growth hormone (GH)	Single-chain polypeptides with disulphide bonds
Lactotroph	~10–25	Prolactin (PRL)	
Basophil cells gonadotroph	~20	Follicle-stimulating hormone (FSH) Luteinising hormone (LH)	Glycoproteins
Corticotroph	~10	Adrenocorticotropic hormone (ACTH)	Peptide
Thyrotroph	5–10	Thyroid-stimulating hormone (TSH)	Glycoprotein

part of a cascade (**endocrine axis**, Figure 45.1), where secretions of the hypothalamus-pituitary-target gland permit signal amplification, flexibility of response to a variety of physiological stimuli and fine regulation of the end hormone product.

The core of the **neuroendocrine system** is represented by the **hypothalamic–pituitary complex**. Within the **hypothalamus**, reside important collections of neuronal cell bodies (termed nuclei) involved in endocrine function (Figure 45.2). A funnel-shaped stalk, the infundibulum, extends from the floor of the hypothalamus to connect with the **pituitary gland** (**hypophysis**), which lies in a bony cavity (sella turcica) in the sphenoid bone. An important anatomical relation to the pituitary gland is the optic chiasm (Figure 45.2); therefore any expanding lesion of the pituitary or hypothalamus can present with visual field defects.

The pituitary gland is composed of two main lobes: the **anterior lobe** (**adenohypophysis**) and the **posterior lobe** (**neurohypophysis**). Developmentally, the anterior gland derives from the ectodermal Rathke's pouch, an extension of the roof of the primitive oral cavity. The posterior gland forms from a neural down-growth of the di-encephalon. The two tissues migrate and fuse to give rise to the pituitary gland.

Hormones of the hypothalamus and pituitary gland

Hypothalamic releasing hormones

Peptide hormones synthesised in the cell bodies of small **parvocellular** neurones are released from axonal endings into capillary loops at the median eminence (Figure 45.2). They are transported via the **hypothalamic-hypophyseal portal vessels** to the capillary plexus within the anterior pituitary, where they act to stimulate or inhibit the release of hormones of specific cell types (Figure 45.3). Damage to the pituitary stalk (physical trauma, surgery, or disease) impairing blood flow to the pituitary can lead to disrupted control of anterior pituitary hormone release.

Anterior pituitary hormones

The anterior pituitary is composed of five different secretory cell types, each of which secretes a different peptide hormone (Table 45.1). These hormones act on peripheral endocrine glands to stimulate hormone secretion (**tropic** effect) or on non-endocrine tissue to exert direct effects (e.g. prolactin on mammary tissue). **Negative feedback**

control, whereby the release of hormone leads to events that inhibit further secretion, at several points in the endocrine axis allows for the maintenance of plasma hormone levels close to the set-point. Additionally, secretion of hypothalamic releasing hormones may be modulated by neuronal input from higher levels of the brain. Note that, unlike other anterior pituitary hormones, prolactin secretion is under tonic inhibitory control by the hypothalamus.

Posterior pituitary hormones

Vasopressin (also called arginine vasopressin [AVP] or antidiuretic hormone [ADH; Chapter 38] because of its main physiological effects) and **oxytocin** are synthesised in the hypothalamus, in the cell bodies of **magnocellular** neurones, located in the supraoptic and paraventricular nuclei (Figure 45.2). Different subsets of the neurones produce either vasopressin or oxytocin. The hormones are transported down the neuronal axons (which comprise the **hypothalamic-hypophyseal neural tract**) to the posterior pituitary, where they are stored (Figure 45.2). The stimuli for release of the posterior hormones are neural signals (**neuroendocrine reflex**).

• Vasopressin release is regulated by plasma osmolality (detected by hypothalamic osmoreceptors) and also blood pressure/volume (detected by baroreceptors), with neural signals sent to hypothalamic nuclei to modulate the secretion of vasopressin from the posterior pituitary accordingly. The main effects of vasopressin in humans are increased renal water reabsorption (via V_2-receptors, Chapter 38) and vasoconstriction (V_1-receptors).

• Oxytocin: suckling or stimulation of the cervix (copulation or parturition) generates neural signals that are relayed to the oxytocinergic neurones in the hypothalamus, with action potentials to the posterior pituitary resulting in the release of oxytocin into the bloodstream; oxytocin acts to stimulate the contraction of the myoepithelial cells that eject milk from the breast, and to stimulate the contraction of the uterus (myometrium). This is a rare example of **positive feedback**.

Endocrine disorders

These can results from hormone deficiency, hormone excess, or hormone resistance. Along with baseline hormone levels, feedback relationships within an endocrine axis form the basis of diagnostic testing (dynamic or provocative testing) in determining where the defect lies. Defects at the level of the peripheral endocrine gland, the anterior pituitary, or the hypothalamus are referred to as **primary**, **secondary** and **tertiary** endocrine disorders respectively.

Pituitary disease: the most common cause is **pituitary tumours**. Pituitary tumours represent ~10% of all intracranial neoplasms and over 99% are benign (non-invasive) tumours known as adenomas. These tumours can either be microadenomas (less than 10 mm in diameter) or macroadenomas. Pituitary adenomas can cause problems in a number of ways:

• hyper-secretion of a pituitary hormone;

• inadequate production of other remaining pituitary hormones;

• exert local effects on anatomically related structures (e.g. headaches, visual disturbances).

Approximately 75% of the adenomas are endocrinologically active, with prolactin-producing adenomas (prolactinomas) being the most common (approximately 40%). Growth hormone-producing adenomas produce acromegaly (adult).

Hypopituitarism: an underproduction of pituitary hormones. The term pan-hypopituitarism refers to the situation when all the pituitary hormones are underproduced. In the clinical situation, hypopituitarism usually varies depending on the dominant hormone that is deficient.

Sue Chan

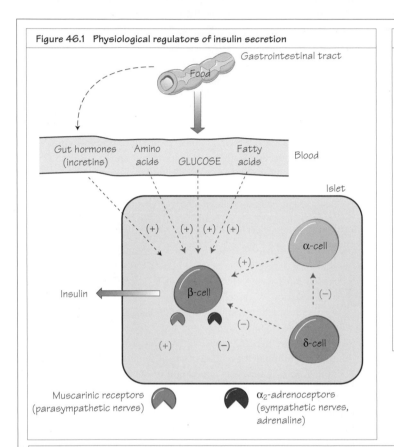

Figure 46.1 Physiological regulators of insulin secretion

Gastrointestinal tract

Food

Gut hormones (incretins) | Amino acids | GLUCOSE | Fatty acids | Blood

Islet

α-cell

(+) (+) (+) (+)

(+)

β-cell

(−)

Insulin

(−)

(+) (−)

δ-cell

Muscarinic receptors (parasympathetic nerves)

α₂-adrenoceptors (sympathetic nerves, adrenaline)

Table 46.2 Diagnostic criteria for diabetes mellitus (WHO)

Diagnostic criteria

The patient has symptoms, and one of the following:
- Fasting plasma glucose ≥7.0 mmol/L (after 8-hour overnight fast)
- Random plasma glucose ≥11.1 mmol/L
- Plasma glucose concentraton >11.1 mmol/L, 2-hour after 75 g glucose in an oral glucose tolerance test (OGTT)
- HbA1c >6.5 % or 48 mmol/ mol*

If the patient is asymptomatic, two independent plasma glucose measurements (with values in the diabetes range) on separate days are required for a diagnosis of DM

Further categories and impaired glucose regulation:

Impaired glucose tolerance, if
Fasting ≤7.0 mmol/L
and
Random or OGTT >7.8 but <11.0 mmol/L

Impaired fasting glycaemia, if
Fasting ≥6.1 mmol/L but <7.0 mmol/L

*HbA1c glycated haemoglobin correlates with average blood glucose level over the last 8–12 weeks (life span of red blood cells)

Table 46.1 Cell types within an islet of Langerhans (typical human adult islet)

Cell type		% of the islet	Hormone(s)	Function	Paracrine effects
α	A	30–40	Glucagon	Counter-regulatory hormone to insulin. Increases blood glucose	(+) Insulin secretion
β	B	50–60	Insulin, amylin	Lowers blood glucose (amylin delays gastric emptying)	(−) Glucagon secretion
δ	D	5–10	Somastatin	Inhibitory effects on digestive processes, islet hormone secretions?	(−) Islet cell secretions
PP	F	1–5	Pancreatic polypeptide	Inhibition of exocrine secretion?	(−) Islet cell secretions
ε		<1	Ghrelin	Promote cell growth and maturation in developing pancreas?	(−) Insulin secretions

Glucose represents an essential energy substrate for many tissues and the maintenance of narrow-controlled blood glucose concentrations (**glucose homeostasis**) is central for a constant provision of glucose to the brain. Glucose homeostasis is dependent on three co-ordinated and simultaneously ongoing processes involving insulin secretion by the pancreas, hepatic glucose output, and glucose uptake by splanchnic (liver and gut) and peripheral tissues (muscle and fat). This involves a complex interplay of hormonal and neural mechanisms in the CNS, the autonomic nervous system and the endocrine pancreas.

Islets of Langerhans

The endocrine pancreas in the adult human consists of approximately one million islets of Langerhans (diameter 50–300 μm), scattered throughout the pancreas and constituting approximately 1–2% of the total pancreatic mass. As well as being highly vascularised (~10% pancreatic blood flow), the islets are richly innervated with nerve fibres of the autonomic nervous system and of the gastrointestinal neuroendocrine system. Within an islet, at least five peptide hormone-producing cells have been identified: **α, β, δ, PP, ε** (also called A, B, D, F, epsilon) (Table 46.1). The majority of islets are composed of insulin-secreting β-cells, intermingled with fewer α-cells and δ-cells. Islets located in the posterior portion of the head of the pancreas are pancreatic polypeptide-rich, with PP-cells representing 80% of the islet cells. More recently, ghrelin-secreting ε-cells have been described in fetal islets; the expression of this cell type becomes rare soon after birth. Islet cells can influence each other through **paracrine** (between adjacent cells) and **autocrine** (act on original secretory cell) communication. Additionally, islets also contain bioactive agents (e.g. neuropeptide Y, galanin) that have been shown to influence exocrine function.

Insulin

Insulin is a 51-amino acid peptide hormone, synthesised initially as the prohormone precursor proinsulin, with subsequent cleavage of the internal C-peptide to give rise to the mature insulin molecule, which comprises an A-chain (21 amino acids) connected to a B-chain (30 amino acids) by two disulfide bonds. The main physiological regulator of insulin release is plasma glucose, influenced by other nutrients, gastrointestinal hormones (**incretins**, e.g. **glucagon-like peptide 1, GLP-1**) and nervous input (Figure 46.1). Insulin, like other peptide **hormones**, has a short plasma half-life of several minutes. At target tissues, the binding of insulin to its receptor results in autophosphorylation via the **receptor's intrinsic tyrosine kinase activity**. This initiates a series of interactions with docking proteins, leading to a cascade of phosphorylation/dephosphorylation reactions. Insulin lowers blood glucose levels by:

- increasing glucose uptake in adipose and skeletal muscle;
- increasing glycogen synthesis, inhibiting glycogenolysis;
- increasing protein synthesis, inhibiting protein breakdown;
- increasing lipogenesis, inhibiting lipolysis;
- inhibiting gluconeogenesis.

Other effects of insulin include uptake of cellular K^+ ions (via Na^+/K^+ ATPase), growth regulation and control of vascular function.

Glucagon

A 29-amino acid peptide, as the primary counter-regulatory hormone to insulin, glucagon increases blood glucose levels by stimulating hepatic glucose output (elevated glyogenolysis and gluconeogenesis) and lipolysis. Glucagon is rapidly secreted when plasma glucose levels fall, and is inhibited by elevated glucose concentrations. Other stimuli include amino acids (such as protein-rich meal), activation of both sympathetic and parasympathetic nervous input.

Somatostatin

Exists in two forms, a 14-amino acid and a 28-amino acid peptide. Its release is glucose dependent. Its physiological role is unclear; suggestions include regulation of the nutrient flow via control of digestion (endocrine) and a tonic inhibitory influence on insulin and glucagon secretion (paracrine).

Diabetes mellitus (DM)

Diabetes mellitus is a metabolic disorder characterised by **chronic hyperglycaemia**. Signs and symptoms include glucosuria (plasma glucose concentration exceeds the transport maximum for renal absorption, with glucose appearing in the urine), polyuria and thirst (due to osmotic diuresis), and fatigue/malaise. The diagnostic criteria are given in Table 46.2. There are two broad categories of DM.

Type 1 (T1DM): an autoimmune condition causing specific destruction of the islet β-cells, with absolute insulin deficiency. Approximately 70–90% β-cell loss occurs before clinical disease is observed. Genetic factors (~30% susceptibility, association with human leucocyte antigen [HLA] haplotypes DR3 and DR4) and environmental triggers (such as viral, toxins) are thought to be important in the aetiology of T1DM. Autoantibodies to glutamic acid decarboxylase (GAD), insulin and insulinoma-associated protein (IA-2) may be detected. Lack of insulin action can lead to excessive hepatic fatty acid β-oxidation with the abnormal production of ketone bodies, causing metabolic acidosis (ketoacidosis). Patients with T1DM require exogenous insulin. This form accounts for 5–15% of all DM, depending on the population.

Type 2 (T2DM): a heterogeneous condition caused by impaired insulin secretion, decreased insulin sensitivity in target tissues (**insulin resistance**), or both. A strong genetic component, together with other risk factors such as obesity and sedentary lifestyle, contribute to the disorder. The mechanisms underlying insulin resistance are not fully established: defects in insulin signalling and abnormal secretion of adipose-derived factors (**adipokines**) such as **resistin** and **tumour necrosis factor-alpha (TNF-α)** may be involved. It is thought that β-cell function progressively declines as the elevated insulin demands exhaust β-cell insulin secretory capacity to overcome peripheral insulin resistance; the resultant hyperglycaemia then manifests with the symptoms of DM described above. The primary treatment for insulin resistance involves diet and lifestyle recommendations: exercise (increases insulin sensitivity of peripheral tissues) and weight loss (if patient is overweight/ obese). Pharmacological management involves drugs to increase β-cell output, including **sulphonylureas** (inhibitors of ATP-sensitive K-channel on β-cells) and meglitinides (post-prandial glucose regulators), while drugs to improve insulin action include **metformin** (a biguanide; activator of AMP kinase) and glitazones (or **thiazolinediones; PPAR-γ agonists**). Incretin-based medicines (such as GLP-1 analogues and dipeptidyl peptidase IV [DPP-IV] inhibitors [gliptins]) which increase insulin release, promote satiety and delay gastric emptying have recently been included in the pharmacotherapy of T2DM. In advanced T2DM, where the patient's insulin secretory response is severely compromised, then exogenous insulin is required. T2DM accounts for 85–95% of cases of DM.

Chronic diabetic complications may be micro- or macrovascular. **Microvascular** complications include retinopathy, nephropathy and neuropathy. Neuropathy is specific to patients with DM due to damage of small vessels (capillary pathology) by hyperglycaemia (e.g. sorbitol) and glycation of proteins. **Macrovascular** complications include ischaemic heart disease, stroke and peripheral vascular disease due to accelerated atherosclerosis.

47 Thyroid gland

Sue Chan

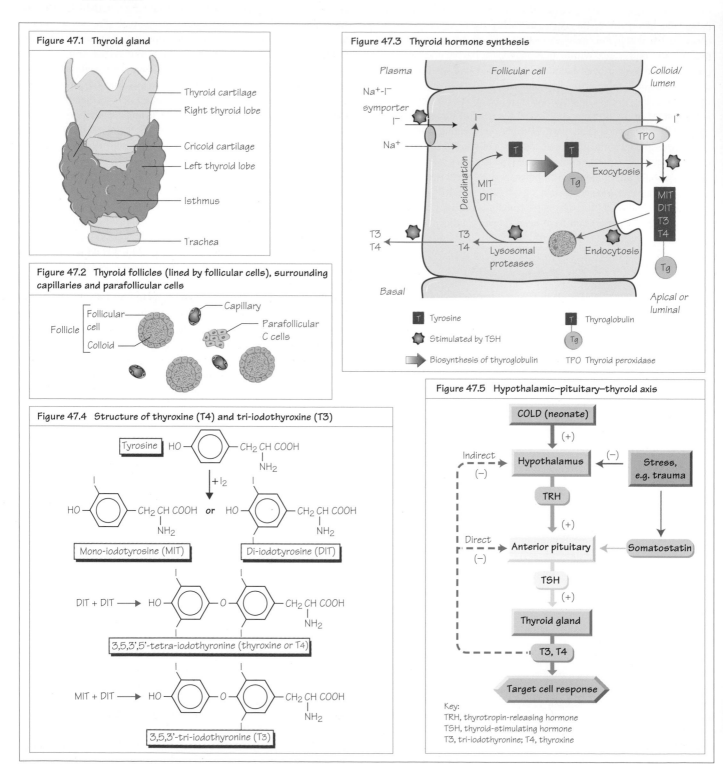

Figure 47.1 Thyroid gland

Thyroid cartilage
Right thyroid lobe
Cricoid cartilage
Left thyroid lobe
Isthmus
Trachea

Figure 47.2 Thyroid follicles (lined by follicular cells), surrounding capillaries and parafollicular cells

Follicle
Follicular cell
Colloid
Capillary
Parafollicular C cells

Figure 47.3 Thyroid hormone synthesis

Plasma   Follicular cell   Colloid/lumen

Na⁺-I⁻ symporter
I⁻
Na⁺
Deiodination
MIT
DIT
T
T
Tg
Exocytosis
T3
T4
T3
T4
Lysosomal proteases
Endocytosis
MIT
DIT
T3
T4
Tg
TPO
I*
Basal
Apical or luminal

T Tyrosine   T Thyroglobulin
Stimulated by TSH   Tg
Biosynthesis of thyroglobulin   TPO Thyroid peroxidase

Figure 47.4 Structure of thyroxine (T4) and tri-iodothyroxine (T3)

Tyrosine   HO—⬡—CH₂CH COOH
                         |
                        NH₂

+I₂

HO—⬡—CH₂CH COOH   or   HO—⬡—CH₂CH COOH
          | |
         NH₂   NH₂

Mono-iodotyrosine (MIT)   Di-iodotyrosine (DIT)

DIT + DIT ⟶ HO—⬡—O—⬡—CH₂CH COOH
                                              |
                                             NH₂

3,5,3',5'-tetra-iodothyronine (thyroxine or T4)

MIT + DIT ⟶ HO—⬡—O—⬡—CH₂CH COOH
                                              |
                                             NH₂

3,5,3'-tri-iodothyronine (T3)

Figure 47.5 Hypothalamic–pituitary–thyroid axis

COLD (neonate)
(+)
Indirect
(−)
Hypothalamus
(−)
Stress, e.g. trauma
TRH
(+)
Direct
(−)
Anterior pituitary
Somatostatin
TSH
(+)
Thyroid gland
T3, T4
Target cell response

Key:
TRH, thyrotropin-releasing hormone
TSH, thyroid-stimulating hormone
T3, tri-iodothyronine; T4, thyroxine

Anatomy

The **thyroid gland** is located anterior to the cricoid cartilage in the anterior neck, composed of two lobes connected by a branch of tissue known as the isthmus (Figure 47.1), which lies over the second and third tracheal rings. The thyroid is a very vascular organ; in conditions of severe hyperplasia, greater blood flow rates may become audible as a noise (bruit). Two pairs of **parathyroid glands** are located on the posterior surface of the thyroid gland.

Histology

The thyroid gland is composed of a large number of **follicles** (Figure 47.2). Each follicle is formed by a single layer of cuboidal epithelial cells (**follicular cells**), which secrete into the interior of the follicle; the lumen is filled with a proteinaceous, viscous material called **colloid**, which acts as a store for thyroid hormones (on the glycoprotein **thyroglobulin**). Scattered around the follicles are larger **parafollicular** or **C cells** that produce **calcitonin**. Within the parathyroid gland, **parathyroid hormone** (**PTH**) is secreted by chief cells, while the function of oxyphil cells remains unknown.

Parathyroid hormone and calcitonin
Parathyroid hormone

Secretion of PTH is stimulated by low plasma calcium levels. PTH acts to raise plasma calcium levels by stimulating calcium resorption of bone, stimulating calcium uptake from the gastrointestinal tract, enhancing renal excretion of phosphate. PTH is required for renal 'activation' of vitamin D into 1,25-dihydroxycholecalciferol, which acts to promote calcium reabsorption from the gut.

Calcitonin

Calcitonin is released in response to high plasma calcium levels. Calcitonin lowers plasma calcium by inhibiting bone resorption and inhibiting reabsorption in the kidney.

Thyroid hormones: thyroxine (T4) and tri-iodothyronine (T3)
Synthesis

Thyroid hormones are the only hormones that require an essential trace element, iodine, for the production of active hormone. The follicular cell actively accumulates iodide (I^-) ions via the Na^+-I^- symporter (driven by the inward Na^+ gradient), expressed on the basement membrane (this process is also called **iodide trapping**, Figure 47.3). At the apical (or luminal) membrane, I^- is transported into the follicle lumen by a transporter called 'pendrin'. I^- is oxidised into an active intermediate by the enzyme **thyroid peroxidase** (or thyroperoxidase, TPO). TPO also catalyses the iodination of tyrosine residues (**organification**) on thyroglobulin (a glycoprotein rich in tyrosine residues), to produce **mono-iodotyrosine** (MIT) and **di-iodotyrosine** (DIT); and the coupling of two DIT molecules to form **thyroxine** (T4), or one MIT with one DIT to give **tri-iodothyronine** (T3) (Figure 47.4). The thyroid hormones are stored as part of the thyroglobulin molecule (colloid), with sufficient amount to supply the body with its normal requirements for 2–3 months.

Release

Small portions of colloid are taken up by endocytosis into the cell. These vesicles fuse with lysosomes, which contain protease enzymes that digest the thyroglobulin to release T4 and T3 (Figure 47.3); the thyroid hormones are then released into the bloodstream (exact mechanism(s) unclear). Approximately 95% of thyroid hormone secreted is T4, the remainder is T3, with negligible amounts of reverse T3 (rT3, formed by coupling of DIT with MIT). As lipophilic molecules, thyroid hormones are poorly soluble in blood plasma and are highly bound (99.9%) to plasma-binding proteins (thyroxine-binding globulin, transthyretin and albumin). **De-iodinase** enzymes in the plasma and peripheral tissues metabolise T4 to the more biological active T3 (about four to five times more potent) and the inactive rT3; in effect, T4 acts as a pro-hormone to T3.

Regulation of thyroid function

The thyroid gland is regulated by thyroid-stimulating hormone (TSH), with thyroid hormones exerting negative feedback control of the endocrine axis (hypothalamic-pituitary-thyroid axis; Figure 47.5). Other stimuli include inhibitory (stress, somatostatin, glucocorticoids) and stimulatory (cold exposure in infants) factors. TSH acts to stimulate the synthesis and release of thyroid hormones, including thryoglobulin synthesis (Figure 47.5). TSH also exerts a '**trophic**' (to nourish, promote growth) effect, stimulating thyroid growth with hyperplasia (increased size) and hypertrophy (increased number) of follicular cells; excess plasma TSH levels can lead to the development of a **goitre** (enlarged thyroid gland).

Actions of thyroid hormones

In tissues, thyroid hormones diffuse across the plasma membrane into cells, and interact with specific nuclear receptors, which are members of the superfamily of ligand-dependent transcription factors, leading to altered gene expression. Non-genomic actions include direct effects on Na^+/K^+-ATPase and Ca^{2+}-ATPase.

• Metabolism: increase basal metabolic rate, oxygen consumption and heat production; stimulate anabolic and catabolic processes of protein, fat and carbohydrate metabolism.

• Cardiovascular system: increase heart rate, cardiac output, blood pressure. As well as direct effects, thyroid hormones act synergistically with catecholamines by upregulating β-adrenoceptors.

• Growth and development: an essential role in normal development and maturation of the brain, and skeletal growth and bone maturation. Thyroid hormones promote growth hormone release from the pituitary, and act in a permissive manner on the actions of growth hormone in growth and development. Lack of thyroid hormone in the developing newborn leads to cretinism (stunted growth and mental retardation).

Thyroid disorders
Hypothyroidism

Thyroid hormone deficiency is a common disorder, estimated to affect 1–2% of all adults in their lifetime. The most common cause worldwide is iodine deficiency, and it may also arise following radioactive iodine therapy or thyroid surgery. Primary failure of the thyroid gland is usually caused by autoimmune destruction or attack of the thyroid gland; Hashimoto's thyroiditis, which accounts for 90% of all hypothyrodism, is a slowly developing chronic autoimmune disease where there is an immune reaction to thyroglobulin and other components of the thyroid gland. Typical symptoms include lethargy, cold intolerance, weight gain and constipation. Treatment is with synthetic thyroid hormones (such as levo-thyroxine).

Hyperthyroidism

Also known as thyrotoxicosis, hyperthyroidism is characterised by elevated plasma T3 and T4 levels, with sweating, tremor, tachycardia and weight loss. There are several causes, the most common of which is Graves' disease, where autoantibodies against the TSH receptor are generated. The thyroid-stimulating immunoglobulins (TSI) activate the TSH receptor, stimulating the thyroid gland to produce and secrete more T3 and T4. Patients present with a goitre. Lymphocytic infiltration and fluid deposition in the orbital soft tissue causes protrusion of the eyeballs (proptosis, exophthalmos). Treatment may include β-blockers for rapid sympathetic relief of β-adrenoceptor-mediated effects (e.g. tremor, tachycardia), antithyroid drugs (e.g. carbimazole; which inhibit TPO activity and hence thyroid hormone synthesis), surgical removal, or radioactive ^{131}I-iodine to destroy the gland.

48 Adrenal glands and steroid hormones

Sue Chan

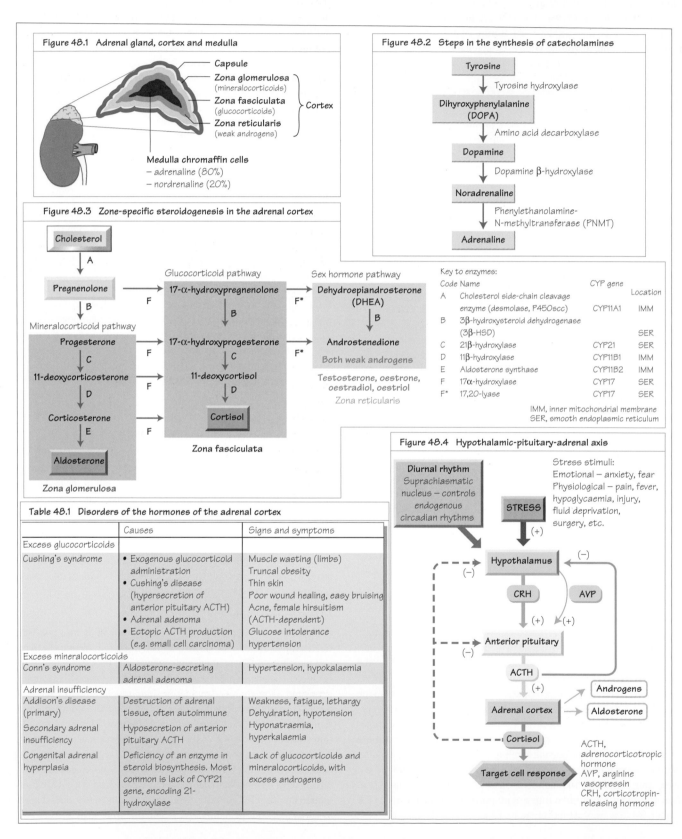

Figure 48.1 Adrenal gland, cortex and medulla

- Capsule
- Zona glomerulosa (mineralocorticoids)
- Zona fasciculata (glucocorticoids)
- Zona reticularis (weak androgens)
- Cortex
- Medulla chromaffin cells
  – adrenaline (80%)
  – nordrenaline (20%)

Figure 48.2 Steps in the synthesis of catecholamines

Tyrosine
↓ Tyrosine hydroxylase
Dihyroxyphenylalanine (DOPA)
↓ Amino acid decarboxylase
Dopamine
↓ Dopamine β-hydroxylase
Noradrenaline
↓ Phenylethanolamine-N-methyltransferase (PNMT)
Adrenaline

Figure 48.3 Zone-specific steroidogenesis in the adrenal cortex

Cholesterol
↓ A
Pregnenolone

Glucocorticoid pathway — *Sex hormone pathway*

Pregnenolone → 17-α-hydroxypregnenolone → Dehydroepiandrosterone (DHEA)
↓ B   F   ↓ B   F*   ↓ B
Mineralocorticoid pathway
Progesterone → 17-α-hydroxyprogesterone → Androstenedione
↓ C   F   ↓ C   F*   *Both weak androgens*
11-deoxycorticosterone → 11-deoxycortisol
↓ D   F   ↓ D   Testosterone, oestrone, oestradiol, oestriol
Corticosterone → Cortisol   *Zona reticularis*
↓ E   F
Aldosterone   **Zona fasciculata**

Zona glomerulosa

Key to enzymes:

Code	Name	CYP gene	Location
A	Cholesterol side-chain cleavage enzyme (desmolase, P450scc)	CYP11A1	IMM
B	3β-hydroxysteroid dehydrogenase (3β-HSD)		SER
C	21β-hydroxylase	CYP21	SER
D	11β-hydroxylase	CYP11B1	IMM
E	Aldosterone synthase	CYP11B2	IMM
F	17α-hydroxylase	CYP17	SER
F*	17,20-lyase	CYP17	SER

IMM, inner mitochondrial membrane
SER, smooth endoplasmic reticulum

Figure 48.4 Hypothalamic-pituitary-adrenal axis

Diurnal rhythm
Suprachiasmatic nucleus – controls endogenous circadian rhythms

Stress stimuli:
Emotional – anxiety, fear
Physiological – pain, fever, hypoglycaemia, injury, fluid deprivation, surgery, etc.

STRESS (+)

Hypothalamus (−)
CRH AVP
(+) (+)
Anterior pituitary (−)
ACTH
(+)
Adrenal cortex → Androgens
→ Aldosterone
Cortisol
↓
Target cell response

ACTH, adrenocorticotropic hormone
AVP, arginine vasopressin
CRH, corticotropin-releasing hormone

Table 48.1 Disorders of the hormones of the adrenal cortex

	Causes	Signs and symptoms
Excess glucocorticoids		
Cushing's syndrome	• Exogenous glucocorticoid administration • Cushing's disease (hypersecretion of anterior pituitary ACTH) • Adrenal adenoma • Ectopic ACTH production (e.g. small cell carcinoma)	Muscle wasting (limbs) Truncal obesity Thin skin Poor wound healing, easy bruising Acne, female hirsuitism (ACTH-dependent) Glucose intolerance hypertension
Excess mineralocorticoids		
Conn's syndrome	Aldosterone-secreting adrenal adenoma	Hypertension, hypokalaemia
Adrenal insufficiency		
Addison's disease (primary)	Destruction of adrenal tissue, often autoimmune	Weakness, fatigue, lethargy Dehydration, hypotension Hyponatraemia, hyperkalaemia
Secondary adrenal insufficiency	Hyposecretion of anterior pituitary ACTH	
Congenital adrenal hyperplasia	Deficiency of an enzyme in steroid biosynthesis. Most common is lack of CYP21 gene, encoding 21-hydroxylase	Lack of glucocorticoids and mineralocorticoids, with excess androgens

Medical Sciences at a Glance, First Edition. Edited by Michael D Randall. © 2014 John Wiley & Sons, Ltd. Published 2014 by John Wiley & Sons, Ltd.

The adrenal glands are situated on the superior pole of the kidney, embedded in the perirenal fat. The **outer cortex**, which is derived from mesodermal tissue, secretes **steroid hormones**, while the **inner medulla**, derived from neuroectodermal tissue, secretes the **catecholamines adrenaline** and **noradrenaline** (Figure 48.1). The adrenal gland is a highly vascular organ, where the arteriolar network gives rise to a small number of medullary arteries that pass directly through the cortex to the medulla, and an abundance of tiny thin-walled blood vessels called sinusoids, into which cortical cells secrete steroid hormones. Consequently, secretions of the adrenal cortex bathe the cells of the medulla before leaving the gland via the venous system.

Hormones of the adrenal medulla

The adrenal medulla can be described as a modified ganglion of the sympathetic nervous system (Chapter 21); **chromaffin cells** secrete adrenaline and noradrenaline into the bloodstream, innervated by nerve fibres of the splanchnic nerve with acetylcholine (ACh) as the neurotransmitter. ACh acts on nicotinic receptors on the chromaffin cell membrane to increase the rate of catecholamine synthesis and release. The expression of the enzyme that converts noradrenaline to adrenaline, phenylethanolamine-N-methyltransferase (Figure 48.2), is maintained by glucocorticoids, so the vascular arrangement within the adrenal gland ensures that chromaffin cells bathed in steroid-rich blood secrete adrenaline as the primary hormonal product of the adrenal medulla.

Hormones of the adrenal cortex

The adrenal cortex is made up of three zones (Figure 48.1), each zone expressing a distinct complement of enzymes involved in steroidogenesis of a different type of steroid hormones (**zone-specific steroidogenesis**, Figure 48.3).
• Outer **zona glomerulosa**, a thin layer of cells lying underneath the capsule, which secretes **aldosterone**.
• Middle **zona fasciculata**, the widest band of cells, which secretes the glucocorticoids (such as **cortisol**) and small amounts of adrenal androgens.
• Inner **zona reticularis** secretes the adrenal androgens **dehydroepiandrosterone** (**DHEA**) and **androstenedione**.
Many of the enzymes belong to the cytochrome P450 (CYP) monooxidase family. The steroid hormones are synthesised from **cholesterol**, which is mainly derived from plasma low-density lipoprotein (LDL), with smaller amounts from *de novo* synthesis from cellular acetate. The rate-limiting step in steroidogenesis is the transfer of the cholesterol from the outer mitochondrial membrane to the inner mitochondrial membrane; this is where cholesterol side-chain cleavage enzyme (desmolase, P450scc) is located, the enzyme involved in the conversion of cholesterol to the first steroid, pregnenolone. Steroidogenic acute regulatory (StAR) protein is thought to play a key role as a cholesterol-shuttling protein. Pregnenolone then exits the mitochondria and is transferred into the microsomal compartment, to be converted to a variety of other steroids, each steroid shuttling between the two subcellular compartments as it progresses along its biosynthetic pathway (Figure 48.3). As lipophilic molecules, steroid hormones are not stored; levels of circulating hormone are controlled primarily by its rate of synthesis. A deficiency of an enzyme involved in steroid biosynthesis can lead to the deficiency of products downstream of the enzyme, with corresponding accumulation of precursors upstream; the most common form of congenital adrenal hyperplasia (CAH, >90%) affects 21-hydroxylase (Figure 48.3, Table 48.1).

Glucocorticoids

Cortisol is the primary glucocorticoid in humans, and also has mineralocorticoid activity. Its metabolic effects generally oppose those of insulin, exerting catabolic effects in muscle and adipose, while in liver it stimulates glycogen synthesis. Cortisol causes elevation in plasma glucose levels, primarily by stimulating hepatic gluconeogenesis and, to a lesser extent, decreasing glucose uptake in skeletal muscle and adipose. At high levels, glucocorticoids exert an anti-inflammatory/immunosuppressive action; synthetic steroids (such as prednisolone) with relatively low mineralocorticoid potencies have thus been developed, and are used to control inflammatory or immune conditions. Cortisol is permissive on the actions of catecholamines on carbohydrate metabolism, and on cardiovascular regulation.

Cortisol production and release is controlled by the hypothalamus and pituitary, forming the **hypothalamic-pituitary-adrenal axis** (Figure 48.4). Superimposed on this basic negative-feedback control are two additional factors that influence plasma cortisol levels by changing the set-point, **diurnal rhythm** and **stress**, which both act on the hypothalamus (Figure 48.4). The diurnal pattern of **adrenocorticotrophic hormone** (**ACTH**) release dictates the diurnal rhythm of cortisol levels: at its lowest concentration at midnight, rising to a peak between 6am and 8am, and falling throughout the rest of the day. In response to stressors (emotional, e.g. anxiety, or physiological, e.g. fluid deprivation or injury), cortisol and sympathetic nervous activity act together to adapt to the stress situation, with mobilisation of biochemical resources (energy molecules), preparing the body to a state of physical and behavioural readiness. However, chronic activation of the stress response can lead to harmful states, with muscle-wasting, immune suppression, gastric ulcers and hyperglycaemia. ACTH also acts in a trophic manner, where elevated ACTH levels can lead to hypertrophy of the zona fasiculata and reticularis (e.g. CAH), and atrophy of the adrenal cortex with low ACTH levels (adrenal insufficiency, adrenal suppression with chronic use if high-dose steroid medication). Conditions of excess (**Cushing's syndrome**) and deficient (**Addison's disease**) glucocorticoids are described in Table 48.1.

Aldosterone

Aldosterone is produced exclusively by adrenal glomerulosa cells, due to their expression of aldosterone synthase (Figure 48.3). Aldosterone production is primarily controlled by levels of angiotensin II, part of the **renin-angiotensin system** (Chapter 32), and plasma K^+ levels, with minor influence by ACTH. Aldosterone regulates renal Na^+, and hence water, reabsorption with K^+ excretion, acting on late distal tubule and collecting duct (Chapter 39). Dysregulation of aldosterone production may lead to systemic hypertension and hypokalaemia (**Conn's syndrome**; Table 48.1).

Adrenal androgens

DHEA and its sulphated form, with a small amount of androstenedione, are weak androgens. Secretion begins at age 5–6, at very low level, with a surge at puberty, peaking at ages 25–30 years, then slowly tapers off. In women, it contributes to 50% of circulating active androgens, influencing pubic and axillary (arm pit) hair growth, and also sex drive. Under conditions of androgen excess (such as ACTH-dependent Cushing's syndrome, CAH), masculinisation of females can occur (*in utero*: ambiguous external genitalia; adult: excessive facial/body hair [hirsutism], acne). In men, adrenal androgens contribution is negligible against the background of testosterone secretion from the testes. Adrenal androgen production is regulated by ACTH, but the androgens do not exert any feedback control on the endocrine axis (Figure 48.4).

49 The genital system

Deborah Merrick

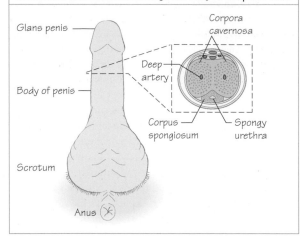

Figure 49.1 Male external genitalia, surface anatomy with associated cross-section through the body of the penis inset

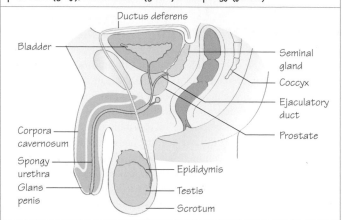

Figure 49.2 Male external and internal genitalia, median section showing the four parts of the male urethra: preprostatic (orange), prostatic (grey), intermediate (green) and spongy (yellow)

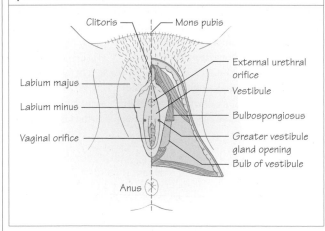

Figure 49.3 Female external genitalia, surface anatomy and perineal musculature shown with vestibule orifices illustrated

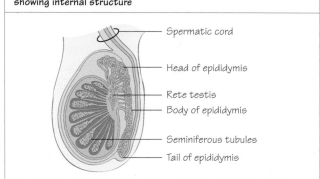

Figure 49.4 Testis and epididymis, lateral view of left testis showing internal structure

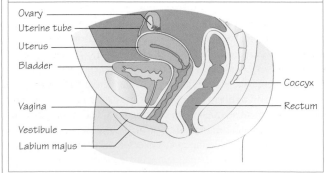

Figure 49.5 Female external and internal genitalia, median section showing relative position of vagina, uterus (anteverted and anteflexed) and ovaries

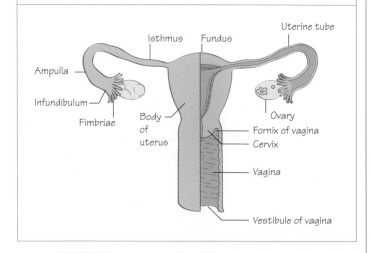

Figure 49.6 Female internal genitalia, illustrating relative positions of the vagina, uterus, uterine tubes and ovaries

The reproductive system comprises a series of organs that are involved in the production and maturation of gametes. The organs also function to unite the gametes, during sexual reproduction. Anatomically, the reproductive system can be divided into external and internal genitalia.

External genitalia
Male
Penis: organ permitting the exit of urine and semen from the body. It is the principal organ of copulation and is anatomically described in its erect position. It has a fixed root, body and glans penis, and is composed of three bodies of erectile tissue: the paired **corpora cavernosa** and the **corpus spongiosum** (Figure 49.1). The root is composed of the **crura** and **bulb** (containing erectile tissues) along with **ischiocavernosus** and **bulbospongiosus muscles**. Distally the corpus spongiosum expands to form the glans penis. The prepuce (foreskin) covers the glans penis to a variable extent.

Urethra: a muscular tube conveying urine and semen to the external urethral orifice at the tip of the glans penis. The urethra in males is long and subdivided into four distinct regions (Figure 49.2):
- preprostatic (intramural): extends through neck of bladder;
- prostatic: descends through prostate;
- membranous (intermediate): passes through perineal membrane;
- spongy (penile): courses through corpus spongiosum.

Scrotum: a cutaneous sac containing the **testes** and **epididymides**, located posteroinferior to the penis. The dartos muscle attaches to the skin of the scrotum, causing it to wrinkle when cold. The cremaster muscle elevates the testes, holding them closer to the body to minimise heat loss.

Female
The terms vulva and pudendum are terms often used to describe the female external genitalia as a whole, and include the following.

Mons pubis: fatty eminence covered with pubic hair extending anterior to the pubic symphysis, tubercle and superior rami.

Labia majora and minora: paired folds of skin. The more prominent labia majora pass from the mons pubis towards the anus (Figure 49.3). They are filled predominantly with subcutaneous fat, the terminal part of the round ligament of the uterus, and are covered in pubic hair. The smaller labia minora are hairless, consisting of spongy connective tissue containing erectile tissue. The labia minora unite anteriorly to form the prepuce and frenulum of the **clitoris** (Figure 49.3). The clitoris is an erectile organ composed of a root (two crura), body (two corpora cavernosa) and glans.

Vestibule: the space bounded by the labia minora containing the openings of the vagina, urethra, and ducts of the greater and lesser vestibular glands (Figure 49.3). The bulbs of the vestibule are paired erectile masses located beneath the bulbospongiosus muscles either side of the vaginal orifice.

Vasculature of the external genitalia: arterial supply is from branches of the internal and external pudendal arteries. Venous drainage accompanies the arteries and the veins are named accordingly. Lymphatic drainage is via the superficial inguinal, deep inguinal, internal iliac and external iliac lymph nodes.

Internal genitalia
Male
Testes and epididymides: suspended in the scrotum by the spermatic cords (Figure 49.4). The testes are oval shaped, producing sperm and hormones (e.g. testosterone). Sperm is formed in the seminiferous tubules, which connect to the epididymis via the rete testis (Figure 49.4). The epididymis is located on the posterior aspect of the testis; it has a head, body and tail. It appears as a solid structure, but is in fact formed from a single elongated duct with multiple convolutions. The tail of the epididymis is continuous with the **ductus deferens**, which ascends in the spermatic cord to enter the pelvis (Figure 49.2). Before termination, the ductus deferens enlarges (ampulla) before joining the duct of the seminal gland to form the ejaculatory duct.

Seminal glands (vesicles): secrete a thick alkaline fluid that mixes with sperm as it enters the ejaculatory duct and urethra. The glands are located superior to the prostate (Figure 49.2).

Prostate: surrounds the prostatic urethra and is composed of fibromuscular and glandular parts, which secrete a thin milky fluid that plays a role in sperm activation. It provides approximately 20% of the volume of semen (fluid containing secretions from the testes, seminal glands, prostate and **bulbourethral glands**). The bulbourethral glands produce mucus-like secretions, which enter the spongy urethra during sexual arousal (Figure 49.2).

Female
Vagina: a musculomembranous tube connecting the vestibule of the vagina inferiorly to the cervix of the uterus superiorly (Figure 49.5). The vaginal walls are usually collapsed with anterior and posterior walls in close contact; with the exception of the superior aspect, where the cervix holds the walls apart. The vaginal fornix is the recess surrounding the protruding cervix. The vagina functions to receive the penis during intercourse, acts as the inferior portion of the birth canal and is a passageway for menstrual fluid.

Uterus: a muscular, hollow, pear-shaped organ possessing a body and cervix inferiorly. The body comprises the fundus, isthmus and the uterine horns (Figure 49.6). The uterine body wall is composed of three layers: perimetrium (outer-serous), myometrium (middle-muscular) and endometrium (inner-mucous). The cervix is narrow and cylindrical in shape, composed of supravaginal and vaginal parts (Figures 49.5 and 49.6). In non-gravid (non-pregnant) women, the body of the uterus lies on the urinary bladder and the cervix lies between the bladder and rectum. This position can change in relation to the fullness of the bladder/rectum and also during pregnancy.

Uterine tubes: extend from the uterine horns to open into the peritoneal cavity, in close proximity to the ovaries (Figure 49.6). Each tube has four parts: infundibulum (distal), ampulla, isthmus and uterine (proximal). The **ovaries** are almond-shaped structures that expel the oocyte into the peritoneal cavity during ovulation. It is the distal portion of the uterine tubes (fimbriae) that captures the oocyte before passing it to the ampulla.

Vasculature of the internal genitalia: the testes and ovaries receive their blood supply via the testicular and ovarian arteries respectively, which arise from the abdominal aorta. The remaining internal genitalia receive blood supply from branches of the internal iliac arteries. Veins accompany these arteries and have similar names. Lymphatic drainage is chiefly into the lumbar (caval/aortic), internal iliac and external iliac lymph nodes.

50 Reproductive physiology

Michael D Randall

Figure 50.1 A summary of the hormonal changes associated with the menstrual cycle

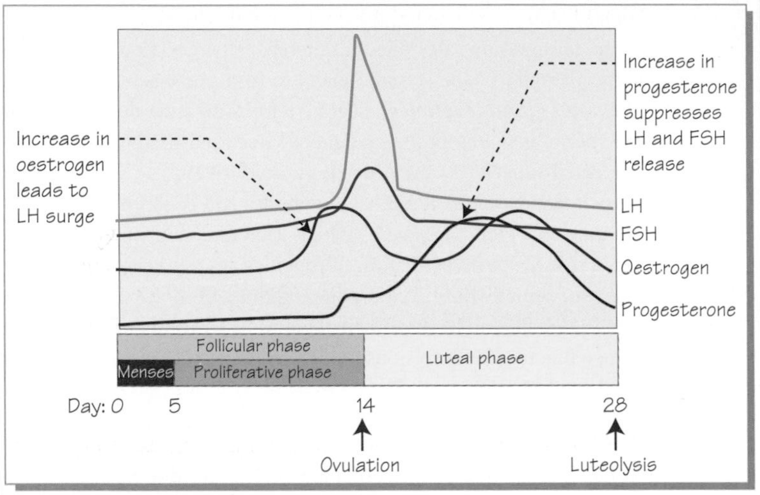

Increase in oestrogen leads to LH surge
Increase in progesterone suppresses LH and FSH release
LH
FSH
Oestrogen
Progesterone
Follicular phase
Menses
Proliferative phase
Luteal phase
Day: 0
5
14
28
Ovulation
Luteolysis

Figure 50.2 The maturation of a primordial follicle leading to ovulation and the formation of the corpus luteum

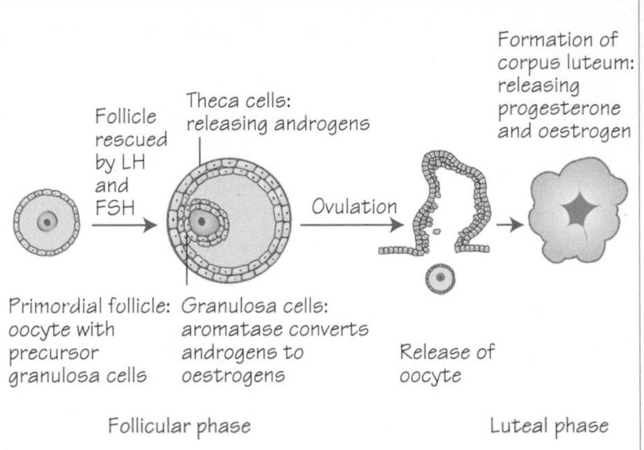

Follicle rescued by LH and FSH
Theca cells: releasing androgens
Ovulation
Formation of corpus luteum: releasing progesterone and oestrogen
Primordial follicle: oocyte with precursor granulosa cells
Granulosa cells: aromatase converts androgens to oestrogens
Release of oocyte
Follicular phase
Luteal phase

Figure 50.3 A summary of the control of testes via the gonadotrophins in males

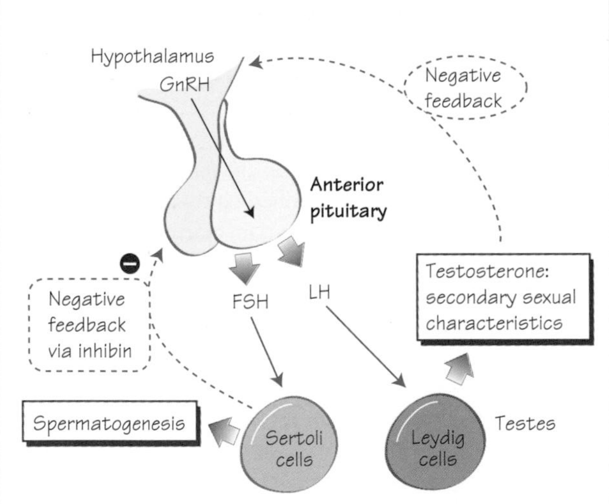

Hypothalamus
GnRH
Negative feedback
Anterior pituitary
Negative feedback via inhibin
FSH
LH
Testosterone: secondary sexual characteristics
Spermatogenesis
Sertoli cells
Leydig cells
Testes

Figure 50.4 A summary of the control of follicular development and the ovaries via the gonadotrophins in females

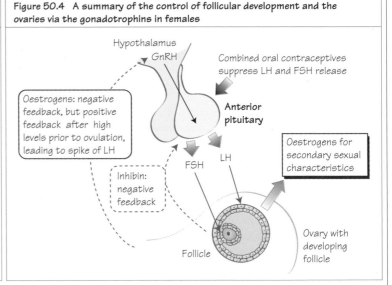

Hypothalamus
GnRH
Combined oral contraceptives suppress LH and FSH release
Oestrogens: negative feedback, but positive feedback after high levels prior to ovulation, leading to spike of LH
Anterior pituitary
FSH
LH
Oestrogens for secondary sexual characteristics
Inhibin: negative feedback
Follicle
Ovary with developing follicle

Reproductive physiology is tightly regulated via hormonal control by the steroidal sex hormones. The process starts with puberty at around 10–13 years in females and slightly later in males.

In males, puberty is associated with maturation of the reproductive organs, with enlargement of the testes and penis. This is regulated via the release of glycoprotein **gonadotrophins** from the anterior pituitary gland in response to **gonadotrophin-releasing hormone (GnRH)** from the hypothalamus (Figure 50.1). The gonadotrophin, **luteinising hormone (LH)** acts on **Leydig cells** of the testes to stimulate the release of the androgens, including testosterone. The release of testosterone leads to the development of secondary sexual characteristics in males (body and facial hair, voice, muscular physique) and libido. Another gonadotrophin, **follicle-stimulating hormone (FSH)**, acts on the **Sertoli cells** in the seminiferous tubules of the testes to promote spermatogenesis. Testosterone also feeds back to inhibit both the hypothalamus and the anterior pituitary. The Sertoli cells exert negative feedback on FSH release via the release **inhibin**, which acts at the anterior pituitary.

In females, adrenache is the maturation of the adrenals, leading to the production of various steroid hormones (e.g. dehydroepiandrostone [DHEA] and androstenedione), which sensitise towards gonadotrophin stimulation. This then leads to gonarche with breast bud development in response to oestradiol. Puberty in females is similarly regulated via LH and FSH, such that increased pulses of the hormones lead to the initiation of the **menstrual cycle** with the regular development and release of ova (Figure 50.2). The female sex hormones lead to the development of secondary sexual characteristics in females, such as breast development.

Hormonal regulation of the menstrual cycle

The human female reproductive cycle is characterised by the **menstrual cycle**, which typically lasts 28 (+/–4) days and coordinates ovulation at its midpoint (Figures 49.3 and 49.4). The cycle is under tight hormonal regulation and divided into four phases.

• **Follicular phase** (from the start of menstrual bleeding to day 14): during this time there is maturation of a **primordial follicle**. Many primordial follicles are present in the ovaries from the fetal stage of the female and they contain an **ovum or oocyte**, arrested in meiosis and surrounded by a single epithelial cell layer (precursor granulosa cells). Many of the primordial follicles undergo atresia but some are rescued by **pulses of LH and FSH**. Follicles mature during the reproductive years and this is influenced by LH, which acts on outer theca cells of the developing follicles, which then release androgens. The androgens are then converted by **aromatase** in the **granulosa cells** to oestrogens, and these levels rise throughout the phase. The maturation process is supported by FSH acting on the granulosa cells. The maturation leads to the formation of a **Graafian follicle**, one of which per cycle becomes dominant.

• **Ovulation**: the Graafian follicle grows substantially and ruptures mid-cycle to release the single oocyte into the peritoneal cavity to enter the oviduct. Ovulation is preceded by the appearance of LH receptors on the granulosa cells and by a surge in LH release due to oestradiol, which at high levels has a positive feedback effect.

• **Luteal phase** (day 14–28): post-ovulation the ruptured follicle becomes the **corpus luteum**, in which the granulosa cells respond to LH by producing progesterone and the theca cells produce oestrogen to provide the optimal conditions for implantation for a fertilised ovum. The progesterone causes negative feedback on GnRH, so that LH and FSH levels become minimal and there is no further follicular development.

• **Luteolysis** (day 28): in the absence of fertilisation the corpus luteum starts to break down, with decreased production of progesterone. This leads to menstruation with the breakdown of the vascular uterine wall, which is shed and leads to menstrual period bleeding.

Conception

Ejaculation during sexual intercourse results in the deposition of spermatozoa in the female genital tract. The spermatozoa undergo capacitation, which results in their ability to fertilise the released oocyte. **Capacitation** involves removing glycoproteins from the spermatozoa to increase membrane permeability in preparation for fertilisation. Once a spermatozoon fuses with an oocyte then fertilisation occurs, in which the maternal and paternal chromosomes are combined. The fertilised zygote then undergoes several cell divisions prior to implantation as a blastocyst in the endometrium.

Pregnancy

If fertilisation occurs the corpus luteum must be retained to maintain pregnancy. This is achieved by the hormone **human chorionic gonadotrophin** (hCG), which is released initially by the trophoblast cells of the blastocyst and then the placenta and continues to be produced until around three months of gestation. Implantation is favoured by the increased levels of oestrogen, which prepare the uterus.

Maintenance of pregnancy is dependent on the establishment of the **placenta**, which supplies the fetus with nutrients, oxygen and acts as an immunological barrier. The trophoblast secretes large amounts of progesterone to maintain pregnancy and the placenta releases oestrogens to prepare the mother (e.g. increase in breast size). The levels of oestrogens and progesterone increase throughout pregnancy until birth.

Parturition

The signal for birth includes increased levels of DHEA from the fetal adrenal glands. After nine months of gestation birth is initiated by increased uterine contractions in response to increasing oestrogen levels. There is ripening of the cervix in preparation for birth. The electrical activity coupled to contraction is also conducted via gap junctions connecting the myometrial cells. The process of labour also stimulates the release of oxytocin from the posterior pituitary and this also promotes uterine contractions.

Oral contraceptives

These provide effective contraception.

• **Combined oral contraceptives** contain oestrogens and a progestogen, and prevent follicular development, ovulation and luteinisation by suppressing the release of LH and FSH.

• **Progestogen-only containing** pills increase the viscosity of cervical mucus and so prevent penetration by spermatozoa.

Deborah Merrick

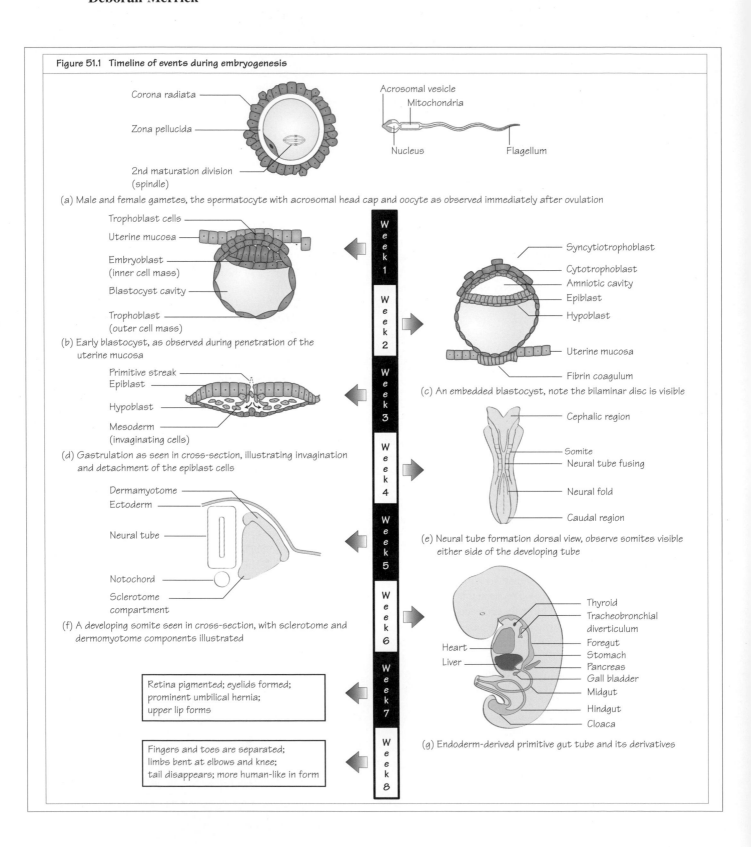

Figure 51.1 Timeline of events during embryogenesis

Corona radiata

Zona pellucida

2nd maturation division
(spindle)

Acrosomal vesicle
Mitochondria
Nucleus
Flagellum

(a) Male and female gametes, the spermatocyte with acrosomal head cap and oocyte as observed immediately after ovulation

Week 1

Trophoblast cells
Uterine mucosa
Embryoblast
(inner cell mass)
Blastocyst cavity
Trophoblast
(outer cell mass)

(b) Early blastocyst, as observed during penetration of the uterine mucosa

Week 2

Syncytiotrophoblast
Cytotrophoblast
Amniotic cavity
Epiblast
Hypoblast
Uterine mucosa
Fibrin coagulum

(c) An embedded blastocyst, note the bilaminar disc is visible

Week 3

Primitive streak
Epiblast
Hypoblast
Mesoderm
(invaginating cells)

(d) Gastrulation as seen in cross-section, illustrating invagination and detachment of the epiblast cells

Week 4

Cephalic region
Somite
Neural tube fusing
Neural fold
Caudal region

(e) Neural tube formation dorsal view, observe somites visible either side of the developing tube

Week 5

Dermamyotome
Ectoderm
Neural tube
Notochord
Sclerotome
compartment

(f) A developing somite seen in cross-section, with sclerotome and dermomyotome components illustrated

Week 6

Thyroid
Tracheobronchial diverticulum
Heart
Liver
Foregut
Stomach
Pancreas
Gall bladder
Midgut
Hindgut
Cloaca

(g) Endoderm-derived primitive gut tube and its derivatives

Week 7

Retina pigmented; eyelids formed; prominent umbilical hernia; upper lip forms

Week 8

Fingers and toes are separated; limbs bent at elbows and knee; tail disappears; more human-like in form

Embryology is the developmental study of the embryo during the **first eight weeks following fertilisation**. During the process of fertilisation, male and female gametes fuse to produce a diploid **zygote**. In the days and weeks that follow this remarkable event, tissues and organs of the embryo are derived from three primitive germ layers.

Fertilisation

Fertilisation is the process by which a female oocyte (egg) and male spermatozoa (sperm) fuse. For fertilisation to occur, the spermatozoa must undergo capacitiation and the acrosomal reaction. **Capacitiation** occurs in the female genital tract by the removal of proteins and glycoproteins from the plasma membrane overlying the acrosomal region. Capacitated spermatozoa can then pass through the corona radiate cells freely (Figure 51.1a). The **acrosomal reaction** occurs after the spermatozoa bind to the zona pellucida and involves the release of enzymes required to penetrate this layer, facilitating fusion of the gametes. Once a spermatozoon enters the oocyte the egg responds by preventing other spermatozoa entering, resuming meiotic division and becoming metabolically active. **Cleavage** is a series of mitotic division that occur once the zygote has reached the two-cell stage. The cells, known as **blastomeres**, become compacted, forming an inner and outer cell mass. The inner cell mass will develop as the embryo proper, while the outer cell mass will form the **trophoblast** (which contributes to the placenta). Fluid penetrates the inner cell mass forming the blastocyst cavity; at this stage the embryo is referred to as a **blastocyst**. By the end of week 1, the blastocyst has begun to **implant** into the uterine mucosa (Figure 51.1b). By the end of week 2, it has become completely embedded and a **primitive uteroplacental circulation** is evident. The inner cell mass (**embryoblast**) differentiates into two layers (epiblast and hypoblast) forming a bilaminar disc (Figure 51.1c).

Gastrulation

This is the process that establishes the three germ layers: **ectoderm, mesoderm** and **endoderm** (Figure 51.1d). It begins with the formation of the primitive streak on the surface of the epiblast. Epiblast cells migrate towards the streak, becoming flask-shaped and detaching, before moving below the epiblast cell layer (a process called invagination). Some invaginating cells displace the hypoblast layer and become the endoderm germ layer. Cells remaining in the epiblast layer form the ectoderm and those cells occupying the region between the endoderm and ectoderm become the embryonic mesoderm. The three germ layers are now established.

Organogenesis

This occurs from week 3 to week 8 of development. During this developmental period the three germ layers give rise to all the organs and tissues of the human body.

Ectoderm derivatives: the ectoderm overlying the **notochord** and **prechordal mesoderm** thickens to form the neural plate. This in turn folds and fuses to form the neural tube, a process that is completed at approximately day 25 (Figure 51.1e). This tube represents the primitive central nervous system. It possesses an extended cephalic region characterised by dilations (vesicles) that will develop into the brain and a thinner caudal part that will become the spinal cord. Other derivatives from the ectoderm germ layer include structures that make contact with our surrounding environment, including the peripheral nervous system, skin and sensory epithelium of the ear, nose and eye. **Neural crest cells** are often referred to as the fourth germ layer. The cells arise at the lateral borders of the neural folds as they fuse; they then migrate and enter the underlying mesoderm. The neural crest cells subsequently give rise to numerous structures, including melanocytes (skin and hair follicles), Schwann cells, connective tissue, and bones of the face and skull.

Mesoderm derivatives: mesodermal cells close to the midline proliferate and form a thickened plate called the **paraxial** mesoderm. Located lateral to this is a thinner region of **lateral plate** mesoderm, which is temporarily connected to the paraxial mesoderm by **intermediate** mesoderm. At the beginning of week 3, the paraxial mesoderm becomes organised into segments called the somitomeres. Cells of the somitomeres contribute to the mesenchyme of the head, forming a large proportion of the neurocranium and voluntary muscles of the craniofacial region. In the occipital region and caudally, the somitomeres further organise into somites at around day 20. Approximately three new somites appear in a craniocaudal sequence every day until 42-44 pairs are present by the end of week 5. After receiving signals from surrounding structures such as the neural tube and notochord, each somite differentiates into a sclerotome and dermomyotome component (Figure 51.1f). Cells derived from the sclerotome give rise to cartilage and bone (e.g. vertebrae) and those cells derived from the dermomyotome form the precursors to muscle and the dermis of the skin. The intermediate mesoderm differentiates into urogenital structures, including nephrotomes, which form an important component of the primitive kidney system. The lateral plate mesoderm splits into somatic and splanchnic layers. Mesodermal cells from the somatic layer give rise to the bones and connective tissue of the limbs, and together with the overlying ectoderm, form the lateral body walls. The splanchnic layer gives rise to the walls of the gut tube in association with cells of endodermal origin. The mesodermal embryonic germ layer also gives rise to the circulatory system, including the heart, arteries, veins, lymph vessels, blood and lymph cells. The spleen and cortex of the suprarenal glands are also mesoderm derivatives.

Endoderm derivatives: the main organ system derived from the endoderm germ layer is the gastrointestinal tract (GI tract), which is formed from a primitive gut tube. The formation of the gut tube is a passive event, caused by embryonic growth and folding. The gut tube is divided into the foregut, midgut and hindgut. The endoderm germ layer provides the epithelial lining of the GI tract, respiratory tract and urinary bladder. Other derivatives include the liver, pancreas and parenchyma of the thyroid (see Figure 51.1g).

Fetal period

This is four times the length of the embryonic period, commencing at week 9. This period is characterised by rapid growth and maturation of the multiple tissues and organ systems. For example, the urogenital system differentiates further between males and females during this period.

Deborah Merrick

Figure 52.1   Anatomy of the central nervous system, illustrating the relative positions of the brain, spinal cord and spinal nerves

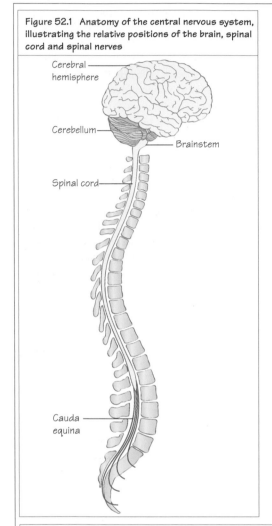

Cerebral hemisphere
Cerebellum
Brainstem
Spinal cord
Cauda equina

Figure 52.2   Lateral view of cerebral hemisphere, right hemisphere with corresponding lobes and sulci indicated

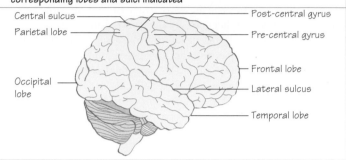

Central sulcus
Parietal lobe
Occipital lobe
Post-central gyrus
Pre-central gyrus
Frontal lobe
Lateral sulcus
Temporal lobe

Figure 52.3   Internal (medial) view of cerebral hemisphere, left hemisphere illustrating the corpus callosum, diencephalon and brainstem

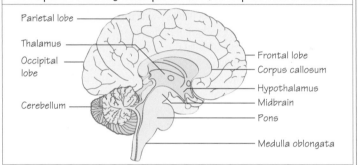

Parietal lobe
Thalamus
Occipital lobe
Cerebellum
Frontal lobe
Corpus callosum
Hypothalamus
Midbrain
Pons
Medulla oblongata

Figure 52.4   Inferior (ventral) view of the brain, the relative positions of the cranial nerves are depicted

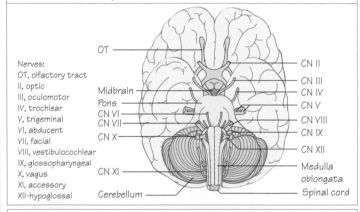

Nerves:
OT, olfactory tract
II, optic
III, oculomotor
IV, trochlear
V, trigeminal
VI, abducent
VII, facial
VIII, vestibulocochlear
IX, glossopharyngeal
X, vagus
XI, accessory
XII-hypoglossal

OT
Midbrain
Pons
CN VI
CN VII
CN X
CN XI
Cerebellum
CN II
CN III
CN IV
CN V
CN VIII
CN IX
CN XII
Medulla oblongata
Spinal cord

Figure 52.5   Ventricular system, the fluid-filled cavities of the brain and the associated subarachnoid spaces filled with CSF (blue); inset showing arachnoid granulations

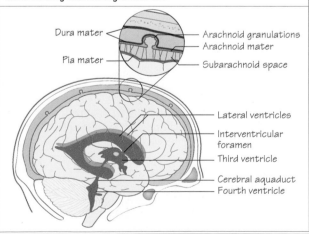

Dura mater
Pia mater
Arachnoid granulations
Arachnoid mater
Subarachnoid space
Lateral ventricles
Interventricular foramen
Third ventricle
Cerebral aquaduct
Fourth ventricle

Figure 52.6   Spinal cord with dissected spinal meninges showing their relative positions

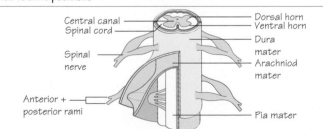

Central canal
Spinal cord
Spinal nerve
Anterior + posterior rami
Dorsal horn
Ventral horn
Dura mater
Arachniod mater
Pia mater

The central nervous system (CNS) allows the coordination and integration of neural signals that control activities of the body, such as respiration. The CNS is also involved in **higher cognitive functions** such as memory and learning. The CNS comprises the brain and spinal cord (Figure 52.1), which are composed of a large number of excitable nerve cells (**neurones**) and specialised tissue (**neuroglia**). Neuronal cell bodies are located within grey matter and the processes of the neurones occupy white matter of the CNS.

Brain

The brain and its membranous coverings are protected by the surrounding neurocranium. The brain is composed of an inner core of white matter surrounded by grey matter. Some specialised grey matter masses (nuclei) are located deep within the white matter.

Cerebrum

The left and right cerebral hemispheres form the largest component of the brain. The cerebral surfaces are thrown into multiple folds (gyri), grooves (sulci) and clefts (fissures). The major sulci separate each hemisphere into frontal, parietal, temporal and occipital lobes, named according to the bones they lie beneath (Figure 52.2). The pattern of gyri and sulci is anatomically important, as some demarcate functional areas of the cortex. For example, the pre-central gyrus corresponds to the primary motor area (Chapter 54) and the post-central gyrus is associated with the primary sensory area of the cortex (Chapter 53). The left and right hemispheres are connected by a large mass of white matter, the corpus callosum. The diencephalon forms the central core of the cerebrum and includes the thalamus and hypothalamus (Figure 52.3 and Chapter 55).

Brainstem

The brainstem is composed of the midbrain (rostral), pons and medulla oblongata (caudal). Cranial nerves III–IV (midbrain), V (pons), VI–VII (pons-medulla junction) and VIII–XII (medulla oblongata) are associated with the brainstem (Figures 52.3 and 52.4).

Cerebellum

This lies posterior to the pons and medulla and is composed of two hemispheres, thrown into folds (folis) united by the vermis (Figure 52.3 and 52.4). The cerebellum connects to the midbrain, pons and medulla oblongata via large bundles of nerve fibres called the superior, middle and inferior cerebellar peduncles, respectively.

Vasculature of the brain

The brain receives approximately one-sixth of the cardiac output via the vertebral and internal carotid arteries. These blood vessels form a collateral circulation by anastomosing at the base of the brain (**circle of Willis**). Cerebral veins draining the brain empty into a series of venous sinuses (Figure 52.5) before returning to the heart via the internal jugular vein.

Meninges and cerebrospinal fluid

Meninges

The meninges are three membranous layers called **pia mater**, **arachnoid mater** and **dura mater** (Figure 52.6). These coverings are termed either cranial meninges (those associated with the brain) or spinal meninges (associated with the spinal cord). The pia mater closely adheres to the surface of the brain and spinal cord (Figures 52.5 and 52.6). The arachnoid mater forms a cobweb-like covering that is separated from the pia mater by the subarachnoid space, which contains **cerebrospinal fluid** (**CSF**). The external cranial dura mater is a thick, two-layered membrane. The outer (periosteal) layer closely associates with the internal aspect of the cranium and the inner (meningeal) layer forms dural infoldings (e.g. falx cerebri). The dural venous sinuses form between the two dural layers where the dural infoldings attach (Figure 52.5). The dura mater surrounding the spinal cord is separated from the vertebral bodies by adipose tissue in the epidural (extradural) space. The meninges form a supporting network for vessels and form a fluid-filled cavity that surrounds and protects the brain and spinal cord.

Ventricular system

This comprises two lateral ventricles and midline third and fourth ventricles (Figure 52.5). Choroidal epithelial cells of the choroid plexuses located within the ventricles secrete CSF (400–500 mL/day). The lateral ventricles connect with the third ventricle via interventricular foramina (of Monro). The third ventricle is continuous with the cerebral aqueduct (of Sylvius), which opens into the fourth ventricle. The fourth ventricle then tapers to become the central canal of the spinal cord. A median aperture (of Magendie) and two lateral apertures (of Luschka) allow CSF to enter the subarachnoid space. CSF is reabsorbed into the venous system via arachnoid granulations (Figure 52.5).

Spinal cord

The spinal cord is continuous with the **medulla oblongata** (Figure 52.1). It is located within the vertebral canal of the vertebral column, surrounded by the spinal meninges and CSF in the subarachnoid space (Figure 52.6). The spinal cord is shorter than the vertebral canal, terminating in the lumbar region in adults (intervertebral disc between L1 and L2 vertebrae). Close to its termination, the roughly cylindrical cord tapers to a cone-shaped structure called the conus medullaris. At its apex, the filum terminale descends to attach to the coccyx, helping to anchor the spinal cord. Thirty-one pairs of spinal nerves (8 cervical, 12 thoracic, 5 lumbar, 5 sacral and 1 coccygeal) attach to the spinal cord via anterior (motor) and posterior (sensory) roots through a series of rootlets. The spinal cord has two enlarged regions (cervical and lumbosacral), which correspond to the innervation of the limbs. Spinal roots arising from the lumbosacral enlargement and conus medullaris form bundles of nerve roots called the cauda equina (Figure 52.1). The cauda equina is located in a distended subarachnoid space called the lumbar cistern. Unlike the brain, the spinal cord has an inner core of grey matter with dorsal and ventral horns that unite through a grey commissure containing a small central canal (Figure 52.6). White matter surrounds the grey matter and can be divided into dorsal, ventral and lateral columns.

Vasculature of the spinal cord

The spinal cord is supplied by three longitudinal arteries (one anterior and two posterior) that are derived from branches of the vertebral, ascending cervical, deep cervical, intercostal, lumbar and lateral sacral arteries. Longitudinal spinal veins (three anterior and three posterior) drain the spinal cord in a similar distribution pattern to the arteries and have a direct continuity with the cranial sinuses.

53 The sensory system

Deborah Merrick

Table 53.1 Sensations mediated by the somatosensory system, with examples of corresponding receptors given

Tactile sensations (touch, pressure, vibration)	Proprioception		Pain
	Conscious	Non-conscious	
Cutaneous mechanoreceptors: Hair follicles *(deformation)* Meissner's corpuscles *(touch, vibration)* Merkel's receptors *(pressure)* Pacinian corpuscles *(vibration)* Ruffini's corpuscles *(stretch)*	Joint mechanoreceptors: Joint receptors*(kinaesthesia)*	Muscle mechano-receptors: Muscle spindles *(limb proprioception)* Golgi tendon organs *(limb proprioception)*	Nociceptors: Mechanical *(sharp pricking pain)* Thermal, mechano-thermal *(slow, burning pain)* Polymodal *(mechanical stimuli, hot or cold burning sensation)*

Figure 53.1 Sensory pathways, fasciculus gracilis and fasciculus cuneatus ascending in the dorsal column (bold lines) and spinothalamic fibres running in the anterolateral quadrant of the spinal cord (dashed lines)

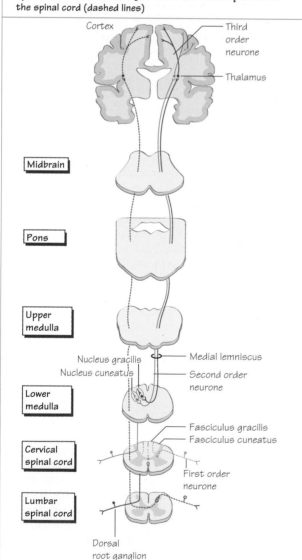

Figure 53.2 Sensory ascending pathways of the spinal cord

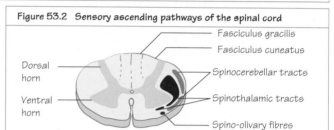

Figure 53.3 Visual cortex, as observed in an internal (medial) view of the brain

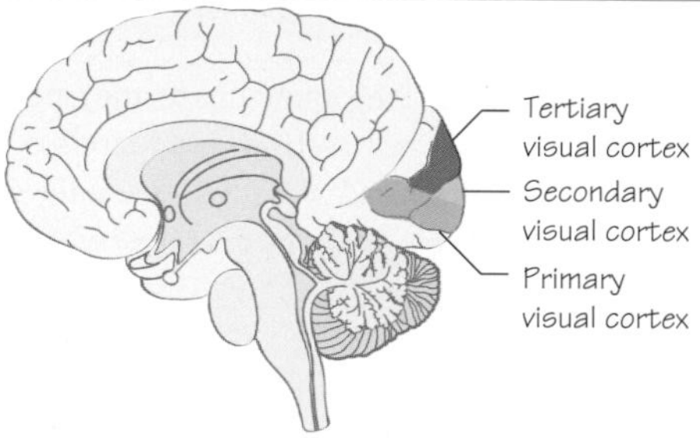

Figure 53.4 Auditory cortex, as observed in a lateral view of cerebral hemisphere

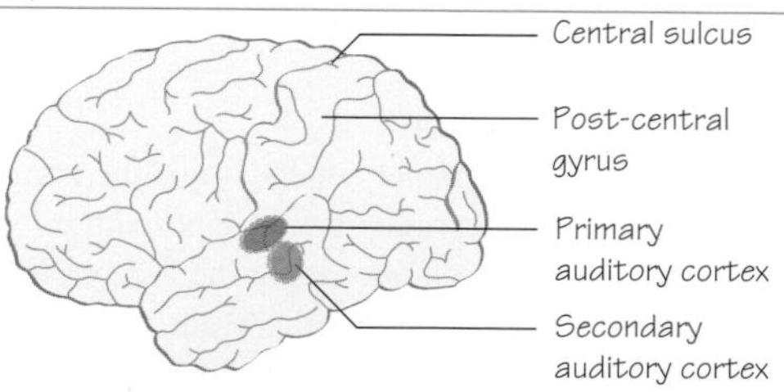

Figure 53.5 Olfactory cortex, as observed in an inferior (ventral) view of the brain

 Medical Sciences at a Glance, First Edition. Edited by Michael D Randall.

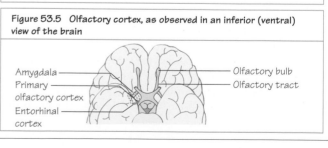

The sensory system monitors the body's internal and external environment. Sensory nerve endings (sensory receptors) respond to a stimulus, which is transmitted to the central nervous system for processing. The sensory system includes somatic, visual, auditory, vestibular, taste and olfactory (smell) systems. The sensory input can be divided into general (somatosensory) and special sensations.

Sensory receptors

These are specialised neuronal structures that make contact with our environment (Table 53.1). The afferents can be classified according to the type of stimulus they respond to. **Chemoreceptors** are sensory receptor that responds to certain chemical stimuli in the environment (e.g. olfactory neurones). **Mechanoreceptors** respond to mechanical pressure or distortion (e.g. hair cells of the cochlear), while **photoreceptors** react to light (e.g. rods and cones of the retina). **Thermoreceptors** respond to changes in temperature (e.g. cutaneous receptors) and **nociceptors** react to potentially damaging stimuli causing the perception of pain (e.g. cutaneous receptors). The sensory stimulus is converted into electrochemical energy of the nerve impulse, in a process called transduction.

Somatosensory system

This relays general sensory information such as touch, pressure and vibration (tactile sensations) through the nervous system via a series of neurones. In its simplest form, this comprises three neurones: first-order, second-order and third-order (Figure 53.1). Neurones segregate themselves into two main general sensory pathways: **spinothalamic** and **medial lemniscus** (dorsal column system).

Spinothalamic: sensory pathway conveying information of pain, temperature, light touch and pressure. The cell bodies of first-order neurones occupy the dorsal root ganglion of spinal nerves (Figure 53.1). Their axons pass into the spinal cord and synapse with cells of the dorsal horn. Second-order neuronal axons pass contralaterally before ascending in the anterolateral quadrant of the spinal cord (Figure 53.2). Most spinothalamic axons terminate in the **ventral posterolateral (VPL) nucleus** of the thalamus. Crude awareness of touch, pressure, pain and temperature are believed to be appreciated here. **Thalamocortical projections** (third-order neurones) pass from the thalamus via the internal capsule and corona radiata to the somatosensory area of the post-central gyrus. The size of the cortical area representative of a particular body region (**homunculus**) is proportional to the region's sensitivity. For example, the hands are disproportionally large due to their heightened sensitivity. The sensation of pain can be divided into 'fast pain' and 'slow pain' experiences approximately 0.1 and 1.0 s following a painful stimulus. Fast pain impulses travel directly to the VPL nucleus before passing to the cerebral cortex. Slow pain fibres end in the reticular formation, activating the entire nervous system.

Medial lemniscus: pathway involved in discriminative touch, conscious proprioception and sensing vibration. Axons from the posterior root ganglion pass into the dorsal columns of the spinal cord. The dorsal column contains two ascending tracts, the fasciculus gracilis and the fasciculus cuneatus. Unlike the spinothalamic system, these fibres remain ipsilateral until the medulla. Long ascending fibres from the sacral, lumbar and lower thoracic region are contained in the fasciculus gracilis. The fasciculus cuneatus comprises upper thoracic and cervical ascending fibres. Fibres synapse with second-order neurones in the nucleus gracilis or nucleus cuneatus of the medulla respectively (Figure 53.1). Axons of these neurones become contralateral, passing over to the opposite side of the spinal cord in the sensory decussation. They ascend (as the medial lemniscus) to synapse with third-order neurones in the VPL nucleus of the thalamus. Axons project to the cerebral cortex as previously described.

Spinocerebellar pathways: terminate in the cerebellar cortex, relaying non-conscious information about limb and joint position (proprioception).

Trigeminothalamic pathway: comparable to the spinothalamic and medial lemniscus pathways, although specific for the head region.

Cuneocerebellar tract: some fibres from the nucleus cuneatus pass to the cerebellum to relay non-conscious information on muscle-joint status related to the upper limb.

Spinotectal tract: sensory fibres ascend and synapse with neurones in the superior colliculus of the midbrain. This pathway is involved in bringing about movement of the eyes and head towards a source of stimulation (spinovisual reflex).

Spinoreticular tracts: pathway involved in influencing the level of consciousness, as second-order neurones synapse with neurones of the reticular formation.

Spino-olivary tract: pathway conveying information from cutaneous and proprioceptive organs to the cerebellum.

Special sensation

Specialised sensations are conducted directly to the brain. Sensory information is relayed via the **thalamus** (relay nuclei) to the cerebral cortex, with the exception of olfaction (smell). Information relating to olfaction is mainly transmitted to the cortex through pathways that do not synapse in the thalamus.

Visual: photoreceptors of the retina (rods and cones) convey visual information to ganglion cells. Axons of the ganglion cells project to the lateral geniculate body of the thalamus via the optic nerve and tract. The lateral geniculate nuclei pass information predominately to the visual cortex for interpretation (Figure 53.3).

Auditory: pressure waves cause vibrations of the basilar membrane that result in mechanical displacement of the cochlear hair cells. This leads to transduction, passing information via the vestibulocochlear nerve and medial geniculate nuclei to the primary auditory cortex (Figure 53.4).

Vestibular: vestibular hair cells, like cochlear hair cells, transduce minute displacements passing information via the vestibulocochlear nerve and vestibular nuclei to multiple brain regions (e.g. cerebellum).

Taste: first-order sensory neurones occupy most of the cell bodies of the geniculate ganglion. They project to the gustatory nuclei before terminating at the ventral posteromedial nucleus of the thalamus. Here projections pass to cortical areas for taste perception.

Olfactory: chemicals with odours are identified by specialised receptors (olfactory cells) located in the olfactory mucosa of the nasal cavity. The cells convey information of smell via the olfactory bulb and tract to several areas of the brain, including the primary olfactory cortex, amygdala and entorhinal cortex (Figure 53.5).

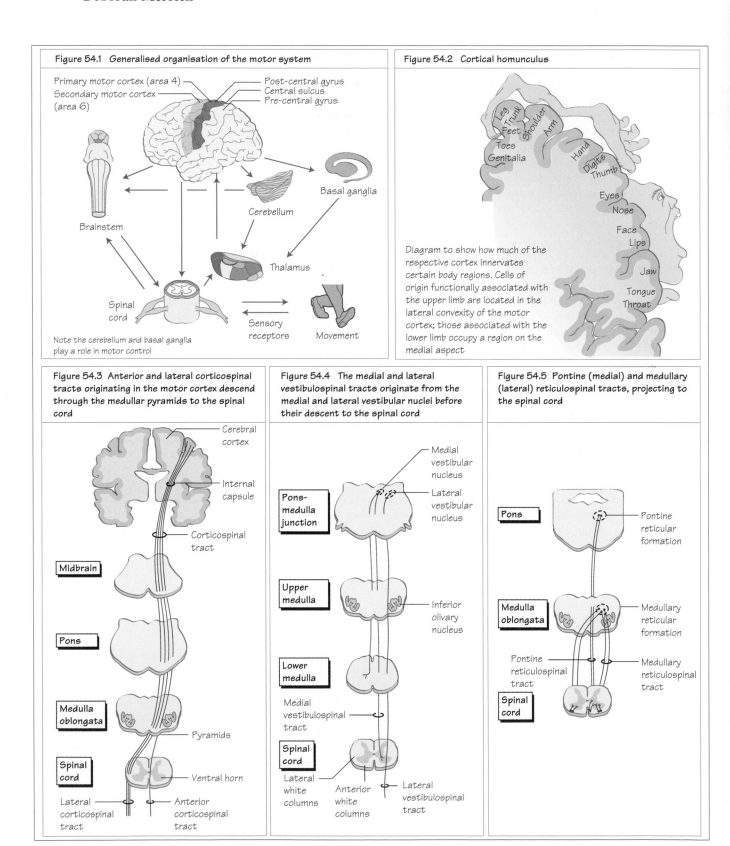

Figure 54.1 Generalised organisation of the motor system

Primary motor cortex (area 4)
Secondary motor cortex (area 6)
Post-central gyrus
Central sulcus
Pre-central gyrus
Basal ganglia
Cerebellum
Brainstem
Thalamus
Spinal cord
Sensory receptors
Movement

Note the cerebellum and basal ganglia play a role in motor control

Figure 54.2 Cortical homunculus

Leg, Trunk, Shoulder, Arm, Feet, Toes, Genitalia, Hand, Digits, Thumb, Eyes, Nose, Face, Lips, Jaw, Tongue, Throat

Diagram to show how much of the respective cortex innervates certain body regions. Cells of origin functionally associated with the upper limb are located in the lateral convexity of the motor cortex; those associated with the lower limb occupy a region on the medial aspect

Figure 54.3 Anterior and lateral corticospinal tracts originating in the motor cortex descend through the medullar pyramids to the spinal cord

Cerebral cortex
Internal capsule
Corticospinal tract
Midbrain
Pons
Medulla oblongata
Pyramids
Spinal cord
Ventral horn
Lateral corticospinal tract
Anterior corticospinal tract

Figure 54.4 The medial and lateral vestibulospinal tracts originate from the medial and lateral vestibular nuclei before their descent to the spinal cord

Medial vestibular nucleus
Lateral vestibular nucleus
Pons-medulla junction
Upper medulla
Inferior olivary nucleus
Lower medulla
Medial vestibulospinal tract
Spinal cord
Lateral white columns
Anterior white columns
Lateral vestibulospinal tract

Figure 54.5 Pontine (medial) and medullary (lateral) reticulospinal tracts, projecting to the spinal cord

Pons
Pontine reticular formation
Medulla oblongata
Medullary reticular formation
Pontine reticulospinal tract
Medullary reticulospinal tract
Spinal cord

The motor system is part of the central nervous system (CNS) and controls voluntary movements. Multiple brain regions work together to ensure coordinated motor control utilising a series of neurones called upper and lower motor neurones (Figure 54.1). Upper motor neurone is a term used to embrace all descending motor pathways from the brain (cerebral cortex and brainstem) which innervate lower motor neurones (of the spinal cord and brainstem). Lower motor neurones have cell bodies that lie in the CNS and function to innervate musculature. The major descending pathways include the corticospinal, vestibulospinal and reticulospinal tracts.

Corticospinal tracts

These are the primary motor pathway involved with voluntary, discrete and skilled movements. The tracts start in the cerebral cortex and terminate in the spinal cord. Approximately one-third of corticospinal fibres arise from the **pre-central gyrus** (area 4), referred to as the **primary motor cortex**. Another one-third of fibres arise from the **secondary motor cortex** (area 6), which is located rostral to the pre-central gyrus. The remaining fibres arise from the post-central gyrus, influencing sensory input to the nervous system.

Pre-central gyrus: site of origin of the fibres controlling motor activity (see Figure 54.1). The pre-central gyrus is organised somatotopically, where a body region corresponds to a particular point of the motor cortex (**homunculus**; Figure 54.2). The homunculus is a distorted image of the human body. Parts of the body that are responsible for fine movement (e.g. digits) occupy a much larger portion of the cortex, compared with body regions that are more coarsely controlled (e.g. trunk).

Corticospinal tracts: axons from pyramidal cells of the fifth layer of the cerebral cortex descend and converge in the corona radiata before passing to the posterior limb of the internal capsule. Fibres are grouped into those associated with the upper and lower extremities. The internal capsule continues into the basis pedunculi of the midbrain. On reaching the pons the tracts get broken up into fasciculi (bundles), which become grouped together to form the **pyramids** in the medulla oblongata (Figure 54.3). The pyramids are swellings that run down the ventral midline of the medulla oblongata. At the point where the medulla oblongata becomes continuous with the spinal cord, most of the fibres (~85%) have crossed the midline (pyramidal decussation). Decussated fibres enter the spinal cord running in the lateral white columns (**lateral corticospinal tracts**). These fibres descend in the spinal cord before terminating in the ventral horn at their target spinal cord level. Fibres that did not cross the midline (**anterior [ventral] corticospinal tract**) continue to descend in the ipsilateral spinal cord within the anterior white columns (Figure 54.3). Most of these fibres cross the midline within the cervical and upper thoracic spinal cord regions, to terminate in the contralateral ventral horn. Only the largest corticospinal fibres synapse directly with motor neurones. Most will synapse with interneurones, which in turn will synapse with alpha motor neurones and some gamma motor neurones. Early in the corticospinal tracts descend some fibres which return to the cortex to inhibit the activity of adjacent cortical regions. Other returning fibres pass to additional brain regions (e.g. reticular formation and olivary nuclei) to inform subcortical areas of the cortical motor activity, in case they are required to react to this via other descending pathways.

Corticobulbar tracts: fibres accompany the corticospinal tracts to the level of the brainstem where they synapse within the reticular formation (near cranial nerve nuclei) or on lower motor neurones associated with the cranial nerves.

Vestibulospinal tracts

These maintain upright posture and balance, resulting from action of the extensor muscles in opposing gravity. **Vestibular nuclei** located in the pons and medulla receive afferent fibres from the inner ear (**vestibular apparatus**) and from the **cerebellum**. Neurones from the lateral vestibular nucleus (**lateral vestibulospinal tract**) send axons uncrossed to the spinal cord where they descend in the anterior white column before terminating by synapsing with interneurones of the ventral horn (Figure 54.4). Neurones from ipsilateral and contralateral medial vestibular nuclei (**medial vestibulospinal tract**) descend in the anterior white column of the cervical spinal cord, terminating in the ventral horn.

Reticulospinal tracts

These mediate control over most movements that do not require dexterity or the maintenance of balance. Neurones derived from the reticular formation in the pons region project ipsilaterally to the spinal cord (pontine reticulospinal tract), descending through the anterior white column (Figure 54.5). Fibres arising from the medulla project contralaterally and ipsilaterally to the spinal cord (medullary reticulospinal tract) and descend in the lateral white column. Both sets of fibres terminate in the ventral horn, facilitating or inhibiting the alpha and gamma motor neurones.

Additional descending tracts: include tectospinal (reflex postural movements in response to visual and auditory stimuli) and rubrospinal tracts (facilitates activity of flexor muscles).

Motor neurones: located in the ventral horns of the spinal cord (and in motor nuclei of the cranial nerves), supplying the skeletal musculature. Collectively known as lower motor neurones, there are two types that supply muscles.

Alpha: large neurones that can innervate between fewer than 10 (where contraction is controlled precisely) to as many as several hundred (large, crude muscle movements) muscle fibres.

Gamma: less numerous in number than alpha, controlling the length and tension of the neuromuscular spindles (proprioceptive organs of skeletal muscle).

Execution of movement: descending pathways can be traced from motor areas of the cerebral cortex to lower motor neurones. However, other parts of the brain also play important roles in the motivation and planning phases, during the formulation of motor commands by the brain (e.g. prefrontal cortex and parietal lobe regions). The coordination of movement requires further input from varying brain regions, including: cerebral cortex, thalamus, subthalamic nucleus, substangia nigra, reticular formation, vestibular nuclei and the cerebellum (Figure 54.1).

Deborah Merrick

Figure 55.1 Relative position of the hypothalamus and thalamus

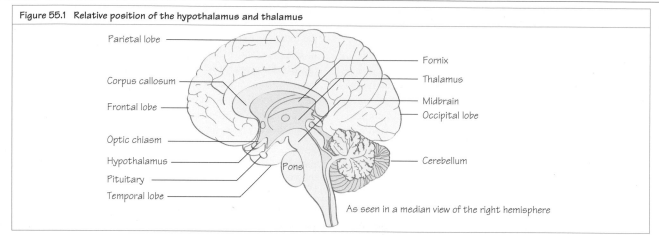

Parietal lobe
Corpus callosum
Frontal lobe
Optic chiasm
Hypothalamus
Pituitary
Temporal lobe
Pons
Fornix
Thalamus
Midbrain
Occipital lobe
Cerebellum

As seen in a median view of the right hemisphere

Figure 55.2 Location of the hypothalamic nuclei

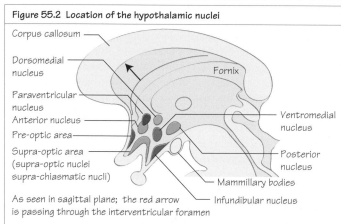

Corpus callosum
Dorsomedial nucleus
Paraventricular nucleus
Anterior nucleus
Pre-optic area
Supra-optic area (supra-optic nuclei supra-chiasmatic nucli)
Fornix
Ventromedial nucleus
Posterior nucleus
Mammillary bodies
Infundibular nucleus

As seen in sagittal plane; the red arrow is passing through the interventricular foramen

Figure 55.3 Location of the main hypothalamic nuclei

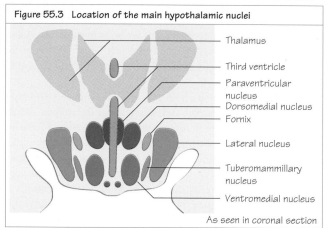

Thalamus
Third ventricle
Paraventricular nucleus
Dorsomedial nucleus
Fornix
Lateral nucleus
Tuberomammillary nucleus
Ventromedial nucleus

As seen in coronal section

Table 55.1

Nuclei	Function	Nuclei	Function
Anterior hypothalamic nuclei	Temperature regulation (response to heat)	Medial hypothalamic nuclei	Reduce food intake (satiety centre)
Posterior hypothalamic nuclei	Temperature regulation (response to cold)	Lateral hypothalamic nuclei	Increase food intake (hunger centre) and water consumption (thirst centre)

Figure 55.4 Arrangement of nuclei within the thalamus

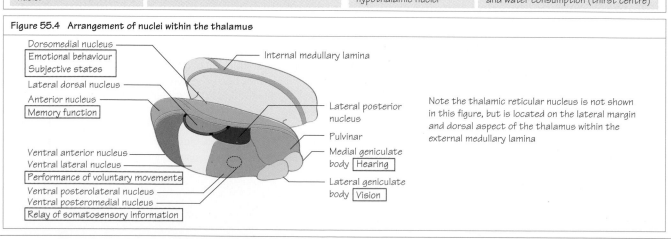

Dorsomedial nucleus
Emotional behaviour Subjective states
Lateral dorsal nucleus
Anterior nucleus
Memory function
Ventral anterior nucleus
Ventral lateral nucleus
Performance of voluntary movements
Ventral posterolateral nucleus
Ventral posteromedial nucleus
Relay of somatosensory information
Internal medullary lamina
Lateral posterior nucleus
Pulvinar
Medial geniculate body Hearing
Lateral geniculate body Vision

Note the thalamic reticular nucleus is not shown in this figure, but is located on the lateral margin and dorsal aspect of the thalamus within the external medullary lamina

Medical Sciences at a Glance, First Edition. Edited by Michael D Randall. © 2014 John Wiley & Sons, Ltd. Published 2014 by John Wiley & Sons, Ltd.

The hypothalamus and thalamus form part of the **diencephalon**, which is located rostral to the brainstem and is divided by the midline third ventricle. The diencephalon is a forebrain derivative, known to function in maintaining **higher order cognition** and **homeostasis**.

Hypothalamus

The hypothalamus is a paired forebrain structure located below the thalamus, forming the floor and inferior walls of the third ventricle (Figure 55.1). It extends from the optic chiasm to the caudal border of the mammillary bodies. Anteriorly is the preoptic area, which is often described as part of the hypothalamus for functional reasons (Figure 55.2). The hypothalamus is bounded laterally by the internal capsule.

Subdivisions/nuclei: the multiple nuclei of the hypothalamus (Figures 55.2 and 55.3) can be divided into the following functional regions:

* anterior, middle and posterior (or);
* medial, lateral and paraventricular.

The nuclei have ill-defined boundaries and therefore some nuclei extend into neighbouring areas. The regions are arranged into regulatory and modulatory centres. For example, the medial hypothalamus contains most of the releasing hormones (which control pituitary function; Chapter 45) and is believed to act in modulating feeding, rage behaviour and control over autonomic functions (Figure 55.3 and Table 55.1). The lateral hypothalamus contains nuclei that are associated with a number of behavioural processes (e.g. drinking, predation).

Connections: located in the centre of the **limbic system**, the hypothalamus receives multiple inputs, including the cerebral cortex, viscera and limbic system. Efferent connections are also multiple and complex in nature. They include descending fibres to the brainstem/spinal cord, pathways of the **limbic system**, anterior nucleus of the thalamus and reticular formation in the tegmentum of midbrain. The hypothalamus communicates with the pituitary gland, which lies inferiorly (Figure 55.2). These two structures are connected via neuronal pathways that pass from the hypothalamic nuclei (supraoptic and paraventricular) to the posterior lobe of the pituitary and by blood vessels that allow communications to the anterior lobe of the pituitary (Figures 55.2 and 55.3). Through these pathways the hypothalamus can influence activities of the endocrine glands.

Function: the hypothalamus is able to influence the autonomic nervous system, and integrate this with the **neuroendocrine system**, ensuring homeostasis. Cells of the hypothalamic nuclei produce releasing factors and release-inhibiting factors that control hormone production of the pituitary gland (anterior lobe). The hypothalamus plays further important roles in temperature regulation, food intake, water balance, emotion and behaviour, and control of circadian rhythms (Figures 55.2 and 55.3).

Thalamus

The medial surfaces of the two midline walnut-shaped thalami form the lateral walls of the third ventricle. They often come into close contact and touch via the interthalamic adhesion (Figure 55.1). Anteriorly, the thalamus forms the posterior boundary of the interventricular foramen and posteriorly it expands to form the pulvinar.

Subdivisions/nuclei: strips of white matter (internal medullary lamina) divide the grey matter of the thalamus into anterior, medial and lateral divisions, each containing a group of nuclei with diverse functions (Figure 55.4). The anterior thalamic nucleus forms connections with the **cingulate gyrus, hippocampal** formation and **hypothalamus**. Its anatomical connections suggest a role in memory function. The nuclei located within the medial part of the thalamus include the large dorsomedial nucleus and several smaller nuclei. The dorsomedial nucleus is connected to the prefrontal cortex, hypothalamic and thalamic nuclei. This part of the thalamus integrates a variety of sensory information and functions in emotional behaviour. The lateral part of the thalamus is divided into a dorsal and ventral tier of nuclei. The former (lateral dorsal nucleus, the lateral posterior nucleus, pulvinar) are thought to connect to other thalamic nuclei, cerebral hemispheres and cingulate gyrus. The ventral tier of nuclei includes the ventral anterior nucleus and ventral lateral nucleus. Both nuclei are intimately involved in control of motor functions (Figure 55.4). The ventral tier also contains the ventral posterior nuclei, which comprise the ventral posteromedial and ventral posterolateral nuclei. The nuclei projections pass to the primary somatic sensory areas of the cortex. Additional thalamic nuclei are also present, including the **medial geniculate** (auditory) and **lateral geniculate** (visual) nuclei (see Figure 55.4).

Connections: these predominantly include those made between thalamic nuclei (excluding reticular nucleus) and the cerebral cortex. Reciprocal fibres pass back from the cerebral cortex to the thalamic nuclei. Thus it is likely that both the cortex and thalamus can modify each other's activities. The thalamus also acts a relay station for sensory-motor axonal loops between the cerebellum and basal nuclei (important for normal voluntary movements).

Function: the thalamus and cerebral cortex are integrally linked, which has resulted in the thalamus often being referred to as the gateway of the cortex. The thalamus acts as a relay for many subcortical areas and is particularly important in processing and relaying a variety of sensory and motor functions. For example, the visual system receives input from the retina, lateral geniculate nucleus (thalamus) and the visual cortex (occipital lobe). However, the thalamus does far more that just relay information; it integrates and regulates the transfer of information in a complex way. The thalamus is also believed to be involved in functions not considered to be sensory or motor related, such as regulating levels of consciousness.

Michael D Randall

The basis of neurophysiology, with the fundamentals of action potential propagation and synaptic transmission are covered in Chapters 19 and 20. The sheer complexity of the human brain is, in part, due to the vast number of synaptic connections made by each neurone and the considerable number of neurotransmitters with a range of actions, such as inhibition and excitation. Neural networks are immensely complex, with inhibitory and excitatory loops, and because a neurone may synapse with 10 000 other neurones and there are 10^{10} neurones in the human brain, this leads to the level of control and sophistication required of the CNS.

Physiological roles of the CNS

Integration of homeostasis as a neuroendocrine role (Chapters 45 and 55): responsible for the regulation of sex hormones (Chapter 50), metabolic hormones (Chapters 47 and 48), maturation (Chapter 45).

Regulation of physiological control of cardiovascular (Chapter 32), renal (Chapters 39 and 45) and respiratory (Chapter 26) systems and bladder control (Chapter 40) by neural mechanisms.

The regulation of appetite: this is a tightly regulated behavioural process that controls the intake of food in relation to metabolic needs. The hypothalamus plays a central role in the control of appetite and involves 5-hydroxytrytamine (inhibitory) and neuropeptide Y (stimulatory) as key transmitters. It is sensitive to a number of hormones such as leptin. Leptin is a peptide hormone produced by adipose tissue and its levels correlate with adiposity; as its levels increase appetite is suppressed. Dysregulation of this system is associated with the development of obesity. The gastrointestinal hormone cholecystokinin also provides a shorter-term inhibitory input.

The biological clock: the brain is the regulator of circadian rhythms. This is controlled via the suprachiasmatic nucleus (SCN) in the hypothalamus, which receives information about day length derived from the visual system. The SCN then regulates the pineal gland, which releases melatonin (levels increasing during dark periods).

Processing of sensory and somatosensory information, which underpins the awareness of the environment (e.g. pain, temperature, vision, hearing, taste balance) (Chapter 53). Perceiving sensory information such as pain leads to the awareness of pain.

Descending pathways, which modulate transmission in the spinal cord.

Spinal cord is responsible for motor output, sensory input and reflexes, which may be modulated via higher control.

Motor roles

• The motor cortex plans and initiations voluntary movements.
• The cerebellum is critical to positional coordination in response to somatosensory information from the spinal cord and other areas of the brain. The cerebellum contains highly sophisticated neural networks of Purkinje cells and granule cells, which carry out complex processing.
• Basal ganglia are deep in the cerebrum and are involved in motor control and dysfunction of this system occurs in Parkinson's disease (Chapter 57). The basal ganglia are also involved in cognitive and affective roles.

Higher functions

The real key to human brain is at the level of the higher functions that underpin the human, such as the ability to have emotions, thoughts, desires, fear, process visual images to lead to awareness of the environment, learning, and having both a short-term and long-term memory. The higher emotions are underpinned by the concept of consciousness.

The limbic system, which includes the hippocampus, amygdala, septal nucleus, cingulated gyrus and fornix, is involved in motivation, emotion, long-term memory and olfaction.

Long-term potentiation (LTP)

This is neuronal mechanism by which increased transmission at a synapse (Chapter 20) leads to an enhancement of activity or re-enforcement such that the effectiveness of the communication is increased. This may be via presynaptic mechanisms enhancing release and post-synaptic mechanisms via receptor and second-messenger upregulation. The excitatory neurotransmitter glutamate acting at NMDA receptors is associated with LTP. This ability to re-enforce communication is thought to underlie memory and the ability to learn.

In contrast to LTP, long-term depression (LTD) also occurs with reduced synaptic activity.

Neuronal plasticity

Both LTP and LTD are examples of neuronal plasticity in which neuronal function can adapt in relation to activity. Plasticity can also occur if neuronal pathways become damaged and adaptations can occur with new connections forming to compensate for any deficit.

Neurotransmitters and function

Our knowledge of the physiology of the CNS is still relatively limited and much of our current understanding comes for pathophysiology and altering function pharmacologically. For example, dopaminergic transmission is implicated in the nigostriatal pathway of the basal ganglia, as it is known that loss of dopaminergic function leads to Parkinson's disease. Conversely, treatment with precursors of dopamine or dopamine agonists provide effective treatments for Parkinson's disease, while dopamine receptor antagonists induce Parkinson-like symptoms. Table 56.1 summarises the actions and activities of some key neurotransmitters and modulators.

Table 56.1 Some key neurotransmitters together with their key sites of action, physiological roles and how their activity may be altered in neurological and psychiatric disorders and drug therapy

GPCR: G-protein coupled receptor

Neurotransmitter	Targets	Examples of neurological roles	Clinical relevance
Noradrenaline	α and β-adrenoceptors, which are all G-protein coupled	• Pre and post-synaptic actions • Involved in arousal and mood • Involved in cardiovascular control centres	• Inhibition of neuronal reuptake of noradrenaline is an effective antidepressant treatment • Stimulation of α_2-adrenoceptors leads to decreased sympathetic output and blood pressure lowering (Chapter 32)
Dopamine	D_1–D_5 dopamine receptors, which are all G-protein coupled	• Involved in mesocortical pathways • High concentrations in limbic system and hypothalamus • Transmitter in nigrostriatal pathway in basal ganglia • Regulation of pituitary secretions • Involved in nausea and vomiting (chemoreceptor trigger zone) • Dopamine reward hypothesis: dopamine release is associated with pleasurable/addictive activities and may contribute towards addiction	• Loss of dopaminergic function leads to movement disorders in Parkinson's disease • Increased dopaminergic activity in the cerebral cortex is associated with schizophrenia • Dopamine receptor antagonists are anti-emetics • Attention deficit hyperactivity disorder responds to inhibition of dopamine reuptake
5-hydroxytryptamine (5-HT) also known as serotonin	5-HT_1–5-HT_7 receptors, which are all G-protein coupled, except 5-HT_3, which is ionotropic	• Raphe nucleus is main site of release and influences many areas • Involved in mood • Suppression of appetite • Involved in nausea and vomiting (chemoreceptor trigger zone)	• Inhibition of the reuptake of 5-HT is an effective antidepressant treatment • 5-HT_3 receptor antagonists are anti-emetics
Acetylcholine	• Muscarinic, are GPCRs. • Nicotinic, which are ionotropic	• Transmitter in cortex, midbrain and brainstem • Associated with memory	• Impairment of cholinergic function is associated with Alzheimer's disease
Histamine	Histamine H_1–H_3 receptors, which are all G-protein-coupled	• Associated with sedation/sleep • Hypothalamus • Vestibular nuclei	• H_1 receptor antagonists are sedating • H_1 receptor antagonists are effective in motion sickness
Melatonin	Melatonin receptors (MT_1–MT_3), which are all G-protein coupled	• Released by pineal gland • Released during darkness	• An effector of the biological clock • Melatonin is advocated for 'jet lag'
Adenosine	A_1–A_3 receptors, which are all G-protein coupled	• Inhibitory actions • Associated with sleep	• Caffeine is an adenosine receptor antagonist and has stimulatory effects
ATP	Purinoceptors • P_{2X} receptors, which are ionotropic • P_{2Y} receptors, are GPCRs.	• P_{2X} receptors are excitatory and may play a role in pain and mechanosensation	
Nitric oxide	Activation of guanylyl cyclase increasing cGMP	• May modulate long-term potentiation and depression	
Endogenous opioids, e.g. endorphins, dynorphin, enkephalins	μ, δ and κ receptors, which are all G-protein coupled and inhibit adenylyl cyclase	• These are peptides that mimic the action of morphine • They can suppression pain pathways and the perception of pain	• Opioids such as morphine are powerful analgesics by reducing pain transmission and its perception • Opioids also lead to euphoria and are highly addictive
Tachykinins, e.g. substance P and neurokinin	• Substance P: NK_1 receptors • Neurokinin A and B: NK_2 and NK_3 receptors • All GPCRs	• Neuropeptides • Substance P is involved in pain and inflammation	
Neuropetide Y	NPY receptors, which are all G-protein coupled	• Hypothalamus • Regulates appetite	
Endogenous cannabinoids, e.g. anandamide	CB_1 receptor and TRPV1 receptors on sensory nerves	• Widely distributed but poorly understood • Stimulates appetite	• Cannabinoid receptor antagonists reduce appetite
GABA	• $GABA_A$: associated with Cl⁻channel • $GABA_B$: G-protein coupled leading to inhibition of adenylyl cyclase	• Principal inhibitory neurotransmitter.	• Enhancement of GABA activity at $GABA_A$ receptors by benzodiazepines leads to sedation, hypnotic and anxioloytic effects • General anaesthetics may enhance the actions of GABA • $GABA_B$ agonists are anti-spastic
Glycine	• Ligand-gated Cl⁻channel	• Inhibitory transmitter in the brain and spinal cord	• Strychnine is an antagonist that causes convulsions by inhibiting the inhibitory effects of glycine
Glutamate	• NMDA/AMPA/kainate receptors: iontropic associated with Ca^{2+} influx • Metabotropic receptors: G-protein coupled	• Excitatory amino acid • Involved in long-term potentiation	

57 CNS disorders and treatments

Michael D Randall

Disorders of CNS can be broadly divided into **neurological** and **psychiatric** conditions. In neurological conditions, control and normal function of neurones is altered, for example there may be changes in neuronal excitability (e.g. epilepsy) or motor control (e.g. Parkinson's disease, multiple sclerosis). Psychiatric disorders involve changes in the 'mind' and may involve alterations in mood (e.g. depression), or perception and behaviour (e.g. schizophrenia).

Epilepsy

There are different forms of epilepsy, including:
- **absence epilepsy**: in which the patient is unaware of their surroundings appears to 'daydream'. This usually presents in childhood.
- **generalised tonic-clonic seizures**: these involve complete loss of consciousness with convulsions, involving uncontrolled movements of the body including the limbs.

Pathophysiology: in general, epilepsy is due to abnormal neuronal discharges, which may or may not spread across the brain. The cause may be due to a structural lesion, secondary to trauma, or due to some unidentified change.

Treatment: drugs are used to prevent seizures and a primary target is to reduce neuronal excitability.
- *Carbamazepine*: thought to cause use-dependent inhibition of Na^+ channels and so reduce excitability.
- *Sodium valproate*: potentiates GABA and causes use-dependent blockade of Na^+ channels.
- *Lamotrigine*: causes use-dependent blockade of Na^+ channels and decreases the release of the excitatory neurotransmitter glutamate.

Parkinson's disease

Parkinson's disease is a relatively common neurodegenerative disease often associated with ageing. It is a disease of movement and is associated with tremor, rigidity and poverty of movement. There may be bradykinesia (slowness of movement), akinesia (lack of movement or rigidity) and dyskinesias (abnormal involuntary movements), and it may be associated with autonomic dysfunction.

Pathophysiology: the disease is characterised by degeneration of dopaminergic neurones in the nigrostriatal pathway in the basal ganglia. Parkinson-like symptoms can be induced by drugs that block dopamine receptors, such as the antipsychotic drugs used in schizophrenia.

Treatment: the aim is to replace dopaminergic neurotransmission.
- *Levodopa:* this is the precursor of dopamine and so will increase levels of dopamine and provide some relief from the symptoms. Administration of L-dopa is associated with widespread side effects due to the peripheral conversion of L-dopa to dopamine by dopa decarboxylase. To reduce these problems, L-dopa is given with an inhibitor of dopa decarboxylase, e.g. carbidopa.
- *Dopamine D_2 receptor agonists (e.g. rotigotine)*: increase dopaminergic activity in the basal ganglia and because the principal peripheral receptor is the dopamine D_1 receptor they have limited peripheral side effects. Their direct agonist activity circumvents the need for the nigrostriatal pathway to synthesis dopamine.

- *Monoamine oxidase B inhibitors (e.g. selegiline)*: MAO-B is involved in the metabolism of dopamine and so inhibition of this enzyme will increase the concentrations of dopamine.
- *Catechol-O-methyltransferase inhibitors*: COMT is also involved in the breakdown of dopamine, and inhibitors of this enzyme will increase levels of dopamine and so enhance dopaminergic function.

Multiple sclerosis (MS)

This is a long-term, debilitating condition that may run a course of relapse and remission.

Pathophysiology: this is an autoimmune inflammatory condition in which the myelin surrounding neurones is damaged and this results in impaired nervous conduction. Common sites of demyelination include the optic nerve, brainstem, cerebellar connections and cervical spinal cord. MS may present with optic neuritis and weakness, and progress to severe disability with ataxia, spasticity and urinary incontinence.

Treatment: current therapies have limited success. They include the following drugs.
- *Beta-interferon:* anti-inflammatory actions and is used in relapse and remitting disease.
- *Glatiramer*: immunomodulating drug.

Stroke

After heart disease and cancer, stroke is the third-biggest killer in the Western world. It is divided into:
- **ischaemic** or **thromboembolic stroke**: thrombus formation in the cerebral circulation leads to impaired blood flow and cerebral infarction. This constitutes about 85% of cases;
- **haemorrhagic stroke**: a burst blood vessel leads to bleeding within the brain. There may be swelling and impaired blood flow leading to infarction.

In both cases the death of brain cells leads to neurological deficits depending on which areas of the brain are affected.

Treatment: ischaemic stroke is managed by restoring blood flow by dissolving the thrombus using thrombolytic drugs that activate plasminogen to plasmin, which digests fibrin. Prevention may involve control of blood pressure, statins and use of anti-platelet (e.g. low-dose aspirin, clopidogrel) drugs to prevent thrombosis. Haemorrhagic stroke may require surgical repair and/or conservative measures.

Pain

This is a normal physiological response to damage or adverse stimuli. It involves transmission of noxious stimuli via pain fibres to the brain, where pain is 'perceived'.

Pathophysiology: tissue damage or inflammation involves a variety of mediators, which may enhance the stimulation of pain receptors. Prostaglandins derived from cyclooxygenase (Cox) enzymes are key mediators as they potentiate painful stimuli.

Migraine is a specific condition associated with severe headaches, which may be unilateral and throbbing, and lasts for 4–72h. There may also be vomiting, photophobia, phonophobia and sensitivity to movement. It is regarded as a neurovascular disease.

Neuropathic pain is a chronic condition where changes in neuronal function or the somatosensory system lead to innocuous stimuli leading to unpleasant sensations.

Treatment: pain management involves the use of analgesics as follows.
• *Non-steroidal anti-inflammatory drugs (NSAIDs)* (e.g. ibuprofen): these are Cox inhibitors that inhibit the production of prostaglandins.
• *Paracetamol*: is a simple analgesic with a poorly defined mode of action.
• *Opioids*: these are morphine-like substances which act at opioid receptors to hyperpolarise neurones and inhibit the transmission of pain in the spinal cord and act centrally to modify the perception of pain.
• *Local anaesthetics*: these block voltage-operated Na^+ channels in pain fibres and so inhibit action potential propagation and the conduction of pain (Chapter 19).
• *Migraine*: treated with analgesics and triptans (e.g sumatriptan). There are $5-HT_{1B/D}$ agonists that abort attacks by inhibiting the release of vasodilator neurotransmitters and constrict dilated arteries.
• *Neuropathic pain*: a number of anti-epileptic drugs and some anti-depressants are used.

Dementia

This is a broad area in which there is progressive impairment of cognitive function in which memory is primarily affected. There may also be behavioural changes.

Pathophysiology:
• **Alzheimer's disease** is the commonest form and involves a pathology of neurofibrillary tangles and neuronal loss.
• **Vascular dementia**: evidence of multiple infarcts.

Management: treatment of Alzheimer's disease has focused on attempting to improve cholinergic function, and acetylcholinesterase (AChE) inhibitors (e.g. galantamine) are used to prevent the breakdown of ACh and prolong its actions.

Depression

This is a common condition associated with low mood and negative thoughts.

Pathophysiology: this is poorly understood, but the commonest theory is the 'monoamine hypothesis', which states that depression is due to an alteration in central levels of noradrenaline and/or 5-hydroxytryptamine (5-HT) (serotonin).

Treatment: mild depression is thought to respond well to behavioural techniques such as cognitive behavioural therapy. Pharmacological treatment is used in more severe or refractory disease and aims to alter or restore brain chemistry. There is a time delay in pharmacological therapy (~2 weeks), which indicates that dug treatments have more complex effects that may be due to alterations in receptor functions and genomic effects. Commonly used antidepressants include the following.
• *Serotonin-selective reuptake inhibitors (SSRIs)* (e.g fluoxetine): these inhibit the cellular reuptake of 5-HT, leading to increased levels in the synaptic cleft. These increases in 5-HT levels are thought to lead to an alteration receptor populations and result in an improvement of symptoms.
• *Tricyclic antidepressants (TCAs)* (e.g. amitriptyline): these inhibit the neuronal uptake of both noradrenaline and 5-HT and are thought to lead to an alteration receptor populations and result in an improvement of symptoms. They also have a number of pharmacological actions, including antagonism of muscarinic, histamine and 5-HT receptors. The antimuscarinic side effects lead to blurred vision, dry mouth, urinary retention and constipation, which limits their use.

Bipolar affective disorder

This is characterised by periods of low mood with manic episodes (which may involve grandiose behaviour, impatience, aggression, excessive enthusiasm, psychomotor agitation).

Treatment: drugs are used to stabilise mood.
• *Lithium*: used for both treatment and prevention. Its mode of action is uncertain but it may interfere with intracellular signalling via inositol triphosphate.
• *Carbamazepine and valproate*: prophylactic mood stabilisers in bipolar disorder and lack the extrapyramidal effects of the antipsychotic drugs.
• *Antipsychotics* such as haloperidol and chlorpromazine: used to control psychotic symptoms.

Anxiety

While a physiological response to stress is normal, when this becomes pathological or the response happens to an apparently innocuous signal, then this becomes anxiety. There may be a central component coupled with somatic symptoms (e.g. tachycardia, palpitations, sweating) due to increased sympathetic activity. Anxiety covers a range of conditions, including panic attacks (which may involve marked symptoms with a fear of impending death), general anxiety disorder and phobias (e.g. social phobias).

Management: this can be symptomatic to relieve the symptoms of increased sympathetic activity and involves the use of β-adrenoceptor antagonists. Other pharmacological approaches include the following.
• *Benzodiazepines* (e.g. diazepam): these enhance the actions of the inhibitory neurotransmitter GABA at $GABA_A$ receptors and are used in the short term as anxiolytics.
• *SSRIs*: some of these antidepressants are used to manage anxiety disorders in the longer term.

Schizophrenia

Schizophrenia presents with psychotic symptoms similar to the manic phase of bipolar affective disorder. The symptoms are grouped as positive (auditory hallucinations, delusions, thought disorder and disorganised communication) or negative (reduced activity with emotional flattening, withdrawal from society and cognitive deficit).

Pathophysiology: poorly understood but based on response to drug treatment, the commonly accepted theory is one of overactivity of dopaminergic neurones in the cortex.

Treatment: pharmacological management is aimed at reducing symptoms and this is achieved by use of antipsychotic drugs
• *Antipsychotics* (e.g. chlorpromazine, haloperidol): these act via antagonism of dopamine D_2 receptors in the cortex. As a side effect they also block dopaminergic transmission in the nigrostriatal pathway and may lead to Parkinson-like symptoms.
• *Atypical antipsychotics* (e.g. risperidone, olanzapine): in addition to D_2 receptor antagonism they also block 5-HT receptors and are associated with fewer movement disorders.

James Lazenby and Chien-Yi Chang

Figure 58.1 The defining features of the major types of pathogens: Bacteria, Viruses, Fungi and Parasites.

This figure depicts some common pathogens with the appropriate scale. In the centre circle a not to scale cartoon illustrates some of the key features of the different types of pathogens. All bacteria have a peptidoglycan layer surrounding an inner membrane, but Gram-negative bacteria also have an external membrane. Some bacteria also have a tough polysacharide capsule for added protection from environmental stresses. Pili and flagella are used for attachment and motility. Bacteria make use of multiple secretion systems to release exotoxins, enzymes and other virulence factors. Lipoteichoic acid (LTA) and Lipopolysaccharide (LPS) are potent activators of innate immune responses. At their most basic, viruses are genetic material (DNA or RNA) surrounded by proteins arranged in regular structural repeating sub-units (the capsid). More complex viruses have an envelope made of a lipid bilayer supported by matrix proteins and studded with glycoproteins used for attachment and receptor mediated endocytosis. Fungi are highly varied but this simple schematic based on the *Candida* sp. illustrates the membrane bound organelles common to eukaryotic cells. *Candida* cells are able to reproduce by budding. Yeast cells possess fimbriae (or pili) for attachment and motility and adhesins that allow them to target specific host cells. They also possess secretory vesicles which can secrete virulence factors like proteases and phopholipases. Parasites can be divided into Protozoa (inside the circle) or the much larger Helminths (outside the circle).

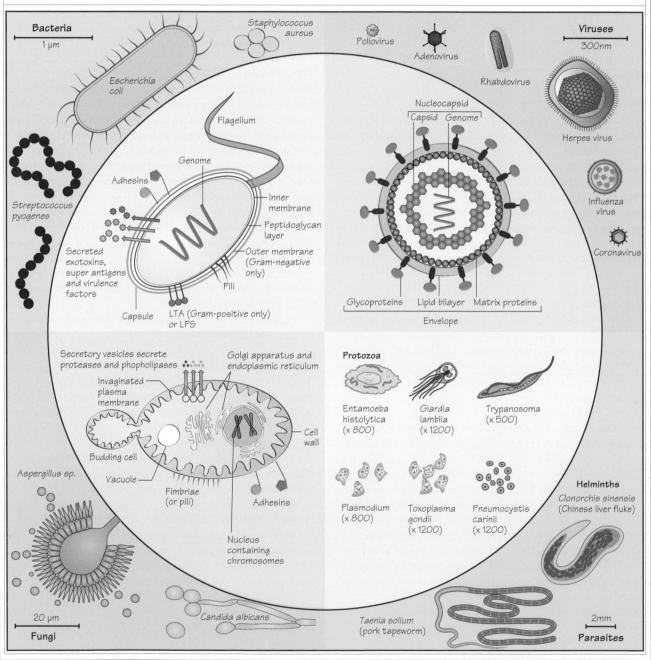

Microbes are widespread in the environment (Figure 58.1). Most of them are free-living and obtain their energy from light and the oxidation of inorganic or dead organic matter. In contrast, a **parasite** lives in or on a living host from which it obtains nourishment. Most parasitic microbes are called **commensal** or **normal** flora and are generally harmless or beneficial to human health. A **pathogen**, however, is any microbial agent that can cause disease in a host. Some microbes are able to invade into the tissues, overcome the host defences and cause disease. They are termed **primary pathogens**. When host defences are impaired or compromised, such as breaking the skin, commensal flora may cause disease and are referred to as **opportunistic pathogens**. The process of invasion of the body is called **infection** and the mechanism of causing infection is called **pathogenesis**. There are five steps to establishing a successful infection.

1 *Attachment and entry*: pathogens attach to the host whereby they gain entry.

2 *Dissemination and multiplication*: once attached or inside the host, the pathogens replicate in number and move away from the initial site of colonisation.

3 *Evasion*: hosts possess mechanisms to protect against pathogens and pathogens have evolved ways to circumvent these defences.

4 *Exit*: in order to continue their life cycle, pathogens also need to leave the original host and spread to fresh hosts. This is often in the normal secretions of the host such as saliva, mucus, or faeces.

5 *Damage*: damage to the host, either directly from the pathogen or as collateral damage from the host response to the pathogen, is often a consequence of pathogen infection.

To identify the organisms causing specific diseases Robert Koch, in 1890, set out criteria known as Koch's postulates.

1 The organism must be present in every case of the disease.

2 The organism must be isolated from diseased host and grown in pure culture.

3 The pure culture must be shown to induce the disease in an experimentally infected host.

4 The organism must be recoverable from the experimentally infected host.

These criteria were well established for living bacterial pathogens but their applicability to pathogens, such as viruses and prions, is problematic.

Bacteria

Bacteria are **prokaryotes** that possess **virulence determinants** for facilitating pathogenesis. For many pathogenic bacteria, colonisation of the host tissues is the initial step of infection and involves interaction between specific receptors on the host cell and different **adhesins** on the bacterial surface. For example, pili (or fimbriae) and flagella provide motility and adhesion in *Vibrio cholerae* and *Campylobacter jejuni*, while *Streptococcus mutans* produces an exopolysaccharide allowing it to adhere to teeth.

Pathogenic bacteria possess several mechanisms to avoid or neutralise host defence systems. For example, to avoid phagocytosis by macrophages *Neisseria meningitis* produces a thick extracellular polysaccharide capsule. *N. meningitidis* also avoids antibody-mediated immune responses by altering of the surface antigens which allows longer survival within a host and makes vaccine development difficult for these organisms.

Many bacteria cause tissue damages by producing toxins. **Endotoxin**, or **lipopolysaccharide** (LPS), a component of the outer membrane of **Gram-negative bacteria**, and **lipoteichoic acid** (LTA), a component of the cell wall of **Gram-positive** bacteria, are potent activators of immune and inflammatory responses. In contrast, **exotoxins** are secreted by pathogenic bacteria and have diverse effects on the host. Shiga toxin produced by *Shigella* inhibits the protein synthesis of host cell while *Staphylococcal* haemolysin forms lytic pores in blood cells.

James Lazenby and Chien-Yi Chang

Viruses

Viruses are **obligate intracellular parasites** and as such cannot make energy or proteins independently. Viruses exist in a latent state until interaction with the appropriate receptor on the host cell whereby they become incorporated. Once inside the cell the biochemical processes of the cell become co-opted to make more viral particles (the **virion**).

Viruses vary widely in size and complexity: at the most basic the virion is essentially the **genome** (either single- or double-stranded DNA or RNA) surrounded by structural proteins, enzymes and nuclear binding proteins (the **capsid**). This is referred to as the **nucleocapsid** and is released from the host cell when the cell lyses. The capsid protects the genetic material of the virus from many environmental challenges and allows these viruses to exist for a long time in the environment and pass through the gastrointestinal tract. Some viruses escape the cell by budding from the cell membrane. In this process, the virus particle is encapsulated in a protein matrix and a lipid bilayer studded with glycoproteins (the **envelope**). These glycoproteins have a variety of roles, such as aiding in attachment to the host cell (e.g. GP120 and GP41 in human immunodeficiency virus [HIV]) or as virulence factors (e.g. haemagglutinin and neuraminidase in influenza). Enveloped virions are very sensitive to inactivation and as such are generally passed from person to person by the exchange of fluids.

Viruses have many virulence mechanisms, mainly to evade host detection and eradication:

- sequestration
- blockade of antigen presentation
- cytokine evasion
- inhibition of apoptosis
- antibody evasion.

Viruses cause damage to the host by disruption of the host cell processes, or lysis of the host cells, or as a result of damage from a persistent and ongoing engagement of host inflammatory or immune responses. For example, HIV causes immunosuppression because its host cells are immune cells, which, when lysed or destroyed, leads to acquired immune deficiency syndrome (AIDS).

Fungi

Fungi are **eukaryotic** organisms, including yeasts and moulds, which occupy a diverse range of environmental niches, but only a small percentage are routinely associated with human disease. Most fungal pathogens are opportunistic and acquired from the environment (with the main exceptions being **dermatophytes** and *Candida albicans*). **Mycoses** (fungal infections) are separated according to the tissue depth of the initial colonisation. Systemic mycoses can affect many different tissues and are often internal, being inhaled into the lungs or spreading through mucosal sites on the body such as the female genital tract. In most cases, there needs to be some depletion of the host defences, such as disruption of the normal microbial flora, or immunosuppression or depletion (for example, pneumonia from *Aspergillus* sp. in chemotherapy patients, or *Pneumocystis jiroveci* pneumonia in those with AIDS). Pathogenic fungi can avoid clearance by killing the engulfing immune cell (e.g. *Candida albicans* can escape clearance by producing long hyphae, which skewer the engulfing macrophage), or avoiding phagocytosis (e.g. *Cryptococcus neoformans* produces a polysaccharide capsule). Damage to the host comes from the breakdown of host tissues by secreted proteases and lipases as well as the secretion of metabolites, such as alkaloids, which can cause acute organ damage.

Parasites

Medical parasitology relates specifically to invertebrate animals capable of causing disease.

- **Protozoa**: protozoa are simple unicellular microorganisms that range in size from 2 to 100 µm. They include amoebae, flagellates and ciliates. Included in this group are the agents responsible for malaria (*Plasmodium sp.*), toxoplasmosis (*Toxoplasmia gondii*) and leishmaniasis (*Leishmania sp.*).
- **Helminths**: metazoa are multicellular macroscopic parasites that include the helminths and arthropods. Helminths can be divided into nematodes (cylindrical-bodied worms such as hook worm or pin worm) and the platyhelminths (flat-bodied worms such as flukes and tapeworms).

Protozoan and helminth infections are virtually always acquired from an exogenous source and can enter the host in a myriad of ways, including oral ingestion (e.g. *Giardia lamblia*, which causes diarrhoea) and penetration though the skin, often via an arthropod vector (e.g. malaria is transmitted by female mosquitoes). The mechanisms by which these parasites attach are also highly varied, with some using adhesins and receptor-mediated attachment like many bacteria and viruses (e.g. *Leishmania mexicana* attaches via CR2 on host cells) and others using mechanical means (e.g. *G. lamblia* attaches using a ventrical disk that clamps on to the host intestinal epithelium). The mechanisms that cause the symptoms of disease are also different. While many protozoan pathogens secrete molecules such as phospholipases and proteases that directly damage the host cell membranes, pathologies from helminth infections are generally the result of the size and longevity of the parasite, which can disrupt host physiological functions, such as blocking bile ducts or compressing parts of the central nervous system. Many parasites utilise mechanisms common to bacterial species to avoid host immune responses, for example, the *Plasmodium* sp. can vary surface antigens, mimic host antigens, directly suppress immune responses and reside intracellularly within the host.

Prions

Prions are transmissible aberrant proteins. Prions are thought to cause a variety of spongiform encephalopathies in mammals, notably **Creutzfeldt-Jakob disease** (CJD) and Kuru in humans. It is thought that the normal cellular prion protein (PrP^c) exists in mammalian tissues and when it comes into contact with the misfolded isoform (PrP^{sc}), the normal version converts and thereby becomes resistant to degradation by proteases, leading to a build up of the aberrant protein, resulting in disease. While prions can be isolated from other tissues, only the brain shows evidence of pathology. It is thought that prions spread by ingestion or injection of brain tissue from contaminated individuals, although there is also a genetic mutation that leads to cases of familial prion disease. Because the prion protein is a host protein, no immune response is initiated and lack of an inflammatory response is a characteristic of prion disease.

Antimicrobial chemotherapy

Bacterial, fungal and viral infections pose significant morbidity and mortality to man and there are a number of drugs that are used to manage infections. Bacterial infections are managed by antibacterial drugs, which include antibiotics. These agents exploit differences between eukaryotic host cells and the prokaryotic bacteria. For example, penicillins target the formation of the bacterial cell wall (by inhibiting the transpeptidases responsible for cross-linking peptidoglycans) and macrolides target the bacterial ribosomes. Viral infections are more difficult to manage by targeting differences in biochemistry, but targets include viral DNA polymerases, neuramidases and HIV reverse transcriptases. Tables 58.1 and 58.2 contain some examples of antimicrobial agents, their modes of action and common usages.

Table 58.1 Commonly used antibacterial agents and their modes of action and uses

Antibacterial agents	Mode of action	Uses
Penicillins, e.g. amoxicillin, phenoxymethyl penicillin, flucloxacillin	Inhibition of cross-linking of peptide side chains	Phenoxymethyl penicillin: tonsillitis. Flucloxacillin: impetigo, cellulitis. Amoxicillin: chest infections, otitis media, UTIs
Cephalosporins, e.g. cefalexin, cefotaxime, cefaclor	Binding to beta-lactam-binding sites and inhibiting cell wall synthesis	Septicaemia, pneumonia, meningitis, biliary tract infections, peritonitis, UTIs
Tetracylines, e.g. tetracycline, doxycycline	Inhibition of protein synthesis, through interfering with tRNA binding	*Chlamydia*, exacerbation of chronic bronchitis (*Haemophilus influenzae*), periodontal disease, acne, respiratory and genital *Mycoplasma* infections. Doxycycline in malaria prophylaxis
Macrolides, e.g erythromycin, clarithromycin	Prevent the translocation movement of the bacterial ribosome along the mRNA and prevent protein synthesis	Suitable alternative in patients who are allergic to penicillin. Respiratory infections, whooping cough, Legionnaires' disease, *Campylobacter* enteritis
Aminoglycosides, e.g gentamicin	Irreversibly bind to the bacterial ribosomes leading to an inhibition of protein synthesis	Gentamicin is used in various infections such as septicaemia, meningitis, acute pyelonephritis and endocarditis
Sulphonamides and trimethoprim	Inhibition of folate synthesis and reduces the precursors of DNA and RNA	Pneumonia in AIDS patients, toxoplasmosis and nocardosis. Acute exacerbation of chronic bronchitis, otitis media and UTIs
Quinolones, e.g. ciprofloxacin, ofloxacin	Inhibition of bacterial DNA gyrase	*Pseudomonas aeruginosa, Haemophilus influenzae, Campylobacter*

Table 58.2 Commonly used antiviral and antifungal agents and their modes of action and uses

Anti-infective agent	Mode of action	Uses
Antiviral, e.g. aciclovir, famciclovir, zanamivir.	Aciclovir: inhibition of herpes virus DNA polymerase. Zanamivir: a neuramidase inhibitor that prevents the entry and release of the viral particles from the host cells	Aciclovir: herpes simplex and herpes varicella. Zanamivir: influenza
Imidazoles, e.g. clotrimazole	Inhibition of P450-dependent demethylase, which converts lanosterol to ergosterol; the accumulation of lanosterol disrupts fungal membrane	Fungal infections
Triazoles, e.g. itraconazole, fluconazole	As for imidazoles	Fungal infections
Other antifungal agents: griseofulvin, terbinafine	Terbinafine inhibits the conversion of squalene to lanosterol, with the accumulation of squalene causing cell death. Griseofulvin: interferes with fungal microtubules and nucleic acid synthesis	Griseofulvin: suitable for tinea infections but not candidiasis

Recognition of pathogens

Lucy Fairclough and Ian Todd

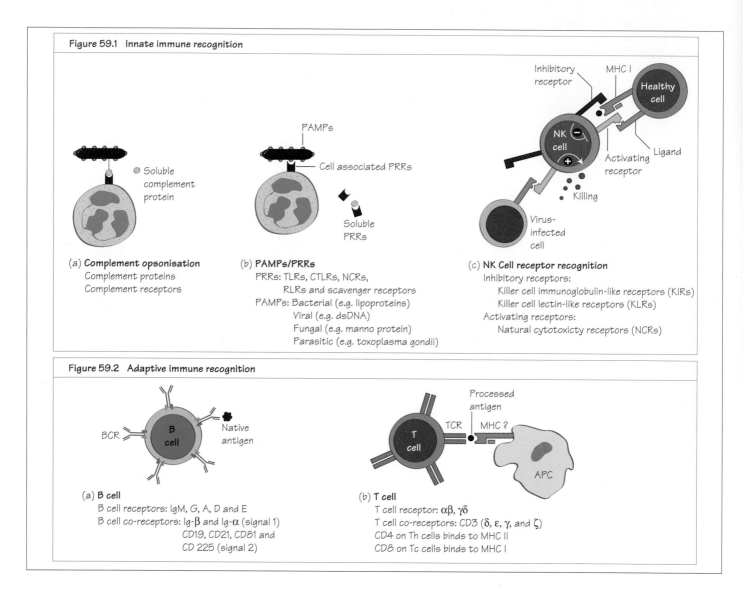

Figure 59.1 Innate immune recognition

(a) **Complement opsonisation**
Complement proteins
Complement receptors

(b) **PAMPs/PRRs**
PRRs: TLRs, CTLRs, NCRs,
     RLRs and scavenger receptors
PAMPs: Bacterial (e.g. lipoproteins)
       Viral (e.g. dsDNA)
       Fungal (e.g. manno protein)
       Parasitic (e.g. toxoplasma gondii)

(c) **NK Cell receptor recognition**
Inhibitory receptors:
     Killer cell immunoglobulin-like receptors (KIRs)
     Killer cell lectin-like receptors (KLRs)
Activating receptors:
     Natural cytotoxicty receptors (NCRs)

Figure 59.2 Adaptive immune recognition

(a) **B cell**
B cell receptors: IgM, G, A, D and E
B cell co-receptors: Ig-β and Ig-α (signal 1)
                    CD19, CD21, CD81 and
                    CD 225 (signal 2)

(b) **T cell**
T cell receptor: αβ, γδ
T cell co-receptors: CD3 (δ, ε, γ, and ζ)
CD4 on Th cells binds to MHC II
CD8 on Tc cells binds to MHC I

The major functions of the immune system are the recognition of pathogens by interacting with microbes and their components, and defence of the body by the elimination of microbes and their components. **Immune recognition** and **defence** are achieved in two ways: by components of the immune system that generate **innate immunity**, and others that generate **adaptive immunity**.

The main features of innate immunity are that it is quickly activated when infection occurs; it remains the same on repeated exposure to the same microbe and is moderately efficient. The main features of adaptive (also known as acquired) immunity are that it is more slowly activated, but its efficacy improves on repeated exposure to the same microbe. Once activated, adaptive immunity is highly efficient and provides specific responses tailored to each individual type of microbe.

Innate recognition

Innate immunity provides a general response to categories of microbe and is triggered by the recognition of both **complement proteins** that have **opsonised** the pathogen, and chemical structures that are characteristic of microbes (termed **pathogen-associated molecular patterns** [PAMPs]). Further recognition is achieved by receptors expressed on **natural killer** (NK) cells.

Complement opsonisation (Figure 59.1(a))

Complement is the name for a collection of about 30 proteins found in the circulation and in tissue fluids that were initially described by their ability to 'complement' the effects of antibodies. Various complement proteins act as activation enzymes, defence molecules and regulatory proteins. Activation of complement proteins is triggered by infection by pathogens and immune activation, and occurs as a cascade or chain reaction with amplification built in. Once activated, fragments of complement bind to the surface of the pathogen, effectively 'opsonising' the pathogen so it can be seen by cells of the immune system expressing complement receptors (such as macrophages).

Pathogen-associated molecular patterns (PAMPs) and pathogen recognition receptors (PRRs) (Figure 59.1(b))

Chemical structures that are characteristic of microbes are often termed pathogen-associated molecular patterns (PAMPs), e.g. bacterial lipopolysaccharide and viral double-stranded RNA. These PAMPs interact with pattern recognition receptors (PRRs) expressed by cells (e.g. **toll-like receptors [TLRs], C-type lectin receptors [CTLRs], NOD-like receptors [NLRs], RIG-like helicase receptors [RLRs]** and scavenger receptors) or soluble PRRs. Cell-associated PRRs enable phagocytosis of PAMPs and associated microbes, activation of cells and consequent release of inflammatory mediators to amplify the immune response. Soluble PRRs can directly attack the microbe and enhance phagocytosis of PRR bound PAMPs, as well as activating the proteolytic cascade resulting in lysis of the microbe.

Cell receptor recognition (Figure 59.1(c))

NK cells recognise target cells via a large repertoire of activating and inhibitory receptors in an antigen non-specific manner and are therefore able to act quickly. There are three main classes of receptor on NK cells: **killer cell immunoglobulin-like receptors (KIRs)** and **killer cell lectin-like receptors (KLRs)** that are largely inhibitory and detect levels of HLA class I, and **natural cytotoxicity receptors** (NCRs) that are exclusively activating receptors. Healthy cells constitutively express HLA class I molecules that bind to inhibitory receptors on the NK cell surface, thereby blocking any stimulatory receptor signalling. However, if HLA class I expression is reduced, when a virus is attempting to avoid detection, this inhibitory signalling is absent and the cell will be killed. Equally, if a cell is under stress and up-regulates the expression of HLA class IB-like molecules such as MIC-A and MIC-B, activating signals, via the NKG2D receptor for example, override inhibitory signalling in the NK cell and the target cell will be killed.

Adaptive recognition

Adaptive immunity involves recognition of **antigens** specific to each type of microbe that are recognised by antigen receptors that are clonally expressed by **lymphocytes**. Thus lymphocytes are the cell type responsible for the properties of adaptive immune recognition.

B cell receptor (BCR) (Figure 59.2(a))

The antigen recognition receptors expressed by B cells are surface immunoglobulins (sIg) that specifically bind native antigens to the B cell surface. All the sIg molecules expressed by a single B cell have identical antigen-combining sites, i.e. a single B cell is specific for a single antigen epitope. When a B cell binds an antigen to its sIg and becomes activated, it differentiates into a plasma cell that secretes antibodies (soluble immunoglobulins) with the same combining sites

(i.e. the same antigenic specificity) as the sIg: thus a B cell produces antibodies that recognise the antigen it originally bound.

The body contains millions of families or **clones** of B cells, each expressing Ig with a different antigen-combining site. Thus an antigen will interact with those clones whose sIg bind it with highest affinity (**clonal selection**). Activation of the B cells that bind antigen results in their proliferation, thus increasing the number of B cells of the specific clones, and some of these are maintained in the body as **memory cells**. However, sIg only has a tail region of three amino acids so cannot signal into the cell. For this reason the BCR does not just contain sIg but also Igβ (CD79b) and Igα (CD79a), which enables signalling. For a B cell to become fully activated, probably as a safeguard mechanism, they require a second signal. One such form of co-stimulation is the BCR co-receptor complex that can engage with molecules such as complement that may be on the same target surface (i.e. a bacterium). The BCR co-receptor consists of CD19, CD21 (CR2), CD81 and CD225.

If the same antigen enters the body again, it will interact specifically with these memory cells, which are reactivated more rapidly and in larger numbers than in the primary response, hence giving the faster and bigger response that characterises adaptive immunity.

T cell receptor (Figure 59.2(b))

The antigen recognition receptors expressed by T cells are called **T cell receptors (TCRs)** and are composed of two polypeptide chains (α and β chains or occasionally γ and δ chains). There is no secreted form of the TCR, i.e. T cells do not produce an equivalent to antibodies secreted by B cells.

Both the α and β chains of the TCR are anchored in the surface membrane. Each chain is about the same size as an immunoglobulin light chain. Indeed, the TCR α and β chains are each composed of two immunoglobulin-like domains with strong structural homologies with immunoglobulin domains; for this reason, the TCR is said to be a member of the immunoglobulin superfamily. In each chain, the domain proximal to the membrane is constant in structure between T cells (C_α and C_β), whereas the domains distal to the membrane are variable in structure between T cells (V_α and V_β) and form a single antigen-combining site; thus the TCR has one antigen-combining site, whereas sIg on B cells has two.

The main function of T cells is to do things to other cells of the body in the context of an immune response. Some T cells, called **T helper (Th)** cells, help other cells of the immune system to fulfil their functions, e.g. Th cells activate B cells to produce antibodies, and stimulate the phagocytic and killing activity of macrophages. Other T cells, called **T cytotoxic (Tc)** cells, kill tissue cells that have become infected by microbes.

The TCR of T cells cannot interact directly with microbes and their antigens, but bind only to fragments of antigenic proteins (i.e. antigen peptides) associated with tissue cells, thereby targeting the T cells to mediate their helper or cytotoxic activities against these cells. Cells that present antigen peptides that T cells can bind to are termed **antigen presenting cells (APC)**. In the cytoplasm of APCs, microbial proteins are broken down into peptides, and some of these antigen peptides than associate with specialised peptide-binding proteins that hold the peptides on the APC surface where they are available to interact with the TCR of T cells. In humans, the antigen-binding proteins are called **HLA** proteins (**human leucocyte antigens**); more generally, in humans and other species, they are termed **MHC** proteins (**proteins of the major histocompatibility complex**).

60 Defence against pathogens

Lucy Fairclough and Ian Todd

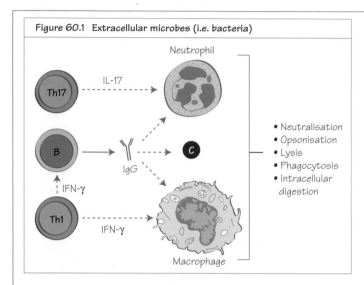

Figure 60.1 Extracellular microbes (i.e. bacteria)

Neutrophil

- Neutralisation
- Opsonisation
- Lysis
- Phagocytosis
- Intracellular digestion

Macrophage

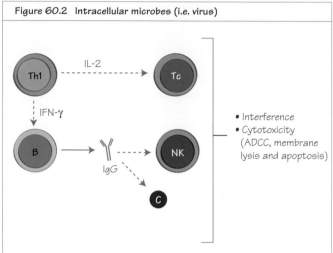

Figure 60.2 Intracellular microbes (i.e. virus)

- Interference
- Cytotoxicity (ADCC, membrane lysis and apoptosis)

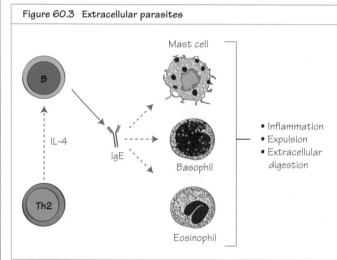

Figure 60.3 Extracellular parasites

Mast cell

- Inflammation
- Expulsion
- Extracellular digestion

Basophil

Eosinophil

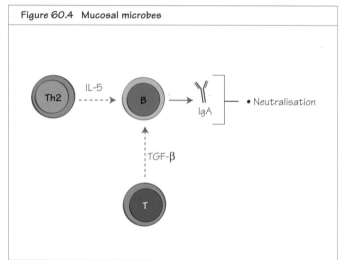

Figure 60.4 Mucosal microbes

- Neutralisation

Immune defence is achieved by components of the immune system that generate innate immunity, and others that generate adaptive immunity. The body is exposed to numerous classes of microbes and the immune system has to manage these different threats to the body. Furthermore, differences in nature, mode of entry, mechanisms of replication and spread in the body of different infective agents mean that a range of defensive mechanisms is necessary.

Extracellular microbes (e.g. bacteria)

(Figure 60.1)

Innate immune defence is mediated by various cell types, including **leucocytes** (e.g. neutrophils) and epithelial cells. These cells produce antimicrobial peptides called **defensins** that are directly damaging to certain microbes.

With regard to the adaptive immune response, B cells secrete antibodies (mainly IgG) that may have defensive effects simply by binding to antigens, e.g. neutralising the activities of bacterial toxins or viruses. Antibodies can also act as intermediaries to activate other defensive components that interact with the **Fc** regions of antibodies. Thus IgM and IgG antibodies can activate the complement system of proteins and virtually all cells of the immune system express Fc receptors (FcR).

Macrophages and neutrophils are phagocytes that engulf microbes and digest them intracellularly. Macrophages are tissue-resident cells derived from blood monocytes; neutrophils circulate in the blood and are recruited into sites of infection and inflammation. The acute phase proteins **C-reactive protein** and **mannose-binding lectin** can opsonise bacteria for uptake by macrophages and neutrophils, and also activate complement.

Macrophages and neutrophils recognise microbes using either pattern recognition receptors (PRRs), or receptors for complement (CR) or antibodies (FcR). This interaction triggers phagocytosis, with the microbe being internalised into a membrane-bound vesicle called a phagosome. Cytoplasmic lysosomes that contain digestive enzymes then fuse with the phagosome, releasing the digestive enzymes on to the surface of the microbe and bringing about its degradation. In addition, the phagocyte produces reactive oxygen species that enter the phagosomes, helping in the degradation and producing a pH appropriate for the activity of the digestive enzymes.

T cells, specifically CD4 T helper cells, play an important role in coordinating and driving the most appropriate immune response. Th17 cells, characterised by secretion of interleukin-17, support neutrophil function, CD4 Th1 cells secrete interferon-gamma supporting macrophage function, whereas.

Intracellular microbes (e.g. viruses)

(Figure 60.2)

Viruses do not have the metabolic machinery for self-replication and so must infect cells in order to replicate. Some defensive strategies of the immune system are directed against free virus particles, destroying them directly or neutralising their ability to infect cells. Other strategies are directed at the infected cells, either blocking virus replication or killing the infected cells.

Strategies directed at intracellular viruses include a combination of mechanisms that target the intracellular phases of virus infection. The early innate response by **interferons** and natural killer (NK) cells limits the growth and spread of the infection. The adaptive response by CD8 cytotoxic T cells takes longer to activate, but its high efficiency may be sufficient to clear the infection.

Virus infection triggers the infected cells to produce and secrete type 1 **interferons** (IFN-α and IFN-β). These bind to receptors on neighbouring cells and trigger an antiviral state in which these cells are resistant to virus replication. This is because interferons induce enzymes that degrade viral mRNA and inhibit protein synthesis. Type 1 interferons also enhance expression of HLA class I, thereby making cells better targets for CD8 cytotoxic T cells, and activate natural killer cells.

NK cells have two mechanisms of recognising cells as targets for killing. The first involves a large repertoire of activating and inhibitory receptors (Chapter 59). The other involves IgG antibodies binding to native viral antigens expressed on the surface of infected cells; NK cells express Fc receptors for IgG that can then bind to the antibodies, thus attaching them to the surface of the infected cells, which they can then kill – this is termed antibody-dependent cellular cytotoxicity (ADCC).

Although NK cells and Tc cells employ different mechanisms to identify virus-infected cells as targets for killing (Tc cells recognise HLA class I-associated peptides (Chapter 59), these two types of killer cell use similar mechanisms to bring about target cell destruction. There are two types of killing mechanism that the killer cells employ,

both of which result in the induction of target cell apoptosis. The killer cells possess granules that contain two types of protein, which are released on to the target cell surface: the **perforins** are similar to the C9 complement protein of the membrane attack complex. They are inserted into the target cell's surface membrane and facilitate uptake of the **granzymes**, which gain entry to the target cell cytoplasm where they activate **caspase** enzymes that initiate the apoptosis pathways. The Tc cells also express a surface protein called Fas-ligand that interacts with Fas protein on the target cell surface; this interaction also activates the apoptosis pathways.

Extracellular parasites (e.g. helminths)

(Figure 60.3)

Extracellular parasites are too large to be engulfed by phagocytes or killed by CD8 cytotoxic T cells and NK cells. They are removed by generating an inflammatory response through the actions of eosinophils, mast cells and basophils. This removal is mediated by IgE, an immunoglobulin isotype produced by B cells.

Eosinophils can mediate extracellular digestion. They express FcR that bind IgG or IgE, and they also express complement receptors. Thus opsonisation of a parasitic worm by antibodies and C3b facilitates binding of numerous eosinophils to the parasite surface. Eosinophils have cytoplasmic granules containing a range of digestive proteins, e.g. major basic protein and eosinophil cationic protein; these are released on to the surface of the parasite to bring about extracellular digestion.

Mast cells are tissue cells that express high affinity-FcR that bind IgE antibodies from surrounding tissue fluid. Thus mast cells become coated with IgE antibodies and therefore acquire the antigenic specificities of these antibodies. When an antigen specifically binds simultaneously to two or more IgE antibodies on a mast cell surface (i.e. the antigen cross-links or bridges the IgE), this triggers the release of inflammatory mediators. Release of inflammatory mediators by mast cells can be similarly triggered by the complement activation peptides C3a and C5a (these peptides also attract and activate neutrophils at sites of inflammation).

Mast cells contain numerous granules in which are stored preformed inflammatory mediators (e.g. histamine, heparin, tryptase); these are released immediately upon mast cell triggering. Mast cell activation also induces the synthesis of newly formed mediators that are released over a longer period of time, e.g. leukotrienes and prostaglandins derived from arachidonic acid, and cytokines.

Mucosal microbes

Mucosal microbes are neutralised by the actions of IgA, an immunoglobulin isotype produced by B cells. IgA is present in blood and internal tissue fluids as a monomer. The dimeric IgA is transported across mucosal epithelium into the mucosal secretions of the gastrointestinal, respiratory and genitourinary tracts. This occurs because of an IgA-binding receptor (the poly-Ig receptor) expressed by mucosal epithelial cells; part of this receptor remains attached to the secreted IgA dimer and is called secretory piece. IgA is also secreted by the mammary gland into milk, and so mother's IgA is transferred to confer protection in the gut of suckling infants. B cells produce IgA under stimulation by IL-5 (produced by CD4 T helper type 2 cells) or TGF-β (produced by CD4 T regulatory cells).

Integration of the immune response

Lucy Fairclough and Ian Todd

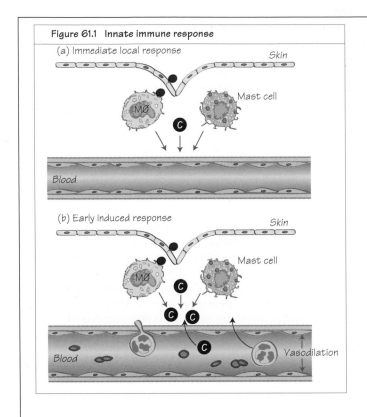

Figure 61.1 Innate immune response

(a) Immediate local response

Skin

MØ

Mast cell

Blood

(b) Early induced response

Skin

MØ

Mast cell

Blood

Vasodilation

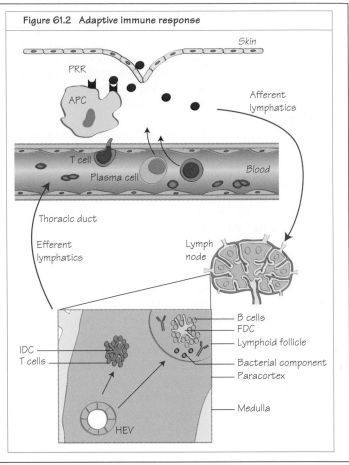

Figure 61.2 Adaptive immune response

Skin

PRR

APC

Afferent lymphatics

T cell

Plasma cell

Blood

Thoracic duct

Efferent lymphatics

Lymph node

B cells
FDC
Lymphoid follicle
Bacterial component
Paracortex

Medulla

IDC
T cells

HEV

The immune system works to generate appropriate responses for removal of pathogens that invade the body. Innate immunity is quickly activated when infection occurs but remains the same on repeated exposure to the same pathogen and is only moderately efficient. Adaptive immunity is more slowly activated due to the requirement for information about the invading pathogen to be taken to naïve T and B lymphocytes in the local secondary lymphoid tissues (e.g. lymph nodes). However, once activated it provides specific responses tailored to each individual type of pathogen.

Innate immunity (Figure 61.1)
Immediate local response (Figure 61.1a)
The first infection by a particular microbe generates a primary immune response. This normally requires pathogens to penetrate surface epi-

thelial barriers of the body, e.g. the epidermis. An immediate local innate response in the infected tissues is generated by components of the immune system resident in those tissues (e.g. macrophages, mast cells and complement proteins). This also generates inflammatory mediators (augmented by the activation of mast cells) that attract further leucocytes and serum proteins into the infected tissues from the bloodstream.

Macrophages are phagocytes that engulf (phagocytose) microbes and digest them intracellularly. Macrophages are tissue-resident cells derived from blood monocytes that phagocytose bacteria using pathogen recognition receptors (PRRs) and after opsonisation with the acute phase proteins: C-reactive protein and mannose-binding lectin. These acute phase proteins can also activate complement, causing generation of the complement peptides C3a and C5a (see below).

Mast cells contain numerous granules in which are stored pre-formed inflammatory mediators. Mast cell activation also induces the synthesis of newly formed mediators that are released over a longer period of time, e.g. leukotrienes and prostaglandins derived from arachidonic acid, and cytokines. Release of these inflammatory mediators can be triggered by the complement activation peptides C3a and C5a, which can also attract and activate neutrophils at sites of inflammation.

Early induced response (Figure 61.1b)

Activation of mast cells (as above) causes release of inflammatory mediators that attract further leucocytes and serum proteins into the infected tissues from the bloodstream. These inflammatory mediators cause vasodilatation that increases the volume of blood reaching the tissues and reduces the rate of blood flow so that leucocytes, especially neutrophils, move more slowly through the blood. In conjunction, there is increased **vascular permeability** that facilitates the movement of neutrophils and complement proteins into the infected tissues. Movement of neutrophils through the tissue to the site of infection is achieved by chemotaxis, with immobilisation and activation when the site of infection is reached.

Chemotaxis involves the directional movement of cells in response to chemical signals (chemoattractants). For example, chemokines produced by activated cells (e.g. macrophages) at the site of infection diffuse through the tissue and bind to receptors, where they impinge on the 'leading edge' of neutrophils. This stimulates new integrin expression at the leading edge of the cell so that it forms new contacts with tissue cells or connective tissue components. Old integrin contacts at the trailing edge of the cell are gradually lost, so the cell moves up the concentration gradient of chemokine towards the site of infection.

Neutrophils, like macrophages, are phagocytes that engulf microbes and digest them intracellularly. However, unlike macrophages they circulate in the blood and are only recruited into tissues during infection and inflammation.

Adaptive immunity (Figure 61.2)

While the above innate response is being generated, antigens are carried from the site of infection to local secondary lymphoid tissues (e.g. **lymph nodes**) in order to generate an adaptive immune response. Some antigens are carried free in the lymph, and some are captured by specialised cells called **antigen-presenting cells** (**APCs**), which are present in most tissues of the body. These APCs migrate to the lymphoid tissues carrying the antigens with them via the afferent lymphatics. In the lymphoid tissues, the antigens activate naïve T and B lymphocytes that specifically recognise them (which will be only a few of all the lymphocytes in these tissues). The specifically activated lymphocytes and antibodies (produced by the B lymphocytes) can then recirculate back to the site of infection. In the tissues, APCs' main function is antigen capture, and in lymphoid tissues, it is antigen presentation.

During the process described above, antigen in the form of immune complexes preferentially localises to **follicular dendritic cells** (**FDCs**) in the B cell-containing follicles or germinal centres. Antigen transported by APCs is presented to CD4 T helper cells in the paracortex which come into close contact with the APCs that become interdigitating dendritic cells (IDC). These T cells then assist in the generation of B lymphoblasts, which then migrate in to the follicle (together with some T cells), where they undergo further maturation and selection through interaction with FDCs in germinal centres. Specific T and B lymphocytes then leave the lymph nodes via the medulla and efferent lymphatics to enter the blood via the thoracic duct.

Once in the blood the effector T and B lymphocytes traffic around the body to the site of infection. Within inflamed tissues, the endothelial cells lining blood vessels are activated by inflammatory mediators to express adhesion molecules that facilitate the adhesion of leucocytes to the blood vessel walls and their migration across the walls. The initial interactions (called capture and rolling) are mediated by selectins (E-selectin and P-selectin expressed by the endothelium, and L-selectin expressed by leucocytes) that bind to highly glycosylated proteins (mucins). This facilitates the interaction of the leucocytes with chemokines on the surface of the endothelium that trigger activation of adhesion molecules called integrins expressed by leucocytes. The integrins form strong interactions with the endothelial cells by binding to ligands called intercellular and vascular cell adhesion molecules (ICAM and VCAM); this is called the activation and flattening stage.

Leucocytes bound to the endothelium pass between adjacent endothelial cells (facilitated by the loss of tight junctions between endothelial cells), again using integrin interactions; this is termed extravasation. As discussed above, the cells move through the tissue by chemotaxis (the directional movement of cells in response to chemical signals) where they assist in removal of the pathogen.

If re-infection with the same type of pathogen occurs soon after the response above, then pre-formed antibodies and effector B and T lymphocytes will be available immediately. A later re-infection will generate a secondary immune response by memory lymphocytes formed during the primary response; these give a faster and bigger response than occurred in the primary response, hence the term adaptive immunity.

In addition to the local inflammatory effects at the site of infection, a body-wide response to infection also occurs, termed the **acute phase response**. This is mediated primarily by systemic effects of the cytokines **interleukin-1**, **interleukin-6** and **tumour necrosis factor**, that are variously produced by activated macrophages, lymphocytes, mast cells and other activated cells. They affect various tissues around the body when released into the bloodstream at significant concentrations. Collectively, these cytokines induce fever by effects on the hypothalamus, promote increased levels of circulating leucocytes (leucocytosis) by release from the bone marrow, and stimulate the liver to produce antimicrobial acute phase proteins such as **C-reactive protein** and **mannose-binding lectin**.

Ian Todd and Lucy Fairclough

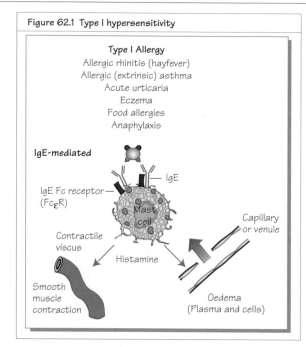

Figure 62.1 Type I hypersensitivity

Type I Allergy
Allergic rhinitis (hayfever)
Allergic (extrinsic) asthma
Acute urticaria
Eczema
Food allergies
Anaphylaxis

IgE-mediated

IgE Fc receptor — (FcεR)
IgE
Mast cell
Contractile viscus
Histamine
Capillary or venule
Smooth muscle contraction
Oedema (Plasma and cells)

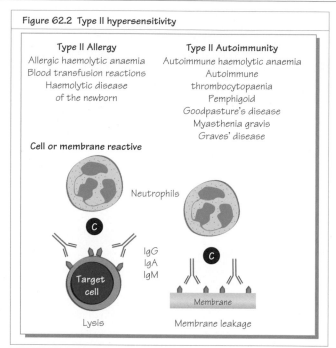

Figure 62.2 Type II hypersensitivity

Type II Allergy
Allergic haemolytic anaemia
Blood transfusion reactions
Haemolytic disease of the newborn

Type II Autoimmunity
Autoimmune haemolytic anaemia
Autoimmune thrombocytopaenia
Pemphigoid
Goodpasture's disease
Myasthenia gravis
Graves' disease

Cell or membrane reactive

Neutrophils
IgG IgA IgM
Target cell
Membrane
Lysis
Membrane leakage

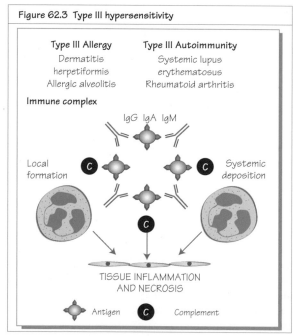

Figure 62.3 Type III hypersensitivity

Type III Allergy
Dermatitis herpetiformis
Allergic alveolitis

Type III Autoimmunity
Systemic lupus erythematosus
Rheumatoid arthritis

Immune complex

IgG IgA IgM
Local formation
Systemic deposition
TISSUE INFLAMMATION AND NECROSIS
Antigen   Complement

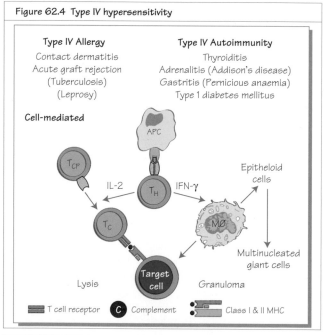

Figure 62.4 Type IV hypersensitivity

Type IV Allergy
Contact dermatitis
Acute graft rejection
(Tuberculosis)
(Leprosy)

Type IV Autoimmunity
Thyroiditis
Adrenalitis (Addison's disease)
Gastritis (Pernicious anaemia)
Type 1 diabetes mellitus

Cell-mediated

APC
T$_{CP}$
IL-2   T$_H$ IFN-γ
Epitheloid cells
T$_C$
MØ
Multinucleated giant cells
Lysis
Target cell
Granuloma
T cell receptor   Complement   Class I & II MHC

Diseases that involve tissue damage as a consequence of inappropriate adaptive immune responses can be categorised on the basis of either the source of the stimulating antigens (allergy or autoimmunity) or the consequent mechanisms of tissue damage involved (hypersensitivity mechanisms types I–IV).

Adaptive immunity to infection involves recognition of foreign (microbial) antigens and damage to the foreign microbes. **Allergy** is a consequence of inappropriate activation of adaptive immunity by non-infective foreign antigens (allergens) resulting in damage to tissues. In **autoimmunity**, tissue damage results from activation of autoreactive lymphocytes that recognise self-tissue components as autoantigens.

Type I hypersensitivity – atopic allergy
(Figure 62.1)
This involves IgE antibodies and mast cells: '**atopy**' refers to a propensity for production of high levels of IgE. Allergen-specific IgE molecules, bound to Fcε receptors on mast cells, are cross-linked by specific allergens, triggering release of preformed inflammatory mediators by degranulation (e.g. histamine) and synthesis of newly formed mediators (e.g. leukotrienes and prostaglandins). These mediators induce inflammation and smooth muscle contraction.

T_H2 **cells** play a central role in the induction type I hypersensitivity, e.g. by secretion of IL-4 that stimulates IgE production by B cells, and IL-5 that stimulates eosinophils. The immediate elicitation phase of a type I hypersensitivity response is generated by mast cell activation, whereas T_H2 cells and eosinophils can be implicated in the late phase reaction that can result in chronic tissue damage.

Different types of atopic disorder are induced by different types of allergen and routes of exposure.
• Allergic rhinitis is commonly triggered by pollen allergens that activate mast cells in the upper respiratory tract – hence the name 'hay fever'.
• Wheezing associated with allergic asthma involves bronchial constriction in the lower respiratory tract, often caused by an allergic response to house dust mite constituents.
• Food allergens may cause local symptoms in the gut (e.g. vomiting, diarrhoea), but once absorbed into the bloodstream may have wider effects, e.g. skin reactions (urticaria, eczema) or potentially life-threatening systemic effects (anaphylaxis) as exemplified in severe nut allergies.
• There are no clear examples of autoimmune diseases that involve type I hypersensitivity.

Type II hypersensitivity – cell or membrane reactive (Figure 62.2)
This involves IgG, IgA, or IgM antibodies that bind to cell surface membranes or connective tissue components. These induce damage by activating complement and/or triggering neutrophils to release digestive products and reactive oxygen species.

Allergic haemolytic anaemia can be induced by drugs that bind to erythrocytes and if antibodies are generated against these drugs, then erythrocyte lysis can result; similarly, autoimmune haemolytic anaemia involves autoantibodies specific for erythrocyte surface autoantigens, and autoimmune thrombocytopaenia involves autoantibody-induced platelet destruction. Naturally occurring antibodies to blood group antigens expressed by erythrocytes (e.g. anti-A and anti-B antibodies) can cause life-threatening reactions to incompatible blood transfusions. The main cause of haemolytic disease of the newborn is maternal IgG antibodies to the rhesus D antigen expressed by the erythrocytes of a D-positive fetus developing in a D-negative woman; these IgG antibodies cross the placenta from the mother to the fetus and cause destruction of fetal erythrocytes.

Autoantibodies to basement membranes cause tissue damage to the skin in pemphigoid (skin epidermal basement membrane) and Goodpasture's disease (kidney glomerular basement membrane).

A special case of type II hypersensitivity (sometimes called type V) involves autoantibodies to membrane-associated receptor proteins.

Myasthenia gravis can involve autoantibodies specific for the acetylcholine (ACh) receptors expressed on muscle cells at the neuromuscular junction (Chapter 22). These autoantibodies block binding of ACh released from nerve endings, and also induce internalisation and degradation of receptors. This results in extreme muscle weakness due to a lack of nerve stimulation of muscle contraction. In Graves' disease, autoantibodies specifically bind to the TSH receptor expressed by thyroid follicular cells and stimulate thyroid hormone production. The action of these 'thyroid-stimulating antibodies' is not regulated (as is TSH itself), leading the overproduction of thyroid hormones and hyperthyroidism (Chapter 47).

Type III hypersensitivity – immune complex disease (Figure 62.3)
This involves numerous soluble antigens and antibodies cross-linking to form a lattice structure known as an **immune complex** (IC) that may precipitate out of solution and/or become lodged in tissues. Immune complexes can activate complement and neutrophils leading to tissue damage.

An example is allergic alveolitis caused by production of antibodies to inhaled fungal spores. Immune complex formation in the walls of the alveoli leads to inflammation and fibrosis. This results in breathlessness due to poor gas exchange across the alveolar walls (as distinct from the wheezing in asthma that is due to constriction of the bronchi). Dermatitis herpetiformis is a skin condition associated with gluten-sensitive gut inflammation (coeliac disease) and involves IgA antibody-containing immune complex deposition.

In the autoimmune disease systemic lupus erythematosus (SLE), autoantibodies are produced to a range of ubiquitous cellular constituents, particularly nuclear components. Among these antinuclear antibodies (ANA) are autoantibodies specific for DNA. Autoantigen/autoantibody immune complexes form in SLE (e.g. DNA/anti-DNA). These deposit in various tissues, causing tissue damage, e.g. in kidney glomeruli, in the skin, joints and central nervous system.

In rheumatoid arthritis much of the damage occurs in joints. Some of this damage is due to immune complexes formed by rheumatoid factors, which are IgM and IgG autoantibodies that are themselves specific for IgG.

Type IV hypersensitivity – cell-mediated hypersensitivity (Figure 62.4)
This involves activation of helper T cells (principally T_H1 **cells**) by their interaction with antigen-presenting cells. The activated T_H1 cells secrete cytokines, e.g. interleukin-2 that can activates T_C cells and interferon-gamma that can activate macrophages (and possibly lead to their dedifferentiation into epithelioid cells and fusion to form multinucleate giant cells). Reactions of this type are seen in the chronic phases of the mycobacterial infections that cause tuberculosis and leprosy.

Contact allergens that induce a **type IV hypersensitivity** reaction seen clinically as contact dermatitis include metals (e.g. nickel, chromium) and plant products (e.g. poison ivy).

In a number of autoimmune diseases the target cells are destroyed principally through the activity of autoreactive T cells.
• Hashimoto's thyroiditis (Chapter 47).
• Addison's disease (adrenalitis) (Chapter 48).
• Pernicious anaemia (Chapter 33).
• Type 1 diabetes mellitus (Chapter 46).

63 Immunodeficiency disorders

Ian Todd and Lucy Fairclough

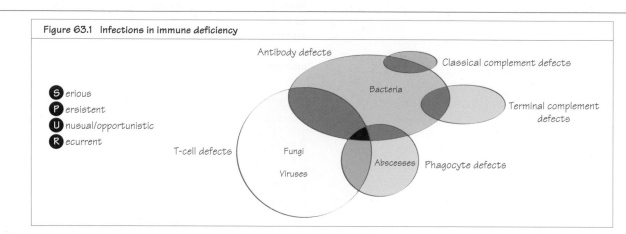

Figure 63.1 Infections in immune deficiency

Antibody defects
Classical complement defects
Bacteria
Terminal complement defects
T-cell defects
Fungi
Viruses
Abscesses
Phagocyte defects

(S)erious
(P)ersistent
(U)nusual/opportunistic
(R)ecurrent

Figure 63.2 Neutrophil functional defects

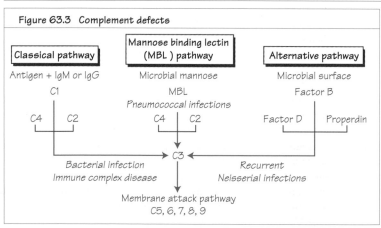

Leucocyte adhesion deficiency
Killing
Chemotaxis
Respiratory burst
Bacteria
Phagocytosis
Chronic granulomatous disease

Figure 63.4 Lymphocyte defects

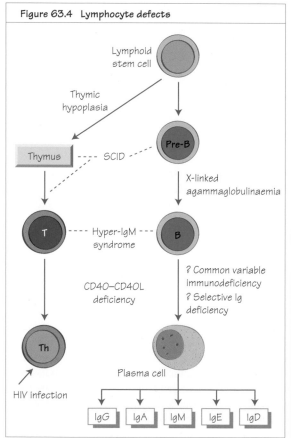

Lymphoid stem cell
Thymic hypoplasia
Thymus
SCID
Pre-B
X-linked agammaglobulinaemia
T
Hyper-IgM syndrome
B
CD40–CD40L deficiency
? Common variable immunodeficiency
? Selective Ig deficiency
Th
Plasma cell
HIV infection
IgG | IgA | IgM | IgE | IgD

Figure 63.3 Complement defects

Classical pathway	Mannose binding lectin (MBL) pathway	Alternative pathway
Antigen + IgM or IgG	Microbial mannose	Microbial surface
C1	MBL	Factor B
	Pneumococcal infections	
C4 C2	C4 C2	Factor D Properdin

C3

Bacterial infection
Immune complex disease

Recurrent
Neisserial infections

Membrane attack pathway
C5, 6, 7, 8, 9

Medical Sciences at a Glance, First Edition. Edited by Michael D Randall. © 2014 John Wiley & Sons, Ltd. Published 2014 by John Wiley & Sons, Ltd.

The nature of immunodeficiency disorders (Figure 63.1)

Immunodeficiency refers to defective immune function that leads to increased susceptibility to infection. These disorders are categorised as primary or secondary.

Primary immunodeficiencies are usually due to inherited mutations in genes with immunological functions. They are mainly very rare conditions. **Secondary immunodeficiencies** are acquired as a consequence of environmental insults and/or as a consequence of other disease processes.

Immunodeficiencies are characterised by infections that tend to be **s**erious, **p**ersistent, **u**nusual (opportunisitic), **r**ecurrent – giving the acronym **SPUR** (Figure 63.1).

The types of infection that occur often reflect the nature of the defects in immune components (Figure 63.1). Thus, bacterial infections are often associated with deficiencies in antibodies, complement, or phagocytes (the latter also leads to abscess formation); T cell defects often involve viral or fungal infections.

Phagocyte defects (Figure 63.2)

Primary deficiencies can affect phagocytes (particularly neutrophils) at various levels, e.g. production, adhesion, chemotaxis and killing activity (intracellular digestion).

Neutrophils are the most plentiful type of white blood cell (50–70% of leucocytes), but are short-lived (about 5 days, but only 1–2 days when activated), and produced in the bone marrow in enormous numbers (about one million per second). Thus any suppression of neutrophil production can have a dramatic effect with greatly increased risk of infection. Defects in neutrophil production can be primary (e.g. Kostmann's disease; cyclic neutropenia), or secondary to other disease processes (e.g. leukaemia, infection) or treatment with antiproliferative cancer chemotherapy.

Two examples of rare primary defects in the function of mature neutrophils are:

- **leucocyte adhesion deficiency** – lack of expression of leucocyte integrins that are necessary for the adhesion of leucocytes (including neutrophils) to activated endothelial cells at sites of infection/inflammation; thus neutrophils cannot migrate from the circulation into infected tissues;
- **chronic granulomatous disease**, which involves defects in enzymes involved in the generation of reactive oxygen species. In this case, neutrophils can migrate to sites of infection but are inefficient at killing pathogens; this generates sites of indolent infection and neutrophil accumulation (known as granulomas).

Complement deficiencies (Figure 63.3)

The complement system of proteins (Chapters 62 and 63) can be activated by three different pathways that coalesce at the activation of the C3 protein. The **Classical Pathway** is activated when C1 protein binds to complexes of antigen with IgG or IgM antibodies. Defects of the Classical Pathway and C3 are also associated with immune complex disease. This is because immune complexes (see type III hypersensitivity in Chapter 62) activate the classical pathway (by binding C1q), leading to C3b association with the complexes. This facilitates binding of immune complexes to complement receptors on erythrocytes and removal of the complexes by liver macrophages. This immune complex clearance cannot happen if there are defects in C1, C2, C3, or C4 resulting in a tendency for immune complexes to accumulate.

Mannose-binding lectin (MBL) is an acute phase protein that can activate the complement system when it binds to microbial polysaccharides. MBL deficiency is particularly common (3% of the population) and is associated with pneumococcal, and other bacterial, infections.

The **Alternative Pathway** is activated when C3b (derived from C3) binds to microbial surfaces and associates with factor B. All three pathways of complement activation result in cleavage of C3 and activation of the Membrane Attack Pathway; the membrane attack complexes (generated from C5–9) damage the lipid membranes of microbes. Neisserial infections are associated especially with defects in the Alternative and Membrane Attack Pathways.

B lymphocyte and antibody deficiencies

Some primary antibody deficiencies inhibit the generation of mature B cells, e.g. X-linked agammaglobulinaemia due to mutations affecting Bruton's tyrosine kinase enzyme. Other primary antibody deficiencies are due to defects in B cell activation and maturation and/or B cell interaction with helper T cells; some become manifest in adults rather than children (e.g. common variable immunodeficiency); they are under diagnosed with the possibility of irreversible tissue damage due to repeated chronic infections (e.g. bronchiectasis) if untreated (e.g. by immunoglobulin replacement).

Selective immunoglobulin deficiencies include IgA deficiency, which is the most common primary immunodeficiency, affecting about 1/600 of the population. Hyper-IgM syndrome is due to defects in immunoglobulin class switching, and includes deficiency of CD40 or CD40-ligand expression, which is required for effective interaction between helper T cells and B cells.

There are several secondary causes of antibody deficiency, including **lymphoproliferative disease**, renal/gut loss of IgG, malnutrition and immunosuppressive drugs.

T cell defects and severe combined immunodeficiencies (SCID) (Figure 63.4)

A number of immunodeficiency disorders affect mainly T cells. A rare primary T cell deficiency occurs in DiGeorge syndrome, which involves impaired development of the thymus and other tissues in the face/neck/chest due to a defect in fetal development.

Adaptive immunity is broadly affected in SCID, leading to generalised susceptibility to infection (bacterial, viral, fungal), essentially from birth. There are many types of primary defect associated with SCID; the most common mutation affects expression of the receptors for the cytokines interleukin-2, 4, 7, 9, 15 and 21. Other types of defect include mutations in genes required for generating T cell and B cell antigen receptors, and in expression of HLA proteins. SCID is often only treatable by bone marrow transplantation (and gene therapy in some cases).

Acquired immunodeficiency syndrome (AIDS) is a well-known secondary T cell immunodeficiency caused by infection with human immunodeficiency virus (HIV). The virus can be transmitted by sexual intercourse; sharing infected needles; infected blood or blood products; from mother to baby at birth or via breast milk.

HIV infects T cells, dendritic cells and macrophages because the surface glycoprotein (gp120) of the virus binds to the **CD4 protein** expressed by these cell types. Dendritic cells pick up the virus in epithelia and transfer it to T cells in lymphoid tissues; CD4 T cells are then the major source of HIV throughout infection.

HIV replicates in activated CD4 T cells and, consequently, lymphoid tissue is the major reservoir of HIV. Infected dendritic cells and macrophages can spread the infection to other tissues (e.g. brain). After the acute phase of infection an immune response by CD8 T cells, CD4 T cells and NK cells contains (but does not clear) the infection; the infection becomes chronic and virus mutation leads to escape from immunological recognition and gradual depletion of the body's CD4 T cells. AIDS develops as CD4 T cells numbers fall below 200/μL of blood (less than 20% of normal levels) and susceptibility to multiple opportunistic infections ensues.

Although a vaccine against HIV is not yet available, **highly active antiretroviral therapy** (HAART) of infected individuals with combinations of reverse transcriptase and protease inhibitors can be very effective in reducing viral loads to undetectable levels, with dramatic improvements in life expectancy.

64 Cancer

Stuart Brown

Figure 64.1 The cell cycle

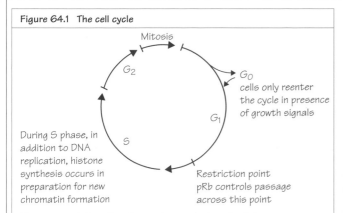

During S phase, in addition to DNA replication, histone synthesis occurs in preparation for new chromatin formation

The stages of the cell cycle are shown. The length of the arrows in each phase gives an approximation of the time taken by each stage i.e if the cell divides in 24 hours S phase is approximately 8 hours and M phase 1–1.5 hours. In addition to pRB control of passage through G_1, p53 is responsible for controlling passage through G_1, G_2 and M phases

---

Figure 64.3 Function of oncogene products

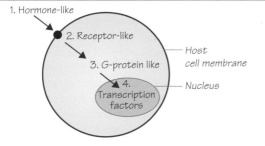

Think! What could stimulate cell division?
Oncogene products mimic the various factors which can cause cell division. They can be (1) hormone-like (e.g. the v-sis oncogene codes for platelet-derived growth factor, (2) receptor-like (e.g. the v-erb B product mimics a modified epidermal growth factor receptor which behaves as if the ligand is always attached, (3) G protein-like (the ras oncogene product mimics the alpha subunit of a trimeric G protein. Point mutations in the ras gene can lead to loss of the GTPase activity necessary to switch the signal off following activation and (4) transcription factors (e.g. the c-myc gene codes for a transcription factor)

Figure 64.2 Cell transformation by RNA tumour virus

(a)   RNA genome
5'–RU$_1$–gag–pol–env–(src)–U$_2$R–3'

Reverse transcription

U$_2$RU$_1$ gag   pol   env   (src)   U$_2$RU$_1$
(LTR)   (LTR)

(b) (i) Sarcoma type

DNA proviral genome

| | GAG | POL | ENV | SRC | | Host |

LTR
Strong promoter

LTR

Expression

Host chromosome

(ii) Leukaemia type   DNA proviral genome

LTR

LTR

Host proto-oncogene

Expression

(a) Following RNA tumour virus infection the RNA genome is reverse transcribed into a double stranded DNA copy. During this process the ends of the genome are modified to produce long terminal repeat sequences which contain all the elements necessary for promoting transcription

(b) The proviral DNA copy of an RNA virus integrates at random into a host chromosome.
(i) The strong promoter activity in the leftward LTR guarantees the viral genes, including the sarcoma gene in the sarcoma viruses, will be transcribed. (ii) Leukaemia virus do not contain an oncogene. However, the rightward LTR will cause over expression of genes close to the viral insert. If a previously silent host proto-oncogene is in that location it will be over-expressed

---

Figure 64.4 Sequential changes to oncogenes and tumour suppressor genes during the formation of colon cancer

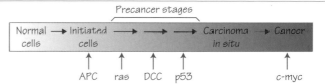

Although the order of the events can vary the first event is usually loss of the APC (apoptosis poyposis coli) tumour suppressor gene on chromosome 5 (5q21). Loss of this controlling gene can trigger polyp formation. Cells in each polyp will contain the abnormal gene. Thus there is a much larger population of 'initiated' cells and hence a much greater chance that one of these cells will undergo further mutagenic events

---

Normal cell growth is controlled by the cell cycle. A series of events ensures a cell grows and divides to produce two identical daughter cells when necessary. Cells enter the cell cycle when instructed by extracellular growth signals. In the absence of these signals cells can enter a special phase known as G_0. Cells in this stage are often referred to as being differentiated and will often be synthesising proteins specific to their cell type. Cells in G_0 may be instructed to enter cell division by extracellular signals.

Tumour cells are derived from normal cells. Genetic changes in normal cells can alter the behaviour of those cells. Thus cancer is a genetic disease. It is very common in the Western world. Approximately 1 in 4 people will be diagnosed with cancer in their lifetimes. One thousand people a day are diagnosed with cancer; that's one every 2 minutes.

The cell cycle (Figure 64.1)

When a cell is instructed to divide by an extracellular growth signal it enters into the cell cycle. The events are divided into four phases.

• *G1 phase:* cells will check the environment to ensure sufficient nutrients are available to sustain growth. They also check the integrity of the DNA molecules for any damage. There is a specific point, the **restriction point** or R point, through which a cell will not pass if DNA damage is detected.

• *S phase:* the DNA present in the chromosomes is replicated.

• *G2 phase:* the integrity of the replicated DNA is checked and the cell prepares for mitosis.

• *M phase:* in the **mitotic phase** chromosomes condense and the cell divides to produce two daughter cells each containing a faithful copy of the parental DNA.

Oncogenes

RNA tumour viruses can cause cancer in humans. Two broad classes of RNA tumour virus exist: acute acting, originally called sarcoma viruses, and those that act in a chronic manner, called leukaemia viruses. They have an RNA genome that is reverse transcribed by **RNA-dependent DNA polymerase** (Figure 64.2a) into a proviral double-stranded DNA molecule that integrates into a host chromosome after the virus infects a host cell. New virus components are synthesised and new virus particles assemble at the cell membrane and bud from the host cell, thus the host cell is not lysed by new viral growth.

The RNA virus genome contains genes essential for growth. The genes are called **gag, pol**, and **env genes** (Figure 64.2b). The gag gene codes for the core viral proteins ('gag' actually stands for 'group-specific antigen'. The viruses were identified using antibodies to detect the core proteins and divided into groups according to which antibodies detected them). The 'pol' gene codes for the viral-specific reverse transcriptase enzyme and the 'env' gene codes for the viral envelope proteins. Sarcoma viruses were also found to contain another gene, called 'src' for sarcoma gene. This gene is known as an **oncogene** as it can be responsible for initiating the cell transformation process.

Different viral oncogenes are present in different sarcoma viruses. Surprisingly, genes similar to these are found in our human genome. They are termed **proto-oncogenes** and are usually silent in differentiated cells. Cells infected by sarcoma virus produce viral oncoproteins that initiate cancer cell formation. However, cell transformation can also be initiated by the presence of a leukaemia-type RNA tumour virus. If the replicated DNA copy of an RNA viral genome integrates next to a silent host oncogene it can cause it to be overexpressed. The reverse transcription process generates identical sequences at both ends of the proviral DNA not originally present in the viral RNA, called long terminal repeats (LTRs). These sequences contain elements that promote transcription, i.e. strong promoter regions and enhancer regions.

There are many different types of oncogene now known, coding for a variety of different gene products; they can activate cell division or inhibit apoptosis (Figure 64.3). The different types of gene product can be divided into five major groups.

• *extracellular growth signals*, e.g. v-sis gene product from the Simian sarcoma virus mimics platelet-derived growth factor;

• *growth factor receptors*, e.g. the v-erb B gene product from the erythroblastosis virus mimics the epidermal growth factor receptor, except that it acts as if a ligand is constantly bound;

• *G protein-like*, e.g. ras (**rat** sarcoma) oncogene product. One of the first oncogenes to be discovered in humans. When stimulated, G proteins become active by binding GTP. This is immediately broken down by a GTPase activity, present in the protein, to limit the signal. Point mutations in many oncogene products of this type result in the loss of GTPase and hence the growth signal is always on;

• *transcription factors*, several oncogene products mimic transcription factors and switch on growth genes;

• *cancer may result from the absence of cell death*. Alteration of gene expression involved in programmed cell death, apoptosis, will lead to excess cell mass, e.g. overexpression of bcl-2 or mutation of bax genes can alter apoptosis.

Tumour suppressor genes (TSG)

Originally termed antioncogenes as they oppose the action of oncogenes, tumour suppressor genes have two primary functions: they act to regulate passage through the cell cycle (hence the term 'gatekeeper genes') and they can help maintain DNA integrity (hence the term 'caretaker genes'). These genes are usually recessive, i.e. inactivation or loss of both alleles is necessary to lose their function. The retinoblastoma gene (pRB, 13q14) was identified from studies on families with children who developed retinoblastoma. From this the **'2-hit' hypothesis** was developed, which stated that children may develop the disease in two ways: either they lose both pRb genes early in life or they may have inherited only one normal pRb gene and hence only have to lose the function of that gene in one cell. The latter group develop the tumours earlier in life and often in both eyes. These properties are mimicked in other common tumours such as breast cancer. Women who inherit an abnormal breast cancer gene, BRCA1 or 2, will develop the disease earlier in life and often in both breasts. Clearly it is far more likely to lose one normal gene from a population of cells containing one normal gene than two normal genes in the same cell.

The pRB gene product controls passage through the restriction point in G_1 (Figure 64.1). It is crucial for normal cell cycle control, and in its absence cells will cycle inappropriately. In the presence of appropriate extracellular growth signals, pRb is gradually hyperphosphorylated during the G_1 phase and this initiates events leading to S phase.

TSG activity may be lost by loss of the protein product rather than loss of gene expression. DNA tumour viruses produce proteins which can interact with TSG proteins and prevent their action. This explains how cervical carcinoma can be caused by a papilloma viral infection (HPV). Two early gene products produced by the virus not only bind to the pRB protein, but degrade it. Hence the cell behaves as if it has lost the pRb gene and loses cell cycle control.

p53 (17p13) is a TSG that has a major impact on the incidence of human cancer. p53 genes are mutated or deleted in more than 70% of all human tumours. p53 displays both gatekeeper and caretaker activities. It is responsible for monitoring cell cycle restriction points and is also involved in monitoring DNA integrity and regulating DNA repair when necessary. It is responsible for halting passage through G_1 if DNA is damaged, for example (Figure 64.1). Levels of p53 are strictly maintained in normal cells.

Cancer formation

Cancer is a genetic disease but it is not caused by a single gene defect. Normal cells accumulate mutations and deletions in oncogenes and TSGs until they are sufficient to transform the cell. Cancer cells may contain tens of mutations when fully developed. TSGs such as p53 are responsible for maintaining DNA integrity and repair. A cell that cannot repair DNA will accumulate many more mutations than one with a normal DNA repair system.

Cancer is not caused by a single gene defect. Colon cancer has been extensively studied with regard to the types of mutation that occur during cancer development and is representative of many other tumours. The stages that the normal cells undergo are (Figure 64.4):
- **hyperplasia**: increase in normal cell number;
- **metaplasia**: transformation of one cell type into another that would not normally be in that tissue;
- **dysplasia**: alteration of the size, shape and organisation of the cells;
- **pre-invasive cell formation**: polyp formation;
- **neoplasia**: literally new growth. Neoplasia is used to mean abnormal new growth or cancer.

The cells that develop into a primary tumour as a result of mutations will continue to accumulate more mutations. As a result, individual cells in the primary tumour may develop properties that allow them to leave the primary site and invade through a basement membrane into lymph and blood vessels (intravasation). They then travel through the bloodstream until they find a new site to colonise (extravasation). This is the process of metastasis. The formation of secondary tumours at distant sites from the primary is probably responsible for approximately 90% of cancer deaths.

Michael D Randall

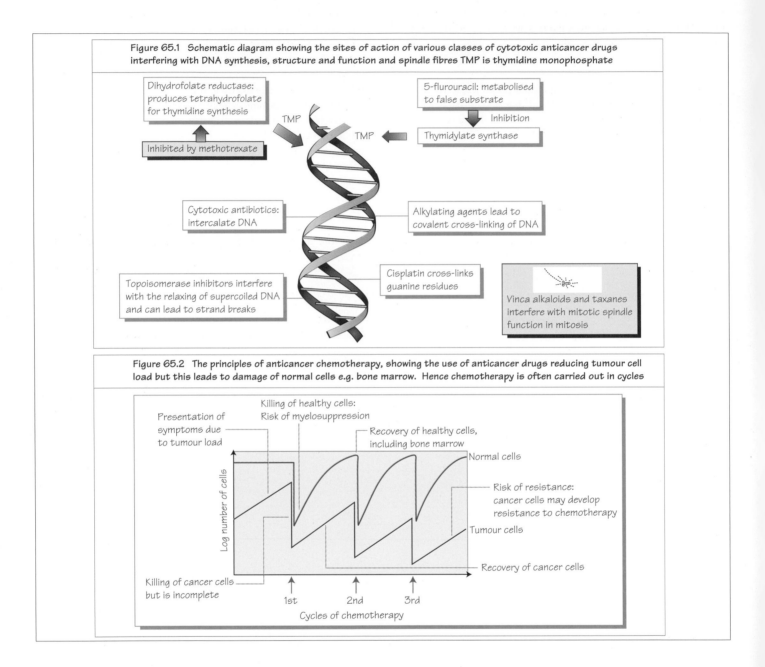

Figure 65.1 Schematic diagram showing the sites of action of various classes of cytotoxic anticancer drugs interfering with DNA synthesis, structure and function and spindle fibres TMP is thymidine monophosphate

Dihydrofolate reductase: produces tetrahydrofolate for thymidine synthesis

Inhibited by methotrexate

TMP

TMP

5-flurouracil: metabolised to false substrate

Inhibition

Thymidylate synthase

Cytotoxic antibiotics: intercalate DNA

Alkylating agents lead to covalent cross-linking of DNA

Topoisomerase inhibitors interfere with the relaxing of supercoiled DNA and can lead to strand breaks

Cisplatin cross-links guanine residues

Vinca alkaloids and taxanes interfere with mitotic spindle function in mitosis

Figure 65.2 The principles of anticancer chemotherapy, showing the use of anticancer drugs reducing tumour cell load but this leads to damage of normal cells e.g. bone marrow. Hence chemotherapy is often carried out in cycles

Presentation of symptoms due to tumour load

Killing of healthy cells: Risk of myelosuppression

Recovery of healthy cells, including bone marrow

Normal cells

Risk of resistance: cancer cells may develop resistance to chemotherapy

Tumour cells

Recovery of cancer cells

Killing of cancer cells but is incomplete

Log number of cells

1st   2nd   3rd

Cycles of chemotherapy

Anticancer chemotherapy is used to manage a range of cancers and may be used to reduce the size of a tumour or prevent the spread of cancer via **metastasis**. In the case of haematological cancers, anticancer chemotherapy may be used to reduce the cancerous cell load prior to bone transplantation (in certain leukaemias) or eradicate the disease (in certain lymphomas).

Chemotherapy works on the principle of **cytotoxicity**, in which chemicals are used to kill cells, and many of the agents target rapidly dividing cells by attacking the biochemical processes associated with DNA replication and cell division (Figure 65.1). Therapeutically, this leads to the killing of **rapidly dividing cells**, which is often a characteristic of cancer cells. However, this also results in damage to rapidly dividing 'normal' cells such as epithelial cells and bone marrow cells. The latter adverse effect leads to **myelosuppression** and results in anaemia, reduced platelet counts (risk of bleeding) and reduced white cells counts (risk of infection). Myelosuppression is usually the key limiting factor and so chemotherapy is often carried out in cycles, in which the patient receives a dose of chemotherapy to kill the cancer cells and there is then a delay of typically 3 weeks before the next dose, as this allows the bone marrow time to recover (Figure 65.2). By carrying out the treatment in cycles there is a substantial reduction in cancer cell load, followed by a period to allow recovery of the bone marrow. During this time the cancer cells remaining can proliferate, but the next cycle brings about another substantial reduce in cancer cell load and this is repeated. Anticancer drugs are classed by the site and mode of action.

Antimetabolites

These interfere with the synthesis of purines and /or pyrimidines.
• **Dihydrofolate reductase (DHFR) inhibitors** (e.g. methotrexate): act by inhibition of DHFR, which is the enzyme that catalyses the conversion of dihydrofolate to tetrahydrofolate. This results in the inhibition of synthesis of the nucleoside thymidine, which is essential for DNA synthesis. These are regarded as antifolate agents.
• **Pyrimidine analogues** (e.g. 5-flurouracil): 5-flurouracil is metabolised to fluorodeoxyuridine monophosphate, which is a false substrate that inhibits thymidylate synthase and so prevents the conversion of dUMP to thymidine monophosphate TMP required for DNA synthesis.
• **Purine analogues** (e.g. 6-mercaptopurine) are activated by hypoxanthine phosphoribosyltransferase to toxic metabolites and inhibit the synthesis of purines essential for DNA and RNA.

Chemical modification of DNA

• **Alkylating agents** (e.g. cyclophosphamide): these are highly reactive agents that chemically modify DNA by alkylation, which leads to the covalent cross-linking of DNA and so interferes with DNA replication, transcription and repair.
• **Platinum compounds** (e.g. cisplatin): cause cross-linking of guanine residues, resulting in DNA damage.
• **Cytotoxic antibiotics**: these chemically interact with DNA via intercalation.
  • In the case of doxorubicin the intercalation between DNA bases prevents the actions of topoisomerase II (which normally relaxes DNA supercoils) and so prevents transcription. This also leads to DNA fragmentation and inhibition of repair.
  • Mitomycin is a bifunctional alkylating agent that cross-links DNA and causes damage.

Topoisomerase inhibitors (e.g. etoposide)

• Topoisomerases are a group of enzymes that 'relax' supercoiled DNA, an essential step in DNA replication. Topoisomerase inhibitors complex with topoisomerase II and DNA, leading to a break in the DNA strand. This leads to inhibition of DNA replication and RNA transcription.

Mitotic inhibitors

These are important for the process of cell division and may be targeted by:
• **vinca alkaloids** (e.g. vincristine): these inhibit mitotic spindle formation by inhibition of tubulin polymerisation;
• **taxanes** (paclitaxel): these stabilise the spindles by inhibiting depolymerisation and so prevent mitosis.

Clinically, the above anticancer drugs are often used in combination, such that drugs with different sites of action are used. This means that lower doses can be used to limit toxicity and also reduce the risk of resistance, which can complicate the use of anticancer chemotherapy.

Targeted therapy

Recent advances in our understanding of cancer have led to newer, more selective approaches.
• **Oestrogen receptor antagonists** (e.g. tamoxifen): some breast cancer cells are sensitive to oestrogen and in patients with oestrogen-sensitive cancers tamoxifen is used to inhibit the oestrogen-dependent activation of these cells.
• **Aromatase inhibitors**: these prevent the conversion of androgens to oestrogen via aromatase and so have anti-oestrogenic effects. Once again these are beneficial in oestrogen-sensitive breast cancers.
• **Trastuzumab**: a monoclonal antibody that targets the human growth factor receptor-2 (HER2) and is used in metastatic breast cancers that express the HER2.
• **VEGF antibodies** (e.g. bevacizumab): these target vascular endothelial growth factor that is associated with angiogenesis, which leads to neovascularisation (and therefore nutrient supply) to tumours. Therefore agents interfere with the formation of blood supply to tumours.
• **Rituximab**: this is a monoclonal antibody against CD-20, which is a cell surface marker on leukocytes associated with non-Hodgkin's lymphoma.
• **Tyrosine kinase inhibitors** (e.g. imatinib): chronic myeloid leukaemia (CML) is associated with the abnormal Philadelphia chromosome codes for the *bcr-abl* protein. This protein has tyrosine kinase activity and so promotes cell proliferation. Therefore tyrosine kinase inhibitors selectively interfere with proliferation in the mutant cells. Imatinib is used in the chronic phase of CML and leads to better patient outcomes compared with the use of conventional chemotherapy and bone marrow transplantation.
• **Epidermal growth factor (EGF) tyrosine kinase inhibitors** (e.g. erlotinib): these interfere with signalling associated with cell activation. Therefore these agents target mutant cells expressing this specific tyrosine kinase activity, e.g. erlotinib is used in some lung and pancreatic cancers.

Adverse effects

Many of the anticancer drugs have severe toxic effects. As described above, meylosuppression is inevitable with cytotoxic agents and this can be overcome by using colony-stimulating factors (CSFs), which can promote the synthesis of certain white cell lines in haemopoiesis (Chapter 33). Nausea and vomiting is also a very common adverse effect and is associated with certain agents. This may be managed with anti-emetic drugs that target either peripheral afferent nerves or the central effects of toxins in the chemoreceptor trigger zone in the brain. Such anti-emetic drugs include histamine H_1 receptor antagonists, dopamine receptor antagonists and 5-HT$_3$ receptor antagonists.

Resistance to chemotherapy

Anticancer chemotherapy may fail due to the development of resistance. Modes of resistance include:
• increased efflux of drug from the cells through increased expression of multidrug resistance 1 (MDR1);
• increased DNA repair, especially for alkylating agents and cisplatin;
• loss of hormone-dependent cell growth.

Appendix 1: Cross references to *Medicine at a Glance (Davey)*

Chapter in *Medical Sciences at a Glance*	Clinical relevance and significant chapters in *Medicine at a Glance*	
Medical Sciences at a Glance, 1ˢᵗ edition (Randall, 2014)	*Medicine at a Glance*, 3rd edition (Davey, 2010)	*Medicine at a Glance*, 4ᵗʰ edition (Davey, 2014)
Part 1 Cellular structure and function		
Chapter 1 Cells		
Chapter 2 Organisation of cell membranes		
Chapter 3 Cell organelles		
Chapter 4 Protein biochemistry	Alzheimer's disease (Chapter 197) Prion diseases (Chapter 197)	Alzheimer's disease (Chapter 204) Prion diseases (Chapter 204)
Chapter 5 Lipid biochemistry	Hyperlipidaemia (Chapter 80)	Hyperlipidaemia (Chapter 82)
Chapter 6 Carbohydrate biochemistry	Glycation (Chapters 151 and 152)	Glycation (Chapters 156 and 157)
Chapter 7 Basic mechanism of drug action	Adverse drug reactions (Chapter 231)	Adverse drug reactions (Chapter 243)
Part 2 Cellular metabolism		
Chapter 8 General principles of cellular metabolism		
Chapter 9 Enzymes		
Chapter 10 Central metabolic pathways		
Chapter 11 Fat metabolism	Ketoacidosis (Chapters 138 and 152)	Ketoacidosis (Chapters 143 and 157)
Chapter 12 Glucose metabolism	Type 1 diabetes mellitus (Chapters 151 and 152) Type 2 diabetes mellitus (Chapters 151 and 152)	Type 1 diabetes mellitus (Chapters 156 and 157) Type 2 diabetes mellitus (Chapters 156 and 157)
Chapter 13 Amino acid metabolism		
Part 3 Molecular and medical genetics		
Chapter 14 Principles of molecular genetics		
Chapter 15 DNA and RNA		
Chapter 16 Gene expression		
Chapter 17 Medical genetics		
Part 4 Nerve and muscle		
Chapter 18 Cell excitability	Hyperkalaemia (Chapter 136) Hypokalaemia (Chapter 136)	Hyperkalaemia (Chapter 141) Hypokalaemia (Chapter 141)
Chapter 19 Nervous conduction		
Chapter 20 Synaptic transmission		
Chapter 21 Autonomic nervous system		
Chapter 22 Neuromuscular transmission	Myasthenia gravis (Chapter 203)	Myasthenia gravis (Chapter 210)
Part 5 Respiratory system		
Chapter 23 Structure of the respiratory system		
Chapter 24 Respiratory physiology	Chest X-ray (Chapter 99)	Chest X-ray (Chapter 102)
Chapter 25 Gas transport		
Chapter 26 Control of breathing		
Chapter 27 Acid-base physiology	Arterial blood gases (Chapter 98) Disorders of acid-base balance (Chapter 138)	Arterial blood gases (Chapter 100) Disorders of acid-base balance (Chapter 143)

Chapter 28 Respiratory Pathophysiology	Asthma (Chapter 104) Chronic obstructive pulmonary disease (Chapter 105) Fibrosis (Chapter 110) Lung function tests (Chapter 95) Lung infections (Chapters 102 and 103) Respiratory failure (Chapter 97)	Asthma (Chapter 109) Chronic obstructive pulmonary disease (Chapter 110) Fibrosis (Chapter 115) Lung function tests (Chapter 97) Lung infections (Chapters 107 and 108) Respiratory failure (Chapter 99)
Part 6 Cardiovascular systems		
Chapter 29 Structure of the cardiovascular system		
Chapter 30 Cardiac physiology	Arrhythmias (Chapters 92 and 93) Heart murmurs (Chapter 17) Valve disease (Chapters 86 and 87)	Arrhythmias (Chapters 94 and 95) Heart murmurs (Chapter 17) Valve disease (Chapters 88 and 89)
Chapter 31 Cardiovascular physiology	Oedema (Chapter 14)	Oedema (Chapter 14)
Chapter 32 Blood pressure	Hypertension (Chapter 79)	Hypertension (Chapter 81)
Chapter 33 Blood: 1	Anaemias (Chapters 50, 171 and 172) Aplastic anaemias (Chapter 174) Blood counts (Chapter 181) Haemolytic anaemias (Chapter 172) Iron deficiency anaemia (Chapters 121 and 171) Megaloblastic anaemia (Chapters 171 and 181) Sickle cell (Chapter 173) Thalassaemias (Chapter 173)	Anaemias (Chapters 50, 176 and 177) Aplastic anaemias (Chapter 179) Blood counts (Chapter 186) Haemolytic anaemias (Chapter 177) Iron deficiency anaemia (Chapters 126 and 182) Megaloblastic anaemia (Chapters 176 and 186) Sickle cell (Chapter 178) Thalassaemias (Chapter 178)
Chapter 34 Blood: 2	Anticoagulants (Chapter 184) Antiplatelet drugs (Chapter 184) Disseminated intravascular coagulation (Chapter 183) Leukaemias (Chapters 175 and 176) Lymphomas (Chapter 177)	Anticoagulants (Chapter 189) Antiplatelet drugs (Chapter 189) Disseminated intravascular coagulation (Chapter 188) Leukaemias (Chapters 180 and 181) Lymphomas (Chapter 182)
Chapter 35 Cardiovascular pathophysiology	Acute coronary syndrome (Chapter 81) Atherosclerosis (Chapter 80) Chronic heart failure (Chapter 85) Ischaemic heart disease (Chapters 13 and 82) Stroke (Chapter 194)	Acute coronary syndrome (Chapter 83) Atherosclerosis (Chapter 82) Chronic heart failure (Chapter 87) Ischaemic heart disease (Chapters 13 and 84) Stroke (Chapter 201)
Part 7 Renal system		
Chapter 36 Structure of the renal system		
Chapter 37 Renal physiology: filtration and tubular function	Renal function (Chapter 135)	Renal function (Chapter 140)
Chapter 38 Renal physiology: loop of Henle		
Chapter 39 Regulation of body fluids	Acute renal failure (Chapter 145) Chronic renal failure (Chapter 146)	Acute renal failure (Chapter 150) Chronic renal failure (Chapter 151)
Chapter 40 Bladder function and dysfunction	Benign prostatic hypertrophy (Chapter 149) Dysuria (Chapter 35) Urinary tract infections (Chapter 150)	Benign prostatic hypertrophy (Chapter 154) Dysuria (Chapter 35) Urinary tract infections (Chapter 155)
Part 8 Digestive system		
Chapter 41 Structure of the gastrointestinal system		
Chapter 42 Upper gastrointestinal physiology	Dyspepsia (Chapter 30) Dysphagia (Chapter 29) Gastro-oesophageal reflux disease (Chapter 118) Peptic ulceration (Chapter 119)	Dyspepsia (Chapter 30) Dysphagia (Chapter 29) Gastro-oesophageal reflux disease (Chapter 123) Peptic ulceration (Chapter 124)
Chapter 43 Lower gastrointestinal physiology	Constipation (Chapters 24 and 133) Crohn's disease (Chapter 123) Diarrhoea (Chapters 25 and 133) Inflammatory bowel disease (Chapter 123) Irritable bowel syndrome (Chapter 133)	Constipation (Chapters 24 and 138) Crohn's disease (Chapter 128) Diarrhoea (Chapters 25 and 138) Inflammatory bowel disease (Chapter 128) Irritable bowel syndrome (Chapter 138)

Chapter 44 The liver	Alcoholic liver disease (Chapter 129) Ascites (Chapter 33) Cholestasis (Chapter 126) Hepatitis (Chapter 127) Jaundice (Chapter 30) Liver failure (Chapter 128) Liver function tests (Chapter 122)	Alcoholic liver disease (Chapter 134) Ascites (Chapter 33) Cholestasis (Chapter 131) Hepatitis (Chapter 132) Jaundice (Chapter 30) Liver failure (Chapter 133) Liver function tests (Chapter 127)
Part 9 Endocrine system		
Chapter 45 Hypothalamus and pituitary	Acromegaly (Chapter 154) Pituitary tumours (Chapter 159)	Acromegaly (Chapter 159) Pituitary tumours (Chapter 164)
Chapter 46 Endocrine pancreas	Type 1 diabetes mellitus (Chapters 151 and 152) Type 2 diabetes mellitus (Chapters 151 and 152)	Type 1 diabetes mellitus (Chapters 156 and 157) Type 2 diabetes mellitus (Chapters 156 and 157)
Chapter 47 Thyroid gland	Calcium balance (Chapter 157) Hyperthyroidism (Chapter 156) Hypothyroidism (Chapter 155)	Calcium balance (Chapter 162) Hyperthyroidism (Chapter 161) Hypothyroidism (Chapter 160)
Chapter 48 Adrenal glands and steroid hormones	Addison's disease (Chapter 158) Conn's syndrome (Chapter 158) Cushing's syndrome (Chapter 136)	Addison's disease (Chapter 163) Conn's syndrome (Chapter 163) Cushing's syndrome (Chapter 141)
Part 10 Reproductive function		
Chapter 49 The genital system		
Chapter 50 Reproductive physiology	Hypogonadism (Chapter 160)	Hypogonadism (Chapter 165)
Chapter 51 Human embryology		
Part 11 Central nervous system		
Chapter 52 Structure of the central nervous system		
Chapter 53 The sensory system	Sensory pathways (Chapter 56)	Sensory pathways (Chapter 56)
Chapter 54 The motor system	Motor pathways (Chapter 56)	Motor pathways (Chapter 56)
Chapter 55 Hypothalamus and thalamus		
Chapter 56 Central nervous system function		
Chapter 57 Disorders and treatments	Anxiety (Chapter 228) Bipolar affective disorder (Chapter 228) Dementia (Chapter 197) Depression (Chapter 228) Epilepsy (Chapter 198) Multiple sclerosis (Chapter 199) Parkinson's disease (Chapter 205) Schizophrenia (Chapter 228)	Anxiety (Chapter 240) Bipolar affective disorder (Chapter 240) Dementia (Chapter 204) Depression (Chapter 240) Epilepsy (Chapter 205) Multiple sclerosis (Chapter 206) Parkinson's disease (Chapter 212) Schizophrenia (Chapter 240)
Part 12 Infections and immunity		
Chapter 58 Pathogens	Bacteraemia (Chapter 161) Bacterial infections (Chapter 165) Fungal infections (Chapter 164) Infections (Chapter 41) Malaria (Chapter 166) Prion diseases (Chapter 197) Tuberculosis (Chapter 167) Viral infections (Chapter 162)	Bacteraemia (Chapter 166) Bacterial infections (Chapter 170) Fungal infections (Chapter 169) Infections (Chapter 41) Malaria (Chapter 171) Prion diseases (Chapter 204) Tuberculosis (Chapter 172) Viral infections (Chapter 167)
Chapter 59 Recognition of pathogens		
Chapter 60 Defence against pathogens		
Chapter 61 Integration of the immune response		

Chapter 62 Immunopathology	Allergy (Chapter 75) Alveolitis (Chapter 109) Anaphylaxis (Chapter 74) Eczema (Chapter 216) Systemic lupus erythematosus (Chapter 214)	Allergy (Chapter 77) Alveolitis (Chapter 114) Anaphylaxis (Chapter 76) Eczema (Chapter 223) Systemic lupus erythematosus (Chapter 221)
Chapter 63 Immunodeficiency disorders	HIV infections (Chapter 163) Immunodeficiency (Chapter 170)	HIV infections (Chapter 168) Immunodeficiency (Chapter 175)
Part 13 Cancer		
Chapter 64 Cancer biology	Aetiology (Chapter 186) Breast cancer (Chapter 189) Cancer with unknown primary (Chapter 191) Colorectal cancers (Chapter 131) Lung cancers (Chapter 116) Pancreatic cancer (Chapter 125) Prostate cancer (Chapter 190) Upper GI cancers (Chapter 130)	Aetiology (Chapter 191) Breast cancer (Chapter 194) Cancer with unknown primary (Chapter 196) Colorectal cancers (Chapter 136) Lung cancers (Chapter 121) Pancreatic cancer (Chapter 130) Prostate cancer (Chapter 195) Upper GI cancers (Chapter 135)
Chapter 65 Chemotherapy	Cancer management (Chapter 187)	Cancer management (Chapter 192)

Index

Page numbers in *italics* refer to figures,
page numbers in **bold** refer to tables.

AQA French

Exclusively endorsed by AQA

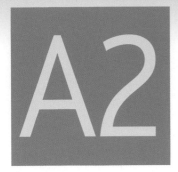

A2

Elaine Armstrong
Lol Briggs
Steve Harrison
Joelle Saunders

Nelson Thornes

Published in 2009 by:
Nelson Thornes Ltd
Delta Place
27 Bath Road
CHELTENHAM
GL53 7TH
United Kingdom

09 10 11 12 13 / 10 9 8 7 6 5 4 3 2

A catalogue record for this book is available from the British Library

978-0-7487-9808-7

Illustrations by: Mark Draisey, Stephen Elford, Eric Smith

Page make-up by eMC Design, www.emcdesign.org.uk

Printed and bound in Spain by GraphyCems

Contents

Introduction

Nelson Thornes has worked in partnership with AQA to ensure this book and the accompanying online resources offer you the best support for your GCSE course.

All resources have been approved by senior AQA examiners so you can feel assured that they closely match the specification for this subject and provide you with everything you need to prepare successfully for your exams.

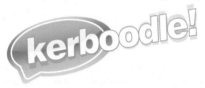

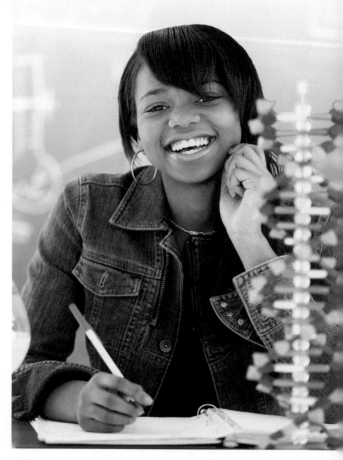

These print and online resources together **unlock blended learning**; this means that the links between the activities in the book and the activities online blend together to maximise your understanding of a topic and help you achieve your potential.

These online resources are available on **kerboodle!** which can be accessed via the internet at **http://www.kerboodle.com/live**, anytime, anywhere. If your school or college subscribes to this service you will be provided with your own personal login details. Once logged in, access your course and locate the required activity.

For more information and help visit **http://www.kerboodle.com**

Icons in this book indicate where there is material online related to that topic. The following icons are used:

💡 Learning activity

These resources include a variety of interactive and non-interactive activities to support your learning.

☑️ Progress tracking

These resources include a variety of tests that you can use to check your knowledge on particular topics (Test Yourself) and a range of resources that enable you to analyse and understand examination questions (On Your Marks...).

📑 Study skills

This icon indicates a linked worksheet (*Feuille*), available online to print out, with activities to develop a skill that is key for language learning, such as expressing opinions in a debate.

🎧 Audio stimulus

This indicates that audio material for listening activities can be found online.

✒️ Audio record

This indicates one of two types of tool that help you develop your speaking skills – either a free-speech recording tool that you can use with speaking activities, or an audio roleplay tool that enables you to interact with pre-recorded native speakers.

📹 Video stimulus

This indicates where audio-visual material can be found online to support listening and other activities.

ℹ️ Research support

This icon appears in chapter 10, the cultural topic, and directs you to online features that are designed to help you develop your research skills.

How to use this book

This book covers the specification for your course and is arranged in a sequence approved by AQA. The ten chapters are arranged in the same sequence as the topics and sub-topics in the AQA specification, so there is always a clear link between the book and the specification. At the beginning of each section you will find a list of learning objectives that contain targets linked to the requirements of the specification.

The features in this book include:

 Le saviez-vous?

An anecdotal insight into facts/figures relating to each sub-topic.

 Pour commencer

An introductory feature designed as an accessible starter activity for each chapter.

 Grammaire

Summary grammar explanations and examples, linked to online worksheets containing fuller explanations and exercises.

(A grammar section can also be found at the back of this book.)

 Compétences

This 'skills' heading directs you to online worksheets that help build key language learning strategies.

Vocabulaire

The most challenging new items of vocabulary from the reading texts on each spread are translated in these boxes.

Expressions clés

Key words and phrases designed to give you prompts for productive tasks.

 Résumé

A summary quiz that tests key language learnt in each chapter (also available as a multiple-choice version online).

AQA Examiner's tips

Hints from AQA examiners to help you with your study and to prepare for your exam.

 Vos enquêtes

Ideas for further research into the themes introduced in the cultural topic (chapter 10).

 WebQuest

Web-based investigation tasks that explore some areas of the cultural topic in greater depth.

Web links in the book

As Nelson Thornes is not responsible for third party content online, there may be some changes to this material that are beyond our control. In order for us to ensure that the links referred to in the book are as up-to-date and stable as possible, the websites are usually homepages with supporting instructions on how to reach the relevant pages if necessary.

Please let us know at **kerboodle@nelsonthornes.com** if you find a link that doesn't work and we will do our best to redirect the link, or to find an alternative site.

A message to students

Congratulations on choosing to study a language to A2 Level – you have made a decision that will give you many opportunities in the future.

Good foreign language skills are in short supply and can be used in many different jobs. Translating, interpreting and the travel industry obviously require linguists, but so too do many other areas of employment – financial services, marketing, engineering, logistics and journalism to name just a few. Or maybe you will use your language skills and understanding of French culture to make your holidays more enriching and enjoyable. Either way, there are many benefits of learning one or more languages to an advanced level.

The new AQA specification in modern languages has been designed to provide a coherent and stimulating course of study, whether as an end in itself or as a stepping stone towards further study at university. The topics have been carefully chosen to enable clear progression and to address your needs and interests as A2 Level students.

In the examination you will be tested in the four essential skills of listening, reading, speaking and writing, including open-ended tasks that require you to express and justify opinions. You will also be tested on your understanding and application of French grammar and structures. In addition, the A2 course gives you the opportunity to explore a variety of themes relating to French culture. This book presents in chapter 10 two contrasting case studies for each of five themes specified by AQA. You can use these studies as starting points for your own research.

This course with its innovative online component has been compiled by experienced teachers and examiners to help you to prepare for the examination with confidence and make the most of your abilities.

The book is clearly laid out to match the topics and sub-topics in the AQA specification. Each sub-topic is presented through a range of texts, recordings and visual material, with new vocabulary introduced and highlighted where appropriate. Essential grammar points are explained clearly and 'skills' features direct students to online support that gives guidance on how to use the language like a native speaker. Open-ended speaking and writing tasks enable you to apply the new vocabulary and structures that you have learnt, including some more challenging tasks designed to extend your skills.

The online component provides additional stimulus material and support for activities in the book, as well as a range of interactive exercises and printable worksheets which you can use both independently and in class. The exercises provide plenty of practice of the grammar and structures presented in the book, together with topic-based activities that will help you prepare for the question types used in Units 3 and 4 of the examination. At the end of each sub-topic you will be able to test yourself through a multiple-choice quiz, focusing again on key vocabulary and structures, and at the end of each topic exam-style questions help you to practise answering the types of questions you can expect in the examination. A new feature for A2 is the inclusion of WebQuests, web-based investigative tasks, within the cultural topic. The WebQuests will enable you to use the internet in a structured way to explore those aspects of French culture that interest you most.

AQA and Nelson Thornes hope that you will find your language study rewarding and enjoyable, and we wish you success for A2 and beyond.

Paul Shannon

AQA Senior Examiner

L'environnement

1 La pollution

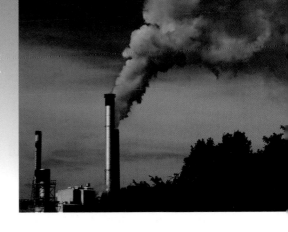

By the end of this chapter you will be able to:

	Language	Grammar	Skills
A **La pollution: fléau de la planète**	■ talk about different types, causes and effects of pollution	■ use present and past tenses of the passive voice	■ formulate questions
B **Comment réduire la pollution?**	■ explore measures to reduce pollution ■ discuss individual and collective action	■ use modal verbs	■ express your own views
C **Le transport**	■ describe transport issues related to pollution	■ use the present subjunctive	■ present alternatives

■ Le saviez-vous?

5,75 millions de véhicules: production totale des constructeurs français en 2003, soit près de 10 % de la production totale mondiale.

Dans le monde entier, 3,65 milliards de tonnes de déchets issus de véhicules seront générés entre maintenant et 2030. De quoi remplir plus de 1000 fois le stade de Wembley.

■ Pour commencer

1 « La moitié de nos besoins provient des énergies fossiles: le pétrole et le gaz. » Choisissez la phrase équivalente:

a Half our energy needs come from fossils in oil and gas.

b We need half of our energy to come from fossil fuels.

c Half of our energy comes from fossil fuels.

2 Donnez un exemple de combustible fossile.

3 Quel est l'intrus?

a les déchets industriels

b la pollution atmosphérique

c les calottes glaciaires

4 Complétez la phrase: La déforestation...

a est indispensable à la vie.

b signifie moins d'oxygène.

c crée l'habitat idéal pour les animaux.

5 Devinez le pourcentage du taux de recyclage des emballages ménagers en France.

a 50%   b 43%   c 61%

A La pollution: fléau de la planète

1
a Traduisez en anglais une phrase de la Charte.

b Prenez le mot POLLUTION. A l'aide d'un dictionnaire, trouvez pour chaque lettre un mot lié au thème de l'environnement. Puis trouvez trois autres mots associés au premier!

Exemple: _____

P = pluie ⟶ inondation

climat   vent

La pollution par les déchets en France

La gestion des déchets coûte de plus en plus cher. En gros, chaque Français paie 120 euros par an pour faire traiter ses poubelles.

Que contiennent les poubelles françaises?

360 kilos d'ordures ménagères sont produits par personne par an, dont:

29 % de déchets putrescibles
25 % de papiers et cartons
13 % de verre
11 % de plastique
 5 % de métaux
17 % de bois, textiles et divers

Les types de pollution et leurs causes

La pollution est un phénomène relativement récent; depuis l'ère industrielle. D'où vient la pollution?

Dans l'air, la pollution atmosphérique vient de la croissance de la consommation d'énergie, du développement des industries, de la circulation routière et aérienne, de l'incinération des ordures ménagères, des déchets industriels, des chauffages des maisons, des fumées des centrales électriques au charbon ou au gaz.

La pollution de l'eau: les océans, les mers et les rivières du monde sont pollués. C'est le résultat d'accidents de pétroliers, de déchets industriels et agricoles, d'égouts, de rejets de navires ou de naufrages. Des maladies chez les végétaux, les animaux et les hommes ont été provoquées par la pollution. Elle peut rompre l'équilibre naturel de certains écosystèmes, voire les détruire.

© *Extraits de L'Ecologuide de A à Z (2004),*
Fondation Nicolas Hulot pour la Nature et l'Homme, www.fnh.org

Vocabulaire

putrescible *biodegradable*
l'ère industrielle *industrial era*
la circulation routière *road traffic*
les ordures ménagères *household waste*
un égout *sewer*
le navire *ship*
le naufrage *shipwreck*
rompre *to break, to upset*
voire *indeed, even*

grimper *to climb*
le réchauffement *warming*
la fonte des calottes glaciaires *melting of the ice caps*
la sécheresse *drought*
bouleverser *to upset*

2
a Lisez les textes. Faites correspondre les expressions équivalentes.

i   l'ère industrielle
ii   la croissance
iii la consommation
iv   la circulation
v   les ordures ménagères

vi   les égouts
vii les usines
viii les navires
ix   un naufrage
x   rompre

a les déchets
b l'utilisation de transport
c casser
d les canalisations pour l'écoulement
e la période où on commence les techniques industrielles
f les bateaux
g l'augmentation
h les endroits où on fabrique des choses
i l'utilisation
j un bateau brisé

b Faites des recherches!
Est-ce que les déchets ménagers chez vous ressemblent à ceux des Français? Ecrivez 50 mots.

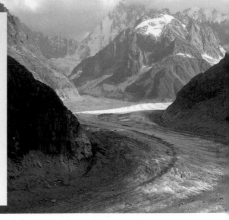

Les effets de la pollution

Depuis le début du 20ème siècle, la courbe des températures n'a pratiquement pas cessé de grimper et la concentration de CO_2 suit une évolution quasi parallèle à celle des températures. Conséquences? Le réchauffement climatique planétaire, une élévation moyenne du niveau des océans, la fonte des calottes glaciaires, sécheresse, montée des eaux. Le visage de notre planète est bouleversé par ces changements climatiques. En conséquence, les canicules, sécheresses, inondations et tempêtes devraient augmenter en intensité et en fréquence.

Les glaciers de montagne constituent un indicateur clé des impacts. En Europe, entre 1850 et 1980, les glaciers alpins ont perdu un tiers de leur surface. Depuis 1980, encore 20 à 30 % de la glace restante a disparu. Si la tendance au réchauffement se poursuit, 95 % des glaciers alpins et la totalité des glaciers pyrénéens pourraient disparaître au cours des cent prochaines années.

La mer de glace près de Chamonix

3 Lisez l'article et choisissez les bonnes fins de phrase.

i   La courbe des températures...

ii   La rapidité de la montée des températures est due...

iii Le réchauffement climatique...

iv   Avec la dégradation de la biodiversité on voit...

v   On a vu...

vi   La totalité des glaciers pyrénéens...

a   la perte et les changements des organismes vivants.

b   risque de ne plus exister.

c   n'a cessé de grimper depuis le début du 20ème siècle.

d   se multiplier les inondations.

e   à la concentration de CO_2.

f   bouleverse notre planète.

4 🎧 Ecoutez l'entretien et notez les détails suivants.

i   L'effet de serre ressemble à:

ii   La température moyenne à la surface de la Terre **avec** et **sans** l'effet de serre naturel:

iii Trois exemples de gaz naturels:

iv   Conséquences du réchauffement:

v   La raison du réchauffement:

5 💡🎧 Ecoutez le reportage et faites les activités interactives.

6 💡 Inondations au Mexique. Ecrivez 10 questions à poser à un journaliste sur place. (Feuille)

7 💡 A l'oral, présentez le problème de la pollution en considérant les aspects suivants (Feuille):

- ce qu'on constate depuis l'ère industrielle
- les causes de la pollution de l'air et de l'eau
- ce que vous pensez du problème des déchets

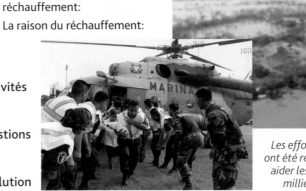

Les efforts de l'armée ont été redoublés pour aider les centaines de milliers de sinistrés

Expressions clés

La pollution est un phénomène qui existe depuis l'ère industrielle.

Les chiffres indiquent un lien entre les émissions de CO_2 et le réchauffement de la terre.

Le réchauffement de la terre est lié aux activités de l'homme.

C'est l'effet de serre qui accélère le réchauffement de la terre.

La pollution atmosphérique vient des fumées émises par les centrales électriques au charbon ou au gaz.

Concernant la pollution de l'eau, on pourrait citer les accidents de pétroliers, les déchets industriels et agricoles et les égouts.

Les déchets ménagers posent un problème.

Avec quelques degrés de plus, le niveau des océans s'élève et le littoral est couvert d'eau.

La planète est bouleversée par les changements climatiques.

Les régions sont dévastées par les inondations, les vents et les pluies.

💡 Grammaire

The passive – *le passif*

The passive voice describes an event without necessarily mentioning who is responsible for it. It is formed using the auxiliary verb *être* (in the appropriate tense) and a past participle. The past participle agrees in number and gender with the subject. See page 116 for more details.

*La récolte **a été** totalement **détruite**.*
(The harvest has been destroyed – *la récolte* is feminine and singular.)

1 Une pollution affligeante:
18 milliards de sacs plastiques sont distribués par an,
10 milliards ne sont pas recyclés.
Quel geste pourriez-vous adopter? Liez les expressions des deux colonnes.

Si je prends l'exemple...		je pourrais...	
a	de l'éclairage	i	favoriser les transports en commun.
b	du jardin	ii	choisir des produits locaux.
c	du chauffage	iii	ne pas utiliser la mise en veille.
d	des déchets	iv	refuser les traitements chimiques.
e	du transport	v	éteindre la lumière en quittant la pièce.
f	des appareils électriques	vi	trier mes déchets.
g	des courses	vii	isoler mon logement.

L'environnement – c'est un grand souci pour nous

Anne

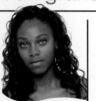

Je pense à l'environnement chaque fois que je fais une balade à la campagne. La forêt est une chaîne vivante; il est très important de ne rien déranger. Moi, j'habite en Bretagne et ce qui me préoccupe, c'est toute la côte. Des milliers de tonnes de déchets toxiques sont rejetés directement en mer par l'industrie.

Thierry

Moi, je trouve formidable la création d'un "Grenelle environnement" qui vise à mobiliser les Français autour des questions liées à l'environnement et à forger une véritable politique de l'environnement. Sur la scène internationale, la lutte contre le changement climatique fait l'objet d'un engagement très ferme de la France et de l'Europe dans la perspective de l'après-Kyoto.

Didier

Je fais partie de Greenpeace. Moi, je trouve qu'il est important de trouver des solutions écologiques. Greenpeace a 3 000 000 adhérents répartis dans 40 pays du monde. Après plusieurs années de lutte, l'organisation a obtenu, pour l'Europe, la fin des campagnes de pêche avec filets dérivants (que l'on nomme également "les murs de la mort").

Catherine

Moi, je pense à l'environnement quand je fais mes courses. Le rôle de la grande distribution est primordial. Des lois essaient d'améliorer la situation mais c'est avant tout à chaque citoyen de prendre conscience du danger et de changer de mentalité. Je suis sensible aussi aux transports routiers et j'essaie d'acheter des produits locaux.

Vocabulaire

la balade *walk*

déranger *to disturb*

un adhérent *member*

le Grenelle *"round table" to bring organisations together*

viser à *to aim at*

lié à *linked to*

primordial *very important, fundamental*

sensible à *aware*

2 a Lisez l'opinion de quatre jeunes. C'est qui?

  i Qui s'occupe du littoral?
  ii Qui parle d'un accord international?
  iii Qui se penche sur les problèmes de l'environnement dans la nature?
  iv Qui est impressionné par les mesures gouvernementales concernant l'environnement?
  v Qui pense aux activités journalières?
  vi Qui est attiré par les grands problèmes planétaires?
  vii Qui estime qu'il faut changer les mentalités des gens?

b Et vous? Répondez aux questions.

  i Vous vous intéressez à quel aspect de l'environnement? Pourquoi?
  ii Que faites-vous pour protéger l'environnement?
  iii Que pensez-vous de Greenpeace?
  iv Selon vous, qu'est-ce qu'un bon citoyen devrait faire?

3 a 🎧 Ecoutez l'extrait d'une émission et notez le numéro des gestes mentionnés.

i | Il faut éteindre les appareils électriques.

v | Il faut fermer le robinet quand on se brosse les dents.

ii | Il faut choisir des appareils économes.

vi | Il faut prendre une douche rapide.

iii | Il faut favoriser l'usage des trains.

vii | Je conduis à une vitesse adaptée.

iv | Il faut éviter les emballages inutiles.

viii | Je regarde les étiquettes sur les emballages.

b Ecrivez des phrases pour décrire quels gestes vous et votre famille pourriez adopter.

4 💡🖥 Regardez la vidéo et faites les activités interactives.

5 💡 Discutez à deux: Chaque image vous fait penser à quoi par rapport à la pollution? Persuadez deux autres personnes que votre point de vue est le bon.

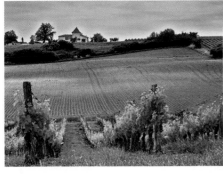
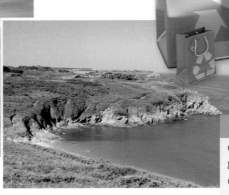

6 a 💡 (Feuille) Ecrivez ce que chaque individu devrait faire pour...

- réduire sa consommation d'énergie
- réduire les déchets
- sauvegarder la nature

b Donnez votre opinion sur le rôle des organismes et du gouvernement.

🧭 Compétences

Express your own views

Useful expressions for putting across your own viewpoint:

Je pense à l'environnement quand...

Ce qui me préoccupe, c'est...

Je me penche sur le problème de l'environnement quand...

Ce problème attire mon attention:...

Je suis conscient(e) du problème de...

Je privilégie l'achat de produits locaux.

Pourquoi ne pas considérer...?

Expressions clés

On doit* lutter pour / contre le gaspillage.

On devrait* trier les déchets.

Il vaudrait* mieux résoudre les problèmes de transport.

Il ne faut pas* gaspiller l'eau.

Il est primordial de protéger les océans.

Il est important de sauvegarder une agriculture saine.

Il est impératif qu'on trouve des solutions concernant les emballages.

Ce qui me préoccupe, c'est le littoral parce que...

Préserver la nature est une urgence pour la survie de...

Une amélioration des transports est nécessaire.

Ne pas gaspiller l'énergie, c'est un défi.

L'habitat subira des conséquences désastreuses.

see modal verbs, present page 110, conditional page 113

C Le transport

transport routier de passagers

transport ferroviaire

transport maritime

transport aérien

transport routier de marchandises

1 a Ecrivez des phrases pour montrer que vous comprenez chaque mode de transport à gauche.

Exemple: _____

Transport routier de passagers: moi, je voyage en voiture quand je fais les courses avec ma mère.

_____

b Mettez, selon vous, les cinq moyens de transport dans l'ordre croissant de leur consommation d'énergie.

Le défi des transports

L'automobile a changé le monde, voyager en avion est devenu produit de consommation courante. Le nombre de porte-conteneurs sur les océans augmente, les camions sur les autoroutes s'allongent. Tout cela veut dire une consommation de produits pétroliers énorme avec *des conséquences environnementales dramatiques:* cinq milliards de tonnes de CO_2 émises par an (émissions importantes de gaz à effet de serre), fragmentation et disparition des milieux naturels et pollutions locales.

Solutions

Il faudrait que nous réduisions nos besoins de transports par un meilleur urbanisme. En France, un tiers des camions circulent à vide.

Il est important que nous changions les véhicules pour qu'ils soient beaucoup moins gourmands en énergie (adaptation des puissances, carburants alternatifs).

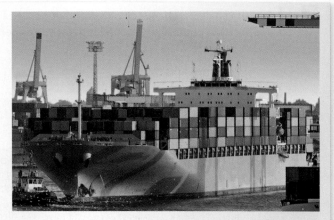

Il est primordial qu'on sache modifier les modes de transport en fonction des usages. On pourrait confier les marchandises au ferroviaire, au fluvial et au maritime et transporter les passagers différemment en ville (transports en commun, vélos, véhicules légers).

2 a Lisez le texte et trouvez l'équivalent des expressions suivantes:

  i   le fret en mer
  ii   un véhicule routier qui transporte les marchandises
  iii un plan pour gérer une ville
  iv   les véhicules qui roulent sans être chargés
  v   plus respectueux vis-à-vis des carburants
  vi   les véhicules qui ne consomment pas autant
  vii les différents moyens d'utiliser les transports

b Reliez les moitiés de phrases.

  i   prendre l'avion
  ii   Les transports
  iii Les émissions de gaz à effet de serre ne sont
  iv   Il faudrait trouver des moyens de
  v   Les solutions écologiques devraient
  vi   Un urbanisme stratégique

  a   qu'une conséquence parmi d'autres.
  b   être favorisées.
  c   est primordial.
  d   sont en hausse.
  e   est devenu très commun.
  f   réduire nos besoins.

Vocabulaire

gourmand *greedy*
sache: *subj. of* savoir *know*
confier à *to entrust*
ferroviaire *using rail*
fluvial *using rivers*

bannir *to banish*
nuisible *harmful*
élaborer *to set out*
puissant *powerful*
atteigne: *subj. of* atteindre *reach*
avoir la cote *to be very popular*

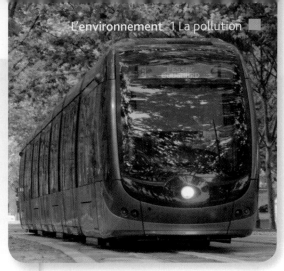

Est-ce qu'on voit une révolution des transports urbains?

Est-ce qu'il est possible de bannir la voiture, nuisible à la santé et à l'environnement, pour favoriser d'autres modes de déplacement? Ce qui se passe en France, c'est que ce sont les lois qui poussent les villes à élaborer leurs plans de déplacements urbains (PDU): ça veut dire organiser la circulation, le stationnement, le déplacement des personnes et des marchandises. Bien sûr, des résistances existent, notamment à cause d'un lobby automobile puissant.

A Paris un ambitieux plan a été adopté pour que la part des transports collectifs, taxis, vélos et marche atteigne 80% des trajets en 2013. Pour le faire: augmenter l'offre de transports en commun. Une ligne souterraine de transport en commun autour de Paris est envisagée avec plus de métros, de trams et de bus, et une ligne fluviale sur la Seine. La plupart des grandes villes développent leurs transports en commun et le tram a la cote.

3 a Lisez le texte et répondez aux questions.

    i   Expliquez le terme PDU.

    ii   Qui est contre? Pourquoi?

    iii Quel est l'objectif de la ville de Paris?

    iv Comment va-t-on réaliser cet objectif?

  b Pourrait-on bannir les voitures en ville? Ecrivez cinq phrases pour et cinq phrases contre.

4 🎧 Ecoutez le texte et écrivez V (vrai) ou F (faux). Corrigez les phrases qui sont fausses.

  a   Vélo'v est un système de location de vélo gratuit.

  b   A Lyon 3 000 vélos sont distribués sur 205 stations.

  c   Le système à Lyon a généré plus de 5,5 millions de locations la première année du lancement.

  d   Une seule compagnie est intéressée par la signature de contrats.

  e   Le maire de Paris aimerait avoir le même système pour les voitures mais ce n'est pas possible.

5 💡🎧 Ecoutez le reportage sur Paris et faites les activités interactives.

6 a 💡 A deux, présentez les bénéfices des différents moyens de transport en ville: bus, tram, vélo, voiture, etc. (Feuille)

  b A deux: que va-t-il se passer si on ne change pas nos habitudes?

  c A deux, choisissez un moyen de transport à privilégier.

7 💡 A l'écrit: décrivez les moyens de transport à Paris. Expliquez comment on essaie de gérer la pollution. Faites une comparaison avec votre ville et évaluez la situation. (Feuille)

8 💡🖊 Ecoutez le dialogue et enregistrez vos réponses.

💡 Grammaire

The subjunctive – *le subjonctif*

Used to express emotive language, such as necessity, obligation, possibility, doubt, fear, regret, happiness. For example, it is used after these phrases:

Il est essentiel que...
Il est important que...
Je doute que...   J'ai peur que...
Il est dommage que...
Je suis heureux que...

It is also used after *il faut que, il vaudrait mieux que,* and some conjunctions such as *bien que, pour que, afin que, sans que.*

See pages 114–5.

Expressions clés

J'aimerais proposer que...

Il faudrait que nous réduisions nos besoins en transport.

Il est important que les véhicules ne soient pas si gourmands en énergie.

On devrait commencer à privilégier les transports en commun.

On pourrait confier les marchandises aux transports ferroviaires.

Il est primordial qu'on sache modifier les modes de transport en fonction des usages.

Il est souhaitable qu'on...

Il s'agirait d'utiliser...

Je voudrais que nous soyons plus intelligents en ce qui concerne...

Je ne crois pas qu'on puisse continuer à utiliser la voiture comme on le fait maintenant.

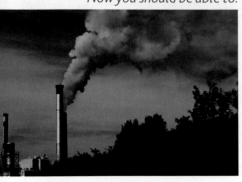

Now you should be able to:

■ talk about different types, causes and effects of pollution

■ explore measures to reduce pollution

■ discuss individual and collective action

■ describe transport issues related to pollution

Grammar

■ use present and past tenses of the passive voice

■ use modal verbs

■ use the present subjunctive

Skills

■ formulate questions

■ express your own views

■ present alternatives

✓ Résumé

1 Expliquez la phrase:

L'environnement est le patrimoine commun des êtres humains.

2 Mettez au passif:

On a annulé les vols.

3 C'est quel phénomène?

L'homme utilise l'énergie et la quantité de CO_2 dans l'atmosphère augmente, provoquant le réchauffement de la terre.

4 Mettez les mots dans le bon ordre:

L'ozone gaz une contre forme couche ultraviolets les est rayons protectrice un qui

5 Complétez la phrase:

Je pense à l'environnement, donc je...

6 Utilisez le subjonctif:

Il faut qu'on ...... (**mettre**) un terme à la destruction de l'environnement. Pour que les gens ...... (**être**) mobilisés autour des questions écologiques, je veux qu'on ...... (**prendre**) des mesures sur les transports.

7 Faites une phrase, en changeant la forme des mots si nécessaire:

falloir réduire l'usage voiture favoriser transport lois élaborer plans de déplacement

8 Formulez une question pour la réponse:

Ce qu'on voit maintenant, ce sont des Vélib' à Paris.

9 Faites une comparaison (**moins / plus / aussi**):

Lyon: 3 000 vélos, 250 stations – les transports collectifs
autre ville: 2 000 vélos, 250 stations

10 Traduisez en français:

It is essential that society understands the importance of the environment.

AQA   Examiner's tips

Listening
Look at the **title of the passage** – it will give you an idea of the content and will encourage your brain to think of relevant vocabulary.

Speaking
Study your two cards **briefly** and choose the one that will give you **most to talk about**.

Reading
Read each question and **follow instructions** correctly. Make sure you answer in the **right language**, French or English!

Writing
If you don't know the exact word you need, use a **similar** one.

L'environnement

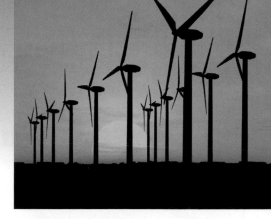

By the end of this chapter you will be able to:

	Language	Grammar	Skills
A Les énergies non renouvelables	■ talk about the different sources of fossil fuels ■ discuss the role of nuclear energy in France	■ revise present tense endings	■ debate controversial issues
B Les énergies renouvelables	■ discuss the need for renewable energy sources	■ revise present and conditional forms (to express necessity)	■ express necessity, consequence and contrast
C Les attitudes changeantes	■ explore changing attitudes to energy consumption	■ use verbs followed by an infinitive	■ evaluate lifestyle using alternative forms of energy

■   Le saviez-vous?

Dans la maison,
1 degré de moins = 7% de consommation énergétique en moins.

1 degré de moins pour tous économiserait l'équivalent de la consommation annuelle de Marseille.

Le point commun entre un rouge à lèvres, du goudron et un chewing-gum, c'est qu'ils sont tous faits avec du pétrole.

■   Pour commencer

1   Comment traduire "la politique énergétique" en anglais?

2   Que faut-il faire pour réduire les gaz à effet de serre?
   a augmenter l'usage du pétrole
   b diminuer l'usage du charbon
   c bannir l'effet de serre

3   Traduisez en anglais:
   Le réchauffement climatique est devenu un enjeu majeur.

4   Que faut-il avoir pour ces énergies?
   a l'éolien
   b l'hydraulique
   c le solaire

5   Quelle est votre réaction à la phrase suivante?
   « La nature a mis 250 millions d'années pour fabriquer le pétrole. Nous sommes capables de l'épuiser en moins de cent ans. »

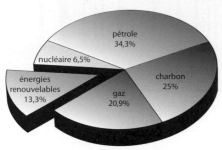

pétrole 34,3%

nucléaire 6,5%

énergies renouvelables 13,3%

charbon 25%

gaz 20,9%

Les sources d'énergie les plus utilisées au monde

1 Lisez le graphique et le texte et répondez aux questions oralement.

a Quelle source d'énergie est la plus utilisée au monde?

b Quelle est la source d'énergie la moins utilisée au monde?

c Quel pays européen favorise la source d'énergie la moins utilisée et pourquoi à votre avis?

L'offre d'énergie en France

La France est pauvre en énergies fossiles contrairement à plusieurs pays européens bénéficiant de matières premières (charbon en Allemagne et en Espagne, pétrole, gaz et charbon au Royaume-Uni, gaz au Pays-Bas, hydraulique en Suisse, etc.). La France est le deuxième producteur d'énergie nucléaire au monde derrière les Etats-Unis.

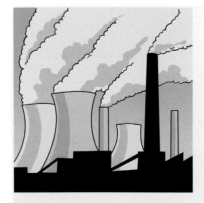

Les énergies non renouvelables

Le pétrole, le gaz naturel et le charbon sont des énergies fossiles et sont à la base de l'électricité issue des centrales thermiques. La nature a mis 250 millions d'années pour fabriquer le pétrole et nous sommes capables de l'épuiser en moins de cent ans. Regarder la télé, jouer sur l'ordinateur, mettre le chauffage, prendre sa voiture, tous ces gestes quotidiens consomment de l'énergie. Bien plus de la moitié de nos besoins en énergie proviennent des énergies fossiles. Mais aujourd'hui ces ressources connaissent une flambée des prix, du fait de leur raréfaction et d'une explosion de la demande mondiale, notamment des pays émergents comme la Chine et l'Inde.

La politique énergétique de la France maintient l'option nucléaire pour les trente ans à venir, mais le nucléaire divise toujours. Le nucléaire produit une énergie très concentrée (un gramme d'uranium produit autant énergie qu'une tonne de charbon) et en plus ne rejette pas de gaz polluants dans l'atmosphère. Les déchets radioactifs produits sont dangereux, car ils émettent des rayons qui peuvent être mortels pour l'Homme. Leur nocivité diminue au cours du temps mais ne devient négligeable qu'au bout de dizaines, de centaines de milliers, voire de millions d'années, selon le type de déchets produits. Dans tous les pays où on utilise l'énergie nucléaire, on cherche activement des solutions pour traiter les déchets sur le long terme.

© Extraits de L'Ecologuide de A à Z (2004), Fondation Nicolas Hulot pour la Nature et l'Homme, www.fnh.org

2 a Lisez l'extrait et faites correspondre les deux parties des phrases.

i Nos besoins d'énergies...	a provient des énergies fossiles.
ii On prévoit...	b deviennent très chers.
iii Plus de 50% de nos besoins énergétiques...	c ne cessent d'augmenter.
iv Les combustibles fossiles...	d soit débattu reste une option énergétique.
v Le nucléaire même qu'il...	e la fin des énergies fossiles.

b Relisez l'extrait et notez les cinq phrases les plus significatives selon vous. Expliquez votre choix à la classe.

Exemple: _____

La politique énergétique de la France maintient l'option nucléaire pour les trente ans à venir, mais le nucléaire divise toujours. – *I find this interesting because I know some countries do not want to continue with the nuclear option.*

Vocabulaire

croître *to grow*

le pétrole *oil*

l'épuisement *exhaustion, running out*

épuiser *to use up*

quotidien *daily*

une flambée des prix *price hike*

la raréfaction *scarcity*

la politique énergétique *energy policy*

la nocivité *noxiousness*

3 💡🎧 Ecoutez le reportage sur les combustibles fossiles et faites les activités interactives.

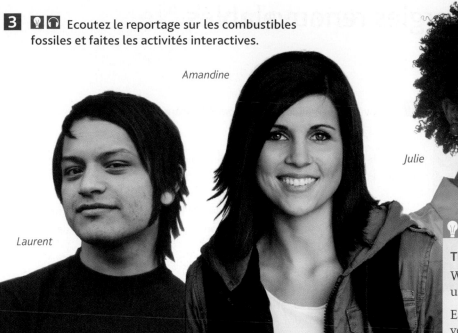

Amandine

Julie

Laurent

💡 **Grammaire**

The present tense – *le présent*

Writing essays involves frequent use of the present tense.

Endings of regular and irregular verbs require practice and need to be learnt by heart. See tables, page 110.

Check that you know the infinitives of the following present tense verbs from the text on page 18:

sont est sommes provient connaissent maintient rejette émettent devient

4 a 🎧 Ecoutez ce que disent trois personnes sur l'énergie nucléaire. C'est qui? Laurent, Amandine ou Julie?

  i   Les coûts vis-à-vis de cette source d'énergie pourraient devenir beaucoup plus importants.

  ii   La politique énergétique a été formée par les expériences du passé.

  iii La France ne veut pas être dépendante de l'étranger pour son approvisionnement en énergie.

  iv   Cette personne est craintive lorsqu'il s'agit du nucléaire.

  v   La France ne suit pas la même politique énergétique que les autres pays européens.

  vi   On prévoit des systèmes pour mieux surveiller l'industrie nucléaire.

  b Répondez aux questions. Trouvez des raisons ou des justifications si possible.

  i   1973 est une date clé. Pourquoi?

  ii   Présentez un argument pour le nucléaire.

  iii Présentez un argument contre le nucléaire.

5 💡 Travail de groupe: débat. (Feuille)
Prenez le point de vue des personnes suivantes:

- une personne qui est pour le nucléaire
- une personne qui vit à côté d'une centrale (thermique ou nucléaire)
- une personne qui est pessimiste vis-à-vis de l'avenir
- une personne qui est optimiste vis-à-vis de l'avenir

6 💡 Ecrivez un article (200 mots) sur votre opinion concernant le nucléaire. Adoptez une position pour ou contre. (Feuille)

Expressions clés

Les combustibles fossiles sont à la base du réchauffement de la terre.

Tout le monde est d'accord sur le fait que l'épuisement de nos combustibles fossiles est prévisible car...

Contrairement à ce que certains pensent, moi je préfère le nucléaire.

Du fait que nous épuisons nos combustibles fossiles, il faudrait...

Ceci permettrait...

Ceci détruit...

Ceci provoque / entraîne...

C'est nuisible / néfaste.

Ceci est reconnu...

Jusqu'à présent on considérait le nucléaire comme avantageux.

Mais en raison du coût...

Quant à la rentabilité, il faudrait penser à...

Les énergies renouvelables

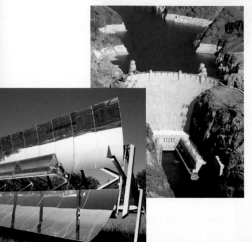

1 Trouvez la bonne définition pour les énergies vertes.

Pour créer de l'énergie avec...

i	les éoliennes	a	on utilise la chaleur du sous-sol de la Terre.
ii	la géothermie	b	on utilise la technique de combustion du bois et des déchets végétaux.
iii	l'hydroélectricité	c	on convertit la force du vent en électricité.
iv	le solaire	d	les rayons du soleil sont captés par des panneaux.
v	la biomasse	e	cette technique utilise la force de l'eau en mouvement.

2 a Lisez *Energies renouvelables* et choisissez trois phrases de la liste (i–vii) qui sont vraies.

Energies renouvelables

Les énergies renouvelables sont issues d'éléments naturels inépuisables: vent, soleil, eau, et matériaux qui peuvent se renouveler comme le bois. Elles s'opposent aux énergies fossiles qui existent en quantité limitée.

L'énergie solaire est constamment utilisable puisque le soleil brillera pendant cinq milliards d'années. Il en est de même du vent, des vagues, de l'eau, et des fleuves.

Aujourd'hui les panneaux solaires photovoltaïques transforment directement les rayons du soleil en électricité. Les capteurs solaires récupèrent la chaleur du soleil. Les éoliennes turbinent le vent et alimentent les réseaux électriques.

L'énergie des chutes d'eau, des marées ou des vagues peut être utilisée pour produire de l'électricité. C'est actuellement la plus efficace des énergies renouvelables exploitées. La chaleur du sous-sol est aussi récupérée dans les installations géothermiques qui utilisent l'eau chaude du sous-sol pour produire de l'électricité ou pour chauffer directement des maisons. La biomasse est également brûlée pour obtenir de la chaleur ou de l'électricité.

La mise en œuvre de certaines énergies renouvelables peut parfois générer des désastres sociaux. La construction de barrages entraîne fréquemment des déplacements de population. L'ouvrage des Trois Gorges en Chine produira autant que dix centrales nucléaires. Mais il aura fallu pour cela inonder 1 000 km² et chasser près de deux millions de personnes. Dans un pays de la taille de la France cela représenterait plus de 60 000 déplacés.

© Extraits de L'Ecologuide de A à Z (2004), Fondation Nicolas Hulot pour la Nature et l'Homme, www.fnh.org

Vocabulaire

inépuisable *inexhaustible*

la vague *wave*

le fleuve *river*

le panneau *panel*

une éolienne *wind turbine*

alimenter *to feed*

la chute d'eau *waterfall*

la marée *tide*

efficace *efficient*

brûlé *burnt*

la mise en œuvre *construction*

le barrage *dam*

entraîner *to bring about*

chasser *to drive out*

la taille *size*

i On met l'accent sur le fait que chaque source d'énergie vient de sources qui s'épuisent.

ii Les énergies fossiles s'épuisent.

iii L'énergie solaire est meilleure que les autres sources d'énergie renouvelables.

iv L'avenir des énergies renouvelables s'annonce bien.

v On explique le fonctionnement de quatre "énergies vertes".

vi Le passage décrit toutes les énergies renouvelables favorablement.

vii La construction de barrages peut avoir un impact négatif.

b Ecrivez des phrases avec vos propres mots sur les idées essentielles du texte.

- Sources des énergies renouvelables
- Un aspect positif de l'énergie solaire
- Un aspect positif de l'usage de l'eau
- Un aspect négatif de l'usage de l'eau

3 a 🎧 Ecoutez le reportage sur les métiers de l'énergie. Vrai ou faux?

i   Le nombre de débouchés dans le secteur des énergies renouvelables augmente.

ii Le nombre d'emplois devrait bientôt atteindre les 15 000 salariés.

iii Pour que Francine puisse travailler dans le secteur de l'énergie solaire, il lui a fallu faire une école d'ingénieurs.

iv Francine préférerait un travail sans autant de déplacements.

v   Arnaud fait seulement installer des installations frigorifiques.

vi Il faut être au point concernant tous les développements technologiques.

vii Il existe de moins en moins de débouchés dans son secteur de travail.

b 🎧 Réécoutez et trouvez pour chaque personne un aspect positif de leur travail.

4 💡 Lisez le texte (en ligne) et faites les activités interactives.

5 💡 A deux: trouvez pour chaque source d'énergie une définition ainsi qu'un aspect positif et négatif. (Feuille)

a   l'énergie éolienne
b   la géothermie
c   l'hydroélectricité
d   le solaire
e   la biomasse

Exemple: _____

A: Explique-moi ce que c'est, l'énergie éolienne.

B: Eh bien, c'est quand on convertit la force du vent en électricité. Un aspect positif, c'est que c'est l'énergie renouvelable la moins coûteuse. Le côté négatif, c'est que les éoliennes ne fonctionnent pas quand il n'y a pas de vent.

_____

6 💡 Comparez deux formes d'énergies renouvelables. Recherchez où, en France, on trouverait des exemples. (Feuille)
Pour vous aider, cliquez sur:

http://www.ecologie.gouv.fr/-Biodiversite-et-paysages-.html
http://www.greenpeace.org/france/campaigns/energie-et-climat
http://www.ademe.fr/particuliers/Fiches/climat/rub6.htm
http://www.defipourlaterre.org

Expressions clés

C'est quand on produit...

C'est lorsqu'on crée...

Cette technique utilise...

On convertit...

On construit...

Ceci permet d'utiliser la force du vent.

Les éoliennes offrent la possibilité de produire une énergie propre, tandis que le nucléaire pose le problème des déchets.

On peut produire de l'électricité en captant l'énergie du soleil, alors que le charbon émet du CO_2 dans l'atmosphère.

D'un côté le nucléaire nous donne de l'énergie sans émissions de CO_2, mais d'un autre côté on doit gérer le problème des déchets radioactifs.

🔧 Compétences

Express necessity, consequence and contrast

The following verbs and phrases are useful to express necessity, consequence and contrast. Revise present and conditional forms of verbs such as *on doit/ on devrait*. See pages 110, 113 and 122 (verb tables).

devoir to have to

falloir to be necessary: *il faut* it is necessary, *il faudra* it will be necessary, *il faudrait* it would be necessary, *il fallait* it was necessary

il est nécessaire de it's necessary to

il est nécessaire que... (+ subj.) it's necessary that...

pouvoir to be able to

entraîner to bring about

permettre à quelqu'un de faire quelque chose to allow someone to do something

prévoir to foresee

être l'opposé / le contraire de to be the opposite of

en être de même pour to be the same for

par contre on the other hand

d'un côté... mais d'un autre côté... on the one hand... but on the other hand...

cependant however   *tandis que* whereas   *alors que* while

C Les attitudes changeantes

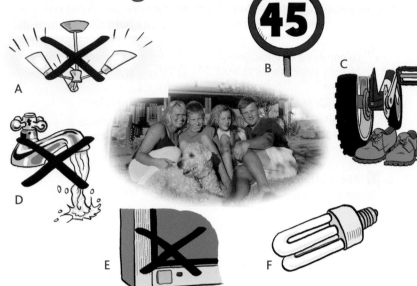

1 a 🎧 Ecoutez les suggestions et notez la lettre de celles qui sont mentionnées.

b Travail de groupe: pourriez-vous ajouter d'autres initiatives?

A

B

C

D

E

F

2 Lisez le texte et répondez aux questions en français.

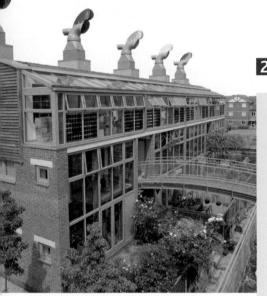

Le projet BedZED au sud de Londres, un village écologique

Vocabulaire

diviser *to divide*

souscrire à *to subscribe*

le gaspillage *waste*

relever le défi *to raise the challenge*

étendu *spread out*

le moindre déplacement *the least movement*

lié à *linked to*

le frein *brake*

la croissance *growth*

préconiser *to recommend*

provenir: proviendra de *to come from: will come from*

La solution passe par l'innovation

Pour éviter la catastrophe climatique, le monde doit, d'ici à 2050 diviser par deux ses émissions de gaz à effet de serre. Pour les pays riches, qui peuvent faire davantage d'effort, c'est par quatre qu'il faudrait diviser les émissions en quelques décennies. Un grand nombre de gouvernements dont celui de la France a décidé de souscrire à cet objectif, souvent baptisé "facteur 4". Technologies propres et moins de gaspillages peuvent encore relever le défi. La majorité des climatologues estiment qu'il ne faut pas réchauffer la planète de plus de 2° C par rapport à sa température préindustrielle. Que signifie ces 2° C pour nos activités quotidiennes? Est-ce qu'on pourrait continuer à faire les mêmes choses?

Les villes actuelles sont très étendues: centres commerciaux, zones résidentielles en périphérie, bureaux dans les centres-villes... le moindre déplacement nécessite l'usage de la voiture. Il faut réussir à maîtriser cette consommation d'énergie essentiellement liée aux transports, au chauffage et à l'éclairage public. La solution consiste à regrouper les lieux de vie, de travail, de commerces et de loisirs. Priorité doit être donnée aux piétons et aux cyclistes et aux transports en commun fonctionnant aux énergies renouvelables.

Dans la première partie d'un rapport sur les freins à la croissance, on préconise la création d'une dizaine d'"Ecopolis", cités tournées vers la qualité environnementale, les nouvelles technologies et pouvant accueillir 50 000 habitants. Ces dix villes intégreraient les technologies vertes. L'énergie proviendra de l'éolien et du solaire. Priorité sera également donnée à la réduction de la consommation d'eau et au tri des déchets. Il faudrait encourager les gens à participer à ces actions.

a De quoi s'agit-il dans le texte?

b Pour sauvegarder notre environnement, que dit-on sur les émissions?

c Que disent la majorité des climatologues?

d Comment sont les villes actuellement?

e Expliquez ce que c'est un écopolis.

3 Ecoutez trois jeunes exprimer leur opinion sur les écovilles. Lisez les phrases a–f. C'est qui: Julie, Annie ou Franck?

a Il vaudrait mieux améliorer les villes qui existent.

b On en a déjà fait l'expérience dans les années 60 sans succès.

c Il faut encourager les innovations si on veut sauvegarder notre environnement.

d Les gens qui conçoivent ces projets ne sont pas ceux qui y vivent.

e Cette personne a déjà vu un bel exemple d'une écoville.

f C'est aussi toutes les facilités qui comptent et pas seulement l'habitation.

4 💡🎧 Ecoutez le reportage sur une ville en Chine et faites les activités interactives.

5 💡 Travail de groupe. Regardez sur la feuille les photos de différentes habitations et posez des questions sur chacune. Présentez les conclusions de votre groupe. (Feuille)

Exemples: _____

Aimeriez-vous habiter dans cet écovillage?

Quels pourraient être les avantages?

Y voyez-vous des inconvénients?

Comment est-ce qu'on vivra à l'avenir, selon vous?

Comment serait votre ville / village idéal(e) sur le plan écologique?

_____

6 💡 Décrivez tous les gestes quotidiens que vous pourriez faire à la maison et dans les lieux publics pour sauvegarder l'environnement. Evaluez s'il y a des différences entre la France et votre pays. (Feuille)

Pour vous aider, cliquez sur: http://www.defipourlaterre.org/agir/

7 💡🖎 Energie et conservation: écoutez les questions et enregistrez vos réponses.

Expressions clés

On pourrait baisser la température / prendre une douche plutôt qu'un bain.

Je fais mon compost.

On a déja eu des villes nouvelles sans âme.

A mon avis, il faut développer les petites villes.

Mieux vaut améliorer ce qui existe déjà.

Je me précipiterais pour aller y vivre.

Il faut tirer les leçons du passé.

On veut des quartiers agréables à vivre.

Il faut beaucoup d'espaces verts.

On désire des commerces de proximité.

Il faut bannir la voiture.

💡 Grammaire

Use verbs followed by an infinitive

When two verbs follow each other, the second is in the infinitive. Sometimes before the second verb there is a preposition, either *à* or *de*. (See pages 117–8.)

These are examples of **dependent infinitives** (see page 118):

faire + infinitive (to cause something to happen)
se faire + infinitive (to have something done to yourself)

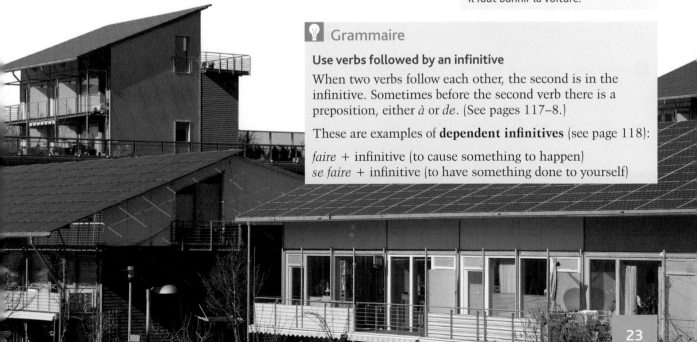

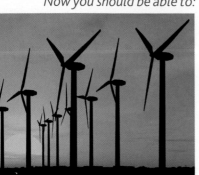

Now you should be able to:

■ talk about the different sources of fossil fuels

■ discuss the role of nuclear energy in France

■ discuss the need for renewable energy sources

■ explore changing attitudes to energy consumption

Grammar

■ revise present tense endings

■ revise present and conditional forms (to express necessity)

■ use verbs followed by an infinitive

Skills

■ debate controversial issues

■ express necessity, consequence and contrast

■ evaluate lifestyle using alternative forms of energy

✓ Résumé

1 Recopiez et remplissez les blancs avec les mots de la case.

Le pétrole est une des énergies ...... L'...... des énergies fossiles est prévisible car leur capacité de ...... est inférieure au rythme de la ...... mondiale.

fossiles   consommation   renouvellement   épuisement

2 C'est quoi?

C'est une énergie renouvelable. Il faut avoir une nacelle pivotante, des pales, un mât, des ordinateurs et des appareillages électriques.

3 Reliez les secteurs i–iv aux buts a–d.
i les combustibles fossiles
ii le transport
iii l'usage efficace à la maison
iv l'industrie propre

a le carburant mieux utilisé
b traiter les déchets
c réduire la partie du fossile
d efficacité énergétique

4 Mettez les mots dans le bon ordre pour faire une phrase:

Une   de   4 à 5 minutes   30 à 80 litres   et consomme   un   d'eau   bain   150 à 200 litres douche

5 Traduisez en anglais:

Partout des initiatives se mettent en place, au niveau de l'Etat, mais rien ne peut aboutir sans action individuelle.

6 Choisissez un geste quotidien pour protéger l'environnement:
a écrire une lettre
b téléphoner à un ami
c trier les déchets

7 Expliquez le terme "Ecopolis".

8 Remplissez les blancs avec la bonne préposition.

Il faut s'habituer ...... trier les déchets et penser ...... l'environnement. J'ai décidé ...... faire de petits gestes quotidiens.

9 Traduisez en français:

You build pleasant areas with small blocks of flats. The essential thing is a good public transport network.

10 Lequel est le verbe au présent?
a choisiront
b choisissent
c choisissaient

AQA   Examiner's tips

Listening
Listen to the passage **all the way through**, then go back and pause the recording to answer each question.

Speaking
Make sure you understand the **overall content** of the card before tackling the printed questions.

Reading
Read the whole text to understand its general meaning before you answer the questions.

Writing
Research sub-topic issues on French websites or in French magazines.

L'environnement

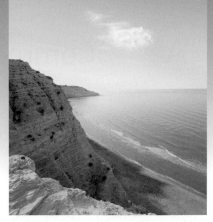

3   Protection de la planète

By the end of this chapter you will be able to:

	Language	Grammar	Skills
A **Comment minimiser les dangers?**	describe the impact of consumerism on the environment and explore how to change behaviour	use interrogative pronouns	recommend future measures
B **Les groupes de pression**	examine the role of pressure groups and their initiatives to promote awareness	use the subjunctive (revisited)	use language to promote a cause
C **Notre responsabilité envers les autres pays**	discuss the need for collaboration and cooperation	use the immediate future and the future tense	express awareness of positive and negative impact

Le saviez-vous?

Seuls 13% des déchets en France sont recyclés.

Un fruit importé par avion consomme 10 à 20 fois plus de pétrole que le même fruit produit localement.

Chaque année, entre 13 et 15 millions d'hectares de forêts tropicales – trois fois la surface de la Suisse – sont coupés.

Pour commencer

1   Qu'est-ce que c'est, une empreinte écologique?
    a   une trace d'animal
    b   une mesure de votre influence directe sur la nature
    c   une brochure sur l'écologie

2   9000 kms, c'est la distance moyenne parcourue par les composants d'un yaourt (lait, fraises, plastiques) avant de rejoindre nos réfrigérateurs. Qu'est-ce qu'on pourrait faire pour minimiser l'impact sur la nature?

3   Donnez un exemple d'animal menacé d'extinction, par exemple à cause de la chasse ou des activités de l'homme.

4   Comment traduire?
    « Vous pourriez faire un don à notre association. »

5   Comment expliqueriez-vous le terme "la biodiversité"?

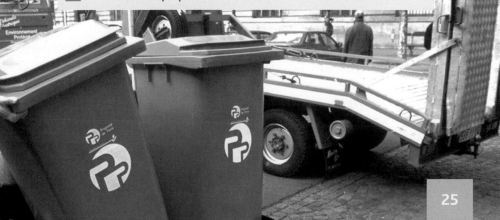

A   Comment minimiser les dangers?

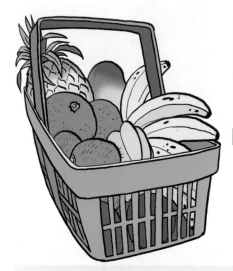

Tracez l'empreinte écologique

Quand on mange une orange, quand on se déplace en véhicule, quand on prend une douche, on consomme des ressources naturelles. Chacun de ces actes s'accompagne d'une consommation de ressources que la planète doit fournir et d'une production de déchets qu'elle doit absorber.

1
a Travail de groupe: mettez dans un ordre logique les étapes de l'empreinte écologique d'un fruit exotique.

   i   l'eau   ii   le travail des gens et des machines   iii   le transport
   iv   l'engrais   v   la réfrigération   vi   l'emballage
   vii   la vente en magasin   viii   la terre pour cultiver

b Comment pourrait-on minimiser l'impact de cette empreinte? Justifiez vos idées.

Qu'est-ce que l'empreinte écologique?

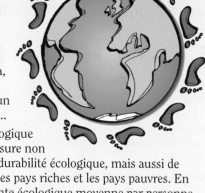

L'empreinte écologique est une estimation de la surface nécessaire à une personne pour produire ce qu'elle consomme et absorber ce qu'elle rejette. Elle s'exprime en hectares, en terrains de football (c'est plus visuel...) ou en nombre de planètes.

La Terre dispose de 11,3 milliards d'hectares « biologiquement productifs ». Cela constitue sa « biocapacité » actuelle. Si on divise ce chiffre par le nombre d'habitants de la planète, on arrive aujourd'hui à un chiffre situé entre 1,7 et 1,8 ha par habitant. C'est ce que la Terre peut donner à chaque personne de manière équitable (et durable).

Or, en moyenne, chaque individu consomme 2,3 ha. Il y a donc déjà un dépassement de la biocapacité terrestre: nous consommons plus que ce que l'écosystème planétaire peut renouveler. En d'autres termes, nous vivons sur nos stocks... De plus, cette consommation est évidemment très inégalement répartie. Un Européen a une empreinte moyenne de 5 ha, un Américain du Nord de 9,7 ha, un Indien de 0,7 ha...

L'empreinte écologique est donc une mesure non seulement de la durabilité écologique, mais aussi de l'inégalité entre les pays riches et les pays pauvres. En France, l'empreinte écologique moyenne par personne est de 7,3 hectares. C'est-à-dire que si tout le monde était comme le Français moyen, il nous faudrait à peu près trois planètes.

Vocabulaire

une empreinte écologique *carbon footprint*

s'exprimer *to be expressed*

disposer de *to have*

équitable *fair*

or *well, but, now*

inégalement *unequally*

réparti *shared out*

la durabilité *sustainability*

l'inégalité *inequality*

2
a Lisez le texte et les phrases. Ecrivez V (vrai), F (faux) ou N (information non donnée).

   i   Calculer une empreinte écologique est devenu une science exacte.

   ii   L'empreinte écologique est un moyen de calculer l'impact d'un individu sur la planète.

   iii   En gros, chaque individu n'a pas encore dépassé ses limites.

   iv   On va organiser une conférence internationale sur le dépassement de la biocapacité terrestre.

   v   Un Indien a un impact plus important qu'un Européen.

   vi   L'inégalité entre les pays pauvres va bientôt disparaître.

   vii   Si on adoptait tous le comportement d'un Français moyen il nous faudrait deux planètes.

b Faites un résumé du texte en anglais en 90 mots.

3 💡 Lisez le texte (en ligne) et faites les activités interactives.

4 a 🎧 Comment minimiser l'impact sur l'environnement? Ecoutez six possibilités et trouvez la bonne image pour chacune.

b Trouvez une raison de privilégier chaque geste. Complétez les phrases avec vos propres mots.

Je devrais privilégier...

i les produits issus de l'agriculture biologique parce que...

ii les fruits et les légumes de saison parce que...

iii les produits durables parce que...

iv les déodorants à bille parce que...

v un sac durable parce que...

vi les commerces de proximité parce que...

5 💡 Pensez à un produit que vous avez acheté récemment. Tracez-en l'empreinte écologique. Aidez-vous d'un dictionnaire. (Feuille)

Exemple: _____

Le cycle d'un jean. Tout d'abord il faut travailler le coton et puis fabriquer le jean...

la culture du coton, la fabrication, l'emballage, le marketing, le transport et la vente en magasin...

_____

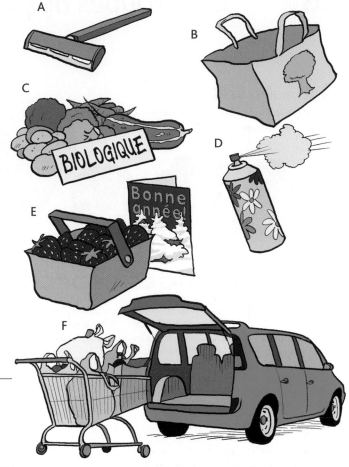

6 💡 Présentez à la classe l'empreinte écologique du produit que vous avez analysé pour l'activité 5. Expliquez comment on pourrait être plus écologique. (Feuille)

Expressions clés

Pourquoi ne pas choisir des fruits de la région?

N'hésitez pas à faire le maximum.

Soyez prudent avec notre planète.

On peut changer ses habitudes.

Vous ne vous rendez pas compte?

Grâce aux petits gestes, on peut faire quelque chose.

Lequel d'entre vous va faire quelque chose?

Il y a trois étapes: la culture, la production, l'utilisation.

Ceci a un effet sur l'environnement.

A cause du transport...

C'est dommageable.

Les groupes de pression

1 🎧 Ecoutez les noms d'animaux à préserver. Regardez les images: quel animal manque-t-il?

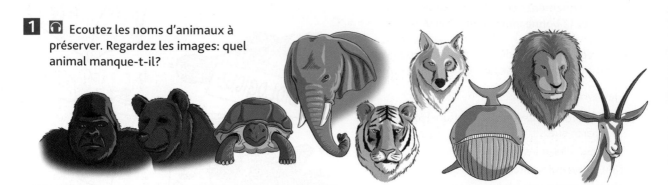

Protection des espèces

La biodiversité, c'est-à-dire la diversité des espèces et des écosystèmes, connaît une érosion. Les espèces disparaissent à un rythme mille fois supérieur au taux d'extinction naturel. Cette crise d'extinction sans précédent est due à l'activité directe ou indirecte des hommes.

Certaines populations d'animaux dans les forêts, dans les océans et sur les côtes, et dans les eaux douces, se sont réduites de 30% depuis les années 1970. Destruction et fragmentation des habitats, surexploitation par la récolte, la chasse, la pêche et le commerce, introduction d'espèces exotiques envahissantes, changements climatiques, pollution et gaspillage sont les

principales causes de disparition. Le WWF à l'ambition de conserver plus de 85% de la diversité biologique sur terre.

En France, les grands carnivores ont longtemps été chassés et avaient quasiment disparu. Revenus naturellement, une centaine de loups vivent aujourd'hui dans les Alpes où ils se reproduisent.

Le lynx a été réintroduit dans les Vosges dans les années 1980 et il est également présent dans les massifs du Jura et des Alpes qu'il a recolonisés progressivement à partir de la Suisse. Le mammifère le plus rare de France, l'ours n'a jamais disparu de nos montagnes et on estime à une vingtaine le nombre d'ours vivant dans les Pyrénées.

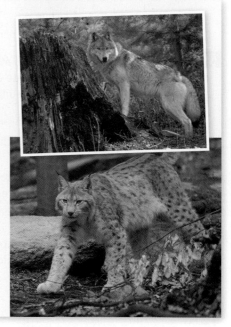

Vocabulaire

une espèce *species*
disparaître *disappear*
les eaux douces *fresh water, lakes*
la récolte *harvest*
la chasse *hunting*
envahissant *invading*
quasiment *almost*
le loup *wolf*
le massif *mountain*
le mammifère *mammal*
un ours *bear*

2 a Lisez le texte et remettez les phrases dans le bon ordre:

    i   Les grands carnivores sont de retour en France.

    ii   Le lynx vient de Suisse.

    iii   Les loups ne sont plus en danger dans les Alpes.

    iv   Le WWF tente de sauvegarder 85% de la diversité biologique sur terre.

    v   Des espèces de faune et de flore sont en disparition.

    vi   L'homme est en partie coupable de cette disparition.

    vii L'ours a toujours été présent en France.

b Traduisez le paragraphe suivant en français.

In order to protect the biodiversity of different species and habitats, it is necessary to rethink some of man's activities which are causing the disappearance of all sorts of species. Due to hunting, many wild animals have almost disappeared. Now some of these animals are returning to France.

3 a 🎧 Ecoutez le message de l'association AVES France. Lisez les phrases: vrai ou faux? Corrigez les phrases qui sont fausses.

  i   L'association veut soutenir les animaux qui risquent de disparaître.
  ii   L'association demande de l'argent.
  iii L'association va publier une liste de tous les animaux.
  iv   Le niveau d'activité des hommes peut rester le même.
  v   Le but de l'association ne sera que d'informer le public.
  vi   L'association va se plaindre chaque fois qu'un ours sera menacé.
  vii Pour aider, il y a quatre choses à faire.

b 🎧 Transcription. Ecrivez en français tout ce que vous entendez à partir de: *Nos missions pour l'ours…* jusqu'à: *… l'aide d'un spécialiste*.
Réécoutez pour vérifier.

c 💡 Regardez la transcription en ligne et vérifiez votre paragraphe. Faites une liste des mots difficiles. Analysez les difficultés.

4 💡 Lisez le texte (en ligne) sur les phoques en France et faites les activités interactives.

5 💡 A deux: choisissez un animal menacé ou une plante menacée et imaginez faire une demande de soutien pour une campagne de protection. Décrivez la situation précaire et expliquez la campagne. (Feuille)

Exemple: _____

Moi, je voudrais faire quelque chose pour sauvegarder le phoque moine en France. Le phoque moine est une espèce menacée. La population mondiale n'est plus que de 200 à 300! Il est aujourd'hui presque impossible d'observer des phoques moines en Méditerranée. Notre but est de sensibiliser le public. Aidez-nous à sauver les phoques! Adhérez aujourd'hui à notre association.

6 💡 Ecrivez un article pour un site web. Persuadez les internautes de soutenir votre action. (Feuille)

a   Donnez une raison pour soutenir votre animal ou cause (disparition possible, vivre en harmonie…).
b   Décrivez le but de votre association (protection de l'animal et de l'environnement, éducation…).
c   Dites ce que l'association fait de l'argent donné (mener des projets, parler avec les gouvernements, surveillance du commerce…).

◥ Compétences

Using language to promote a cause

Enhance your cause by:

- stating a high impact fact
- giving a sense of finality if action isn't taken
- asking for help.

The present subjunctive will be needed if you are expressing fear or a sense of superlative (*le seul, le premier, le dernier*, etc.):

*On craint qu'il y **ait** seulement une espèce survivante.*

*C'est la seule espèce que l'on **puisse** voir dans le monde.*

Expressions clés

Cet animal est une espèce menacée d'extinction.

On commence à prendre conscience du déclin.

Cela contribue également au déclin.

Les causes du déclin sont liées à l'action de l'Homme.

C'est la conséquence de la surexploitation des stocks de poisson.

On peut se rendre compte de la difficulté.

Diverses organisations internationales se mobilisent pour la sauvegarde de l'animal.

La tâche à accomplir est très lourde.

Nous avons besoin de votre soutien.

Notre mission porte sur l'éducation.

Nous souhaitons la protection de l'association.

Vous pourriez adhérer à l'association.

Vous pourriez faire un don / nous sponsoriser.

Aidez-nous à sauvegarder les animaux.

Notre responsabilité envers les autres pays

1 🎧 Ecoutez ce bulletin. Notez tous les chiffres et les dates que vous entendez.

Climat: les principaux pollueurs entament deux jours de débats à Paris

Les 16 principales économies, qui cumulent 80% des émissions mondiales de gaz à effet de serre, se retrouveront jeudi pour deux jours de discussions informelles sur la lutte contre le changement climatique.

Ce rendez-vous va être consacré aux possibilités de réduire les émissions de gaz à effet de serre (GES) par secteurs de production (ciment, sidérurgie, électricité...) et aux transferts de technologie. A la veille de la réunion, les Etats-Unis, instigateurs de ce forum, ont annoncé qu'ils entendaient arrêter la progression de leurs émissions d'ici 2025, pour commencer à inverser la tendance.

Or les Etats-Unis, premiers "pollueurs" avec la Chine, restent le seul pays industrialisé à ce jour à ne pas avoir ratifié le Protocole de Kyoto. L'Union européenne prônera une réduction d'au moins 20% des émissions mondiales d'ici 2030 et visera 50% pour 2050.

On va parler des pays en développement qui sont les plus durement touchés par les effets du changement climatique. Le changement climatique n'est pas équitable, car les pays les plus vulnérables sont ceux qui en sont les moins "responsables". On va donc demander un effort supplémentaire des pays riches pour permettre aux pays les plus pauvres de s'adapter au changement climatique.

L'administrateur du Programme des Nations unies pour le développement, Kemal Dervis,

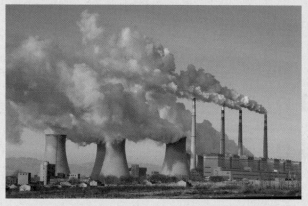

a rappelé que « 70% des gaz à effets de serre déjà émis sont dus à l'activité des pays riches, 28% ont été émis par les pays émergents et seulement 2% par les pays les moins développés ». La Commission européenne a donc proposé la création d'une "alliance mondiale" pour la lutte contre le changement climatique, pour laquelle elle a affecté 50 millions d'euros pour la période 2008–2010.

Certains pays, dans les régions en proie aux sécheresses ou aux inondations ou encore les petits Etats insulaires menacés par la hausse du niveau de la mer, ne disposent pas des ressources nécessaires pour s'adapter alors qu'ils sont déjà confrontés aux impacts du changement climatique.

Vocabulaire

entamer *to open up*

consacré à *dedicated to*

la sidérurgie *steel*

la veille *the night before*

la réunion *the meeting*

ratifier *to ratify, to endorse*

prôner *to preach*

viser à *to aim at*

en proie à *victim of*

la sécheresse *drought*

disposer de *to have*

2 a Lisez l'article et faites une liste en anglais de dix points importants.

b Répondez aux questions en français.

   i   Qui sont les principaux pollueurs?

   ii   Quel est le thème des discussions?

   iii Quel sera le but du forum?

   iv Quelle est l'intention des Etats-Unis?

   v   Quelle est l'intention de l'Europe?

   vi Dans quelle situation se trouvent souvent les pays les moins développés?

c Traduisez le dernier paragraphe de l'article en anglais.

3　a　A l'aide d'un dictionnaire, trouvez l'équivalent en anglais de ces expressions:

　　i　le maïs　　　　　　　iii　d'une décharge électronique
　　ii　la pénurie des denrées de base　　iv　aller au marteau

　　b　🔊 Ecoutez le reportage sur les biocarburants (= *biofuels*) et les déchets électroniques. Choisissez les trois phrases qui sont vraies.

　　i　La production des biocarburants crée une situation difficile pour les pays pauvres.
　　ii　Les pays pauvres n'ont plus de difficultés à cause de la production des biocarburants.
　　iii　Ce n'est pas discutable, on devra continuer la production des biocarburants des pays pauvres.
　　iv　Les Américains font beaucoup pour préserver l'environnement.
　　v　Les Américains sont les principaux producteurs d'une décharge électronique.
　　vi　5% à 80% des 30 000 à 400 000 tonnes de déchets électroniques sont envoyés en Chine, en Inde et au Niger.
　　vii　50% à 80% des 300 000 à 400 000 tonnes de déchets électroniques sont envoyés en Chine, en Inde et au Niger.

4　💡🎧 Ecoutez le passage et faites les activités interactives.

5　💡　A l'oral: préparez une présentation pour une conférence sur la biodiversité. Développez chacune des mesures ci-dessous, en expliquant leurs conséquences. (Feuille)

- Réduire l'appauvrissement de la biodiversité
- Lutter contre la déforestation, contre la surpêche
- Mettre fin à la disparition des espèces
- Instaurer l'établissement d'une alliance mondiale

Exemple: _____

Il faut réduire l'appauvrissement de la biodiversité parce que des millions de personnes vont souffrir d'un manque de nourriture.

_____

6　💡 Ecrivez 300 mots sur l'importance des forêts tropicales dans le monde en considérant les aspects suivants. (Feuille)

- importance pour la diversité des espèces
- importance pour le climat
- conséquences de la destruction

Pour vous aider, cliquez sur:
http://terresacree.org/forevieg.htm

7　💡🎙 Ecoutez le dialogue et enregistrez vos réponses.

💡 Grammaire

Le futur proche et le futur simple

The future tense (*le futur simple*) expresses what will happen at any point in the future.

The immediate future (*le futur proche*) describes an event in the near future. See page 112.

*Les 16 principales économies **se retrouveront** jeudi pour deux jours de discussions.* (= futur simple)

*On **va parler** des pays en développement.* (= futur proche)

▨ Expressions clés

Tout d'abord, je dirais que…

Ce qui me trouble, c'est…

On ne peut pas ignorer ces statistiques choquantes qui montrent que la situation est grave.

Il faut faire le point sur le développement durable.

La disparition des espèces a pris une allure dramatique.

La biodiversité nous apporte beaucoup.

L'impact de la perte de la biodiversité sera énorme.

On dépend de la forêt pour l'alimentation et les médicaments.

Sans ces forêts on est plus vulnérable face aux catastrophes naturelles.

Les arbres sont des maillons essentiels de la chaîne de la vie.

Beaucoup d'experts tirent la sonnette d'alarme.

Il faut mettre ces sujets fondamentaux à l'ordre du jour.

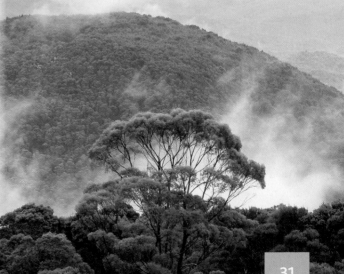

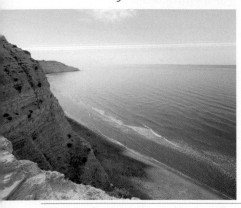

Now you should be able to:

■ describe the impact of consumerism on the environment and explore how to change behaviour

■ examine the role of pressure groups and their initiatives to promote awareness

■ discuss the need for collaboration and cooperation

Grammar

■ use interrogative pronouns

■ use the subjunctive (revisited)

■ use the immediate future and the future tense

Skills

■ recommend future measures

■ use language to promote a cause

■ express awareness of positive and negative impact

✓ Résumé

1 De quoi s'agit-il?

C'est une estimation de la surface nécessaire à une personne pour produire ce qu'elle consomme et absorber ce qu'elle rejette.

2 Remplissez les blancs avec les mots ci-dessous.

Pour transporter mes courses, j'..... les sacs jetables et je choisis les sacs durables. J'..... toujours d'..... avec ..... un sac réutilisable, plié dans ma ..... ou dans mon ..... à main.

moi   sac   essaie   abandonne   amener   poche

3 Choisissez entre **Qu'est-ce qui**, **Qu'est-ce que**, **Qui est-ce qui**:

a ...... la dame a répondu?

b ...... veut aller au marché avec moi?

4 Choisissez entre **Laquelle** et **Lequel**:

a ...... parmi ces hommes est déjà membre de l'association?

b ...... préfères-tu entre toutes ces plantes?

5 Traduisez la phrase en anglais:

Mis à part les croyances et les intérêts purement commerciaux du passé, ce sont surtout l'attitude des pêcheurs et la malnutrition qui sont à l'origine de la disparition du phoque moine.

6 Expliquez le terme "la biodiversité".

7 Traduisez en français:

You could join our association, make a donation and help us protect the animals.

8 Traduisez en français en utilisant le futur proche:

The activists are going to meet next month.

9 Que veut dire le sigle "GES"?

10 Lequel est le verbe au futur?

a meurent

b mourront

c allaient mourir

AQA Examiner's tips

Listening
Read the questions carefully. They may provide clues about vocabulary used in the passage.

Speaking
Prepare a brief answer to the question *De quoi s'agit-il?* **Summarise the subject** of the card in a couple of sentences.

Reading
Illustrations around the text might **help you understand** the content.

Writing
Discuss the exam topics with your friends, so that you have **plenty of ideas** to write about.

La société multiculturelle

L'immigration

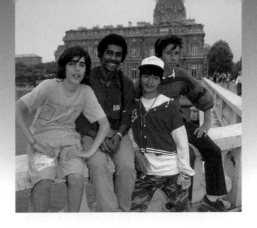

By the end of this chapter you will be able to:

	Language	Grammar	Skills
A **La France, terre d'accueil?**	■ explore the reasons for immigration	■ revise numbers	■ express proportions and statistics
B **Immigration choisie**	■ talk about government policy to curb immigration ■ discuss the benefits and problems of immigration	■ use the future perfect tense	■ defend a viewpoint
C **Immigration au sein de l'Union européenne**	■ talk about immigration within the enlarged European community	■ use indirect speech	■ present oral analysis of advantages and disadvantages of immigration

■ Le saviez-vous?

Quelques chiffres: Au dernier recensement de 2005, on comptait 3,5 millions d'étrangers en France, dont 40% en provenance des Etats de l'Union européenne, 31% du Maghreb, 13,7% du Sud-est asiatique, 7% d'Afrique subsaharienne, 6,5% de Turquie. Au total, les étrangers représentent 5,7% de la population en France.

La Cité Nationale de l'histoire de l'immigration a ouvert ses portes le 10 octobre 2007. Consultez son site Internet www.histoire-immigration.fr où plus de deux siècles d'immigration sont racontés par des films, des textes et des photos.

■ Pour commencer

1 Vous connaissez les mots "immigré" et "émigré". Quelle est la différence entre les deux?

2 Quels sont les trois pays qui constituent le Maghreb?
- le Maroc
- le Sénégal
- la Tunisie
- l'Espagne
- l'Algérie
- l'Egypte

3 Comment s'appelle un homme originaire du Maghreb?

Et une femme?

4 Il y a maintenant combien de pays membres de l'Union européenne?
- 24
- 27
- 29

5 Qu'est-ce qu'un "sans-papiers"?
Une personne qui...
- ne sait pas écrire
- n'a pas d'argent
- n'a pas de titre de séjour

A. La France, terre d'accueil?

1 🎧 Ecoutez l'introduction d'une émission sur l'immigration. Que dit-on sur l'immigration européenne en France?

LES IMMIGRÉS EN FRANCE: UNE SITUATION QUI ÉVOLUE

Par sa situation géographique qui en fait un lieu de croisement des commerces et des populations, et puis par son histoire coloniale, la France est un pays de migration de longue durée et est choisie comme pays de destination à cause de la familiarité avec la langue française.

Les immigrés proviennent de pays de plus en plus lointains; le regroupement familial et les demandes d'asile sont en augmentation, les femmes représentant la moitié des immigrés vivant en France.

Du fait de la taille de leur famille, de la faiblesse de leurs revenus et de leur concentration dans les grandes villes, les immigrés sont plus souvent locataires du secteur social et vivent plus fréquemment dans des logements surpeuplés. Les immigrés sont davantage affectés par le chômage, ils occupent plus souvent des postes d'ouvriers ou d'employés.

Dans les dernières décennies, les origines géographiques des immigrés se sont beaucoup diversifiées. En 1962, les immigrés venus d'Espagne, d'Italie, du Portugal et de Pologne représentaient à eux seuls la moitié des immigrés résidant en France; de nos jours, ils n'en représentent qu'à peine un sur six.

A l'inverse, la part des immigrés nés au Maghreb a doublé: ils représentent désormais presque un tiers des immigrés. De plus en plus d'immigrés viennent d'Afrique subsaharienne, de Turquie ou d'Asie.

Les immigrés sont davantage présents dans les zones frontalières et les régions urbanisées ou industrielles, soit l'Ile-de-France, les régions de l'est et méridionales.

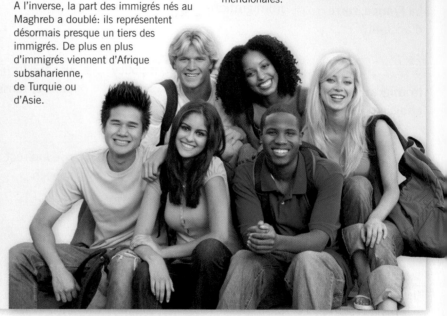

Vocabulaire

le lieu *place*

la durée *period of time*

provenir *to come from*

lointain *far away*

un asile *asylum*

la faiblesse de leurs revenus *their low income*

le/la locataire *tenant*

surpeuplé *overcrowded*

davantage *more*

un ouvrier *worker*

la décennie *decade*

à peine *only just, barely*

à l'inverse *on the contrary*

désormais *from now on*

la zone frontalière *border zone*

2 **a** Lisez le texte et dites si les phrases sont vraies (V) ou fausses (F).

  i   Beaucoup d'immigrés parlent français.

  ii   Les femmes immigrées sont peu nombreuses.

  iii Les salaires des immigrés sont bas.

  iv   Le nombre d'immigrés en provenance du Maghreb s'est multiplié par deux.

  v   Les immigrés s'installent souvent dans les zones rurales.

  vi   Les immigrés viennent de pays de plus en plus éloignés.

b Choisissez la fin de phrase qui convient.

  i   La France est choisie comme pays de destination...
       a depuis peu   b depuis longtemps

  ii   Le regroupement familial et les demandes d'asiles sont...
       a en hausse   b en baisse

  iii Les immigrés occupent des emplois...   a de manœuvres   b qualifiés

  iv   Les immigrés sont souvent...   a propriétaires   b logés en HLM

  v   On trouve un grand nombre d'immigrés...
       a dans le sud de la France   b dans le centre de la France

3 🎧 Ecoutez cet extrait sur le statut des réfugiés politiques.

    a   Donnez quatre raisons pour lesquelles une personne peut être persécutée dans son pays d'origine.

    b   Répondez aux questions suivantes:

        En quelle année la France a-t-elle signé la Convention de Genève?

        Combien de pays dans le monde l'ont désormais signée?

        A quel moment cette Convention a-t-elle été élaborée?

    c   Pensez-vous que cette Convention soit une bonne idée? Pourquoi? Discutez-en avec votre partenaire.

4 💡🎧 Réécoutez l'extrait et faites les activités interactives.

5 💡 A deux, préparez une présentation sur l'origine des immigrés au Royaume-Uni (différentes nationalités, origines, raisons). (Feuille)

    a   Faites une comparaison avec la France.

    b   Comparez vos résultats avec le reste de la classe.

6 💡 A l'écrit: relisez vos réponses à l'activité 3a. (Feuille)

    a   Y a-t-il d'autres raisons pour lesquelles une personne puisse vouloir quitter son pays d'origine?

    b   Ecrivez un paragraphe sur la protection des réfugiés. Pensez-vous qu'il est de notre devoir de les accueillir ou non?

7 💡🔖 Jeu de rôle: écoutez le dialogue et enregistrez vos réponses.

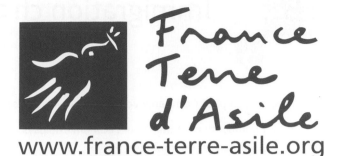

www.france-terre-asile.org

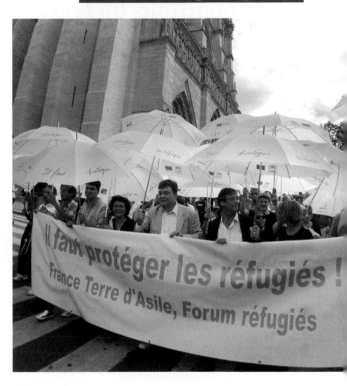

Expressions clés

Les conditions de vie sont difficiles / insupportables.

C'est un pays en conflit.

Il y a une guerre civile dans mon pays.

mourir de faim

la persécution / être persécuté par...

un immigré clandestin

un passeur fait traverser une frontière

les anciennes colonies britanniques / françaises

trouver refuge dans un autre pays

s'exiler de / fuir son pays

s'échapper de, échapper à

gagner sa vie, réaliser un rêve

satisfaire les besoins de sa famille

Je n'ai pas les moyens de nourrir ma famille.

Un réfugié politique doit être accueilli.

🔖 Compétences

Express proportions and statistics

Percentages: *cinq pour cent* = 5%

Decimals: *dix-sept virgule cinq pour cent* = 17,5 %

Proportions:

la moitié	*plus de la moitié*
un tiers	*plus d'un tiers*
un quart	*plus d'un quart*
un sur six	
de plus en plus	*de moins en moins*
au moins	*à peine* *davantage*

Useful verbs: *augmenter, doubler, baisser, chuter, diminuer*

Immigration choisie

1 D'accord ou pas? Comparez vos opinions avec le reste de la classe.

a « L'immigration est utile pour l'économie du pays. »

b « Il faut fermer les frontières. »

c « On doit légaliser tous les sans-papiers. »

Nouvelle loi sur l'immigration: durcissement des conditions du regroupement familial

TEST DE LANGUE: les personnes souhaitant bénéficier d'un regroupement familial doivent "connaître la langue française et les valeurs de la République". Elles doivent donc passer un test. Si leurs résultats sont insuffisants, elles sont soumises à une formation de "deux mois maximum".

REVENU MINIMUM: un immigré se trouvant en France ne peut faire venir sa famille que s'il a des revenus suffisants, que la loi fixe à 1 à 1,33 fois le Smic, hors prestations sociales comme les allocations familiales, selon le nombre de personnes à charge.

CONTRAT D'ACCUEIL ET D'INTÉGRATION: une fois que leurs enfants seront arrivés, les parents devront signer un contrat avec l'Etat. Son non-respect peut entraîner la suppression des allocations familiales.

TESTS ADN: cette proposition a fait grand bruit. La loi prévoit de faire passer un test ADN aux enfants candidats (sur la base du volontariat) au regroupement familial pour s'assurer de leur filiation avec la personne se trouvant déjà en France.

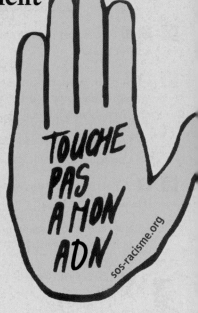

TOUCHE PAS A MON ADN
sos-racisme.org

ADN   Smic   revenu   formation   filiation   allocation familiale   regroupement familial

2 a Reliez les mots et expressions à gauche avec leurs définitions (a–g).

a versée aux familles d'au moins deux enfants

b la descendance des parents en ligne directe

c réunit tous les membres d'un même foyer

d le salaire minimum interprofessionnel de croissance

e ce que rapporte un travail

f la molécule support de l'information génétique héréditaire

g apprentissage qui permet de se perfectionner

b **En vous aidant du texte ci-dessus, trouvez la fin de chaque phrase.**

i Un contrat devra être signé…

ii Les immigrés qui ne parlent pas français…

iii Les enfants qui veulent rejoindre leurs parents…

iv Un immigré doit gagner un certain salaire…

a pour faire venir sa famille.

b devront passer un test ADN.

c dès l'arrivée en France.

d suivront des cours pendant deux mois.

Vocabulaire

le durcissement *hardening*

insuffisant *insufficient*

être soumis à *to be subject to*

hors *except for, apart from*

la prestation sociale *social security benefit*

entraîner *to lead to*

faire grand bruit *to cause an outcry*

prévoir *to plan*

3 Recopiez le dépliant et remplissez les blancs avec des mots choisis dans la liste ci-dessous. Utilisez chaque mot une fois seulement.

unique   autre   99,9%
code-barres   organiques   sang
établir   génétique   os   similaires
molécules   contient   personne

Comment fait-on le test ADN

Les tests ADN permettent d'...... le profil génétique d'une personne à partir de matières ......

1   Prélèvement

Des ...... d'ADN sont extraites à partir de salive ou de ...... , sueur, fragments de peau, ...

2   Analyse

Chaque cellule ...... de l'ADN dont la composition est ...... pour chaque ...... (équivalent d'un ......).

3   Comparaison

Le code ...... obtenu par l'ADN peut être comparé à un ....

4   Identification

S'ils sont ...... , l'identification est sûre à ....

4 a 🎧 Ecoutez le reportage sur une nouvelle loi sur l'immigration. Lisez les phrases (i–v) et choisissez l'expression correcte.

i   Si leur dossier est rejeté, les personnes [**en situation irrégulière / sans papiers**] n'auront plus qu'un seul mois pour contester la décision.

ii   A partir de maintenant, tous [**les étrangers / les immigrés**] qui déposent une demande de régularisation risquent une obligation à quitter le territoire français.

iii   Déposer une demande de [**carte de séjour / titre de séjour**] pose un risque très important.

iv   Beaucoup d'étrangers ne feront même pas [**la démarche / la demande**] de peur d'être frappés par cette mesure.

v   Quelqu'un qui a [**des papiers / des documents**] parfois depuis des années, dépose comme chaque année une demande de [**reconduction / renouvellement**] de son titre de séjour...

b 🎧 Quels termes sont utilisés pour exprimer les idées suivantes?

i   un dossier non accepté par l'administration:
   a   un dossier rejeté   b   un dossier refusé

ii   brusquement:
   a   sur-le-champ   b   du jour au lendemain

iii   annoncer une réponse négative:
   a   notifier un refus   b   signifier un refus

5 💡 A l'oral: « Tests ADN, pour ou contre? » (Feuille)

a   Dites ce que vous pensez des déclarations suivantes:

> La génétique décide qui a le droit ou non de s'établir en France.

> Le but du test est de rechercher une filiation avec la mère, pas avec le père.

> Seul le sang détermine une parenté avec la mère.

b   A votre avis, que va-t-il se passer dans le cas de familles recomposées ou d'enfants adoptés?

c   Accepteriez-vous de passer un test ADN? Pourquoi?

6 💡🎧 Ecoutez l'extrait sur l'exploitation d'immigrés et faites les activités interactives.

7 💡 A l'écrit. La nouvelle loi stipule qu'un immigré ne peut faire venir sa famille en France que s'il a des revenus suffisants. Développez la phrase ci-dessous. (Feuille)

« Les immigrés sont souvent affectés par le chômage et sont parfois exploités. »

💡 Grammaire

The future perfect – *le futur antérieur*

Use the **future** of the auxiliary verb (*avoir* or *être*) plus a **past participle** to say what 'will have happened' by some point in the future.

It is used after expressions such as *quand, une fois que, aussitôt que, après que*, when the verb in the main clause is in the future. See page 113.

Expressions clés

prouver qu'il y a un lien de parenté / un lien biologique

soumettre les immigrés à un test ADN

Cela permet d'éviter qu'un chef de famille ne découvre qu'il n'est pas le père biologique.

Un fichier d'empreintes digitales permettrait...

Le projet laisse entendre que...

Ce qui pose un vrai problème, c'est...

Or, on sait bien que la famille, c'est...

Un enfant appartient à celui qui l'élève.

Cette loi pose des problèmes d'ordre éthique.

Les tests ADN peuvent être utilisés pour...

Immigration au sein de l'Union européennc

1 Expliquez le contenu de cette phrase.

> Etre européen, c'est avoir le droit de circuler, séjourner, s'installer, travailler, étudier dans les autres Etats membres de l'Union.

Paris accélère les expulsions de Roms avant la trêve d'hiver

Depuis septembre 2007, les évacuations de bidonvilles Roms s'intensifient dans la capitale française. Seule une petite partie des Tsiganes sont relogés. Les Roms seraient entre deux et trois mille en région parisienne, avec l'ouverture de trente-trois campements l'année passée.

Les interventions ont lieu au petit matin. Premièrement, les forces de l'ordre « sécurisent » les lieux, afin d'éviter des fuites. Ensuite, les « candidats » au départ sont priés de monter dans des bus. Ils voyageront d'une traite aux frontières de la Roumanie ou de la Bulgarie. Enfin, les campements sont réduits en morceaux, afin que d'autres Roms ne viennent pas les occuper.

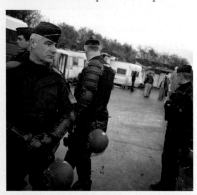

Le gouvernement de Sarkozy a fixé des objectifs chiffrés en matière d'expulsions d'étrangers. Et les Roms constituent un réservoir dans lequel il est facile de puiser, puisqu'ils vivent en communauté, dans des camps situés loin des regards; dans des terrains vagues, sous des autoroutes, dans des sites industriels abandonnés.

Depuis janvier 2007, les Roumains et les Bulgares sont devenus des citoyens européens, donc la France pousse dehors des ayant droit à la libre circulation. Les Roms ont le choix entre l'arrestation ou le départ dit « humanitaire », ce qui fait bondir les ONG locales.

2 a Cherchez les détails suivants dans le texte.

 i pays d'où sont venus les Roms
 ii combien ils sont
 iii nombre de nouveaux campements
 iv date d'adhésion de la Bulgarie et de la Roumanie à l'UE

b Lisez les phrases et écrivez V (vrai), F (faux) ou N (information non donnée).

 i La police intervient à l'aube.
 ii Elle vérifie les papiers des Roms.
 iii Tous les Tziganes sont relogés.
 iv On demande aux Roms où ils veulent habiter.
 v Les Roms ont légalement le droit de rester en France.

c Traduisez en anglais le passage suivant.

 Bien que les Roumains soient devenus des citoyens européens en janvier 2007, le gouvernement continue à vouloir les expulser. Les forces de l'ordre détruisent les bidonvilles et leur demandent de quitter le territoire français en les faisant monter dans des bus qui les ramènent d'une traite à la frontière. Ces opérations font bondir les ONG locales.

d Préparez des questions sur le texte et posez-les à votre partenaire.

Exemples: _____

Qui sont les Roms? Que penses-tu de l'action des forces de l'ordre?

Vocabulaire

la trêve *truce*

le bidonville *shanty town*

les tsiganes, les Roms *gypsies*

au petit matin *early in the morning*

les forces de l'ordre *the police*

la fuite *escape*

être prié de *to be requested to*

d'une traite *without stopping on the way*

réduire en morceaux *to smash to pieces*

puiser *to draw from*

le terrain vague *waste land*

un ayant droit *a person entitled to something*

faire bondir *to enrage*

une ONG: organisation non gouvernementale *NGO, humanitarian organisation*

3 a 🎧 Ecoutez la première partie de l'enregistrement. Recopiez la transcription et complétez-la avec les mots que vous entendez.

> A ...... la nuit dernière, des ...... d'...... ont été tirés sur ...... frontières européennes. En effet, à minuit, ... pays de l'Union européenne .... dans ce qu'on appelle l'espace Schengen. Ce qui .... que les habitants de ces pays .... librement sans ...... d'un pays à l'autre: il n'y a plus de ...... frontières.

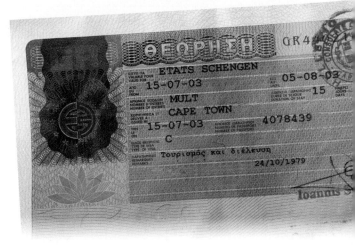

b 🎧 Ecoutez le reste de l'enregistrement et répondez aux questions.

i Combien de pays faisaient partie de l'espace Schengen auparavant?

ii Combien y en a-t-il maintenant?

iii Combien d'Européens pourront voyager librement?

4 💡 Lisez le texte sur les immigrés britanniques en France et faites les activités interactives.

5 a A deux, faites une liste des avantages et des inconvénients de la libre circulation des Européens dans l'espace Schengen. Comparez votre liste avec celle d'un autre groupe.

b 💡 Pouvons-nous accueillir les nouveaux immigrés européens? Préparez un exposé oral en considérant les côtés positifs, les problèmes, les dangers. (Feuille)

6 💡 Imaginez que votre famille annonce que vous allez habiter en France! Ecrivez un e-mail à votre correspondant(e) français(e). Expliquez le projet de vos parents et dites ce que vous en pensez: les avantages et les inconvénients. (Feuille)

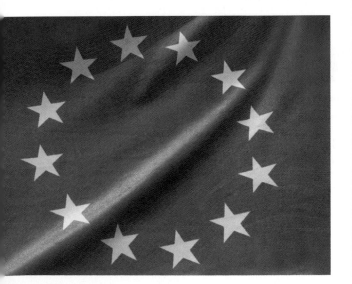

Expressions clés

être bon / mauvais pour l'économie

On pourra voyager sans contrainte.

On aura le droit de circuler librement.

avoir des compétences

enrichir notre culture / c'est enrichissant pour notre culture

plus de contrôles pour franchir les frontières de l'Europe

Le taux de chômage est trop élevé.

Il y a des problèmes de logement.

Il n'y a pas assez de place dans les écoles.

des emplois peu rémunérés

une montée possible de la criminalité et de l'immigration illégale

des problèmes de langues

💡 Grammaire

Indirect speech – *le discours indirect*

We use indirect speech (or reported speech) to report what people have said. See page 117.

- It is introduced by *que*.
- The subject pronouns change.
- The verb tenses change:

present → imperfect
elle est → *qu'elle* **était**

perfect → pluperfect
elle est partie → *qu'elle* **était partie**

future → conditional
elle sera → *qu'elle* **serait**

future perfect → conditional perfect
elle sera partie → *qu'elle* **serait partie**

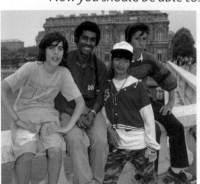

Now you should be able to:

■ explore the reasons for immigration	■ talk about government policy to curb immigration	■ talk about immigration within the enlarged European community
	■ discuss the benefits and problems of immigration	

Grammar

■ revise numbers   ■ use the future perfect tense   ■ use indirect speech

Skills

■ express proportions and statistics	■ defend a viewpoint	■ present oral analysis of advantages and disadvantages of immigration

✓ Résumé

1 Traduisez en français:

Immigrants now come from faraway countries.

2 C'est qui?

C'est une personne qui quitte son pays parce qu'elle est persécutée.

3 Complétez les phrases:

La (½) des immigrés sont des femmes. La part des immigrés nés au Maghreb a (×2). Ils représentent désormais (⅓) des immigrés.

4 Mettez les mots dans le bon ordre:

conscience   vrai   Le   tests   un   recours   aux
ADN   de   problème   pose

5 Mettez les verbes entre parenthèses au **futur** ou au **futur antérieur**, selon le cas.

Dès que leur dossier (**être rejeté**), les sans-papiers n' (**avoir**) plus qu'un seul mois pour contester la décision. Il est possible qu'une fois qu'ils (**déposer**) leur demande de titre de séjour, la Préfecture (**décider**) de ne pas renouveler leurs papiers.

6 Complétez la phrase:

L'esclavage moderne, c'est...

7 Donnez un autre nom pour le travail illégal.

8 Mettez ces phrases au discours indirect, en commençant par: *La journaliste a expliqué que...*

Neuf autres pays de l'Union européenne **sont entrés** dans l'espace Schengen. Les habitants de ces pays **pourront** voyager librement car il n'y **a** plus de postes frontières.

9 Ecrivez une phrase qui veut dire:

Les forces de l'ordre ont détruit les habitations des tsiganes.

10 Complétez la phrase:

Depuis janvier 2007, les Romains et les Bulgares...

AQA Examiner's tips

Listening
Remember that you do not always have to answer in full sentences; **one word will** sometimes be enough.

Speaking
Prepare detailed answers that **justify reasons and opinions** where necessary.

Reading
Questions follow the text in chronological order. If you have answered questions (4) and (6), the answer to (5) will be somewhere in between them in the text.

Writing
Always **draft a plan** before you start to write your answer.

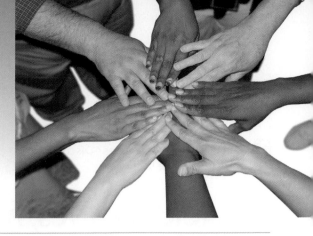

La société multiculturelle

5 L'intégration

By the end of this chapter you will be able to:

	Language	Grammar	Skills
A **Multiculturalisme**	■ talk about factors facilitating integration ■ discuss which culture immigrants should show loyalty to	■ use conjunctions	■ express well-informed and sophisticated opinions in a debate
B **La désintégration de la France**	■ consider factors making integration difficult	■ use demonstrative pronouns: *celui*, *celle*, *ceux*, *celles*	■ give precise descriptions using complex sentences
C **L'intégration des jeunes**	■ talk about the experiences of individual immigrants	■ use relative pronouns with prepositions: *dans lequel*, *auquel*, *duquel*, *dont*	■ express obligation and support someone's rights

 Le saviez-vous?

Toute personne d'origine étrangère ou de couleur de peau non blanche est considérée comme immigrée même si elle est française. Ainsi les immigrés des deuxième et troisième générations se sentent toujours traités comme des étrangers alors qu'ils sont nés en France et sont de nationalité française.

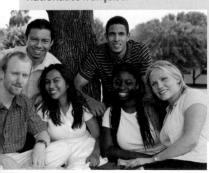

 Pour commencer

Choisissez la bonne réponse.

1 **Le multiculturalisme**, c'est:
a la façon dont vivent les immigrés dans un pays
b l'appartenance à plusieurs cultures à la fois
c la coexistence de plusieurs cultures dans un même pays
d la création de milieux culturels divers

2 **Une émeute** est:
a une révolution
b une révolte
c une réclamation
d une revanche

3 **Un déchirement familial**, c'est:
a une complicité dans la famille
b une dispute dans la famille
c une union de la famille
d une rupture de la famille

4 **La réussite scolaire**, c'est:
a s'amuser à l'école
b bien s'entendre avec les enseignants
c bien travailler à l'école
d se faire beaucoup d'amis

5 **L'école laïque**, c'est:
a la séparation des professeurs et des élèves
b la séparation du gouvernement et de l'école
c la séparation des parents d'élèves et des professeurs
d la séparation de l'éducation et de la religion

Multiculturalisme

1 Que disent ces personnes? Discutez-en avec le reste de la classe.

> Les immigrés ne sont pas tous bien intégrés dans notre société.

> Que peut-on faire pour améliorer la situation?

BLACKS, BLANCS, BEURS À LA MÊME ENSEIGNE

A l'hypermarché Casino d'Argenteuil, en banlieue parisienne, le groupe de grande distribution mise sur la diversité pour préserver la paix sociale.

Au total, les 210 salariés représentent plus de 20 nationalités, à l'image de la population locale: la moitié des 100 000 habitants d'Argenteuil est d'origine étrangère. Facile, compte tenu du taux de chômage à Argenteuil: 14% actuellement? Pas vraiment! Casino a dû diffuser des annonces jusque dans les boîtes aux lettres, car la grande distribution, avec ses horaires à rallonge et ses salaires au Smic, n'attire guère.

Dans les travées, la clientèle est aussi colorée que le personnel. Les promotions du jour s'égrènent de la viande halal, au paquet de croissants boulangers, aux pâtisseries orientales. Au rayon ménage-bricolage-accessoires auto, Dieynaba Diouf a appris à faire face aux clients difficiles. « Certains ne peuvent pas croire que je suis la responsable, » raconte cette jeune femme de 25 ans arrivée du Sénégal en 1999 pour faire un BTS puis une licence.

Une expérience vécue aussi par son collègue et compatriote, Henri Lolonga, 29 ans, chef du rayon électronique-électroménager. Mais il ne s'arrête pas à cela. D'abord recruté en CDD comme vendeur, il a vu son contrat converti en CDI. Puis il est devenu manager commercial. En trois ans, son salaire a doublé. Son credo: « Travailler avec différentes cultures apporte un plus. »

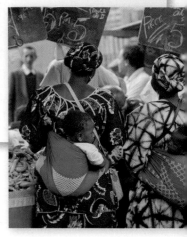

Vocabulaire

le/la beur (verlan, tiré du mot "arabe") *2nd generation North African living in France*

à la même enseigne *in the same boat*

la grande distribution *(chains of) supermarkets*

miser sur *to bank on, to count on*

compte tenu de *considering, in view of*

à rallonge *never-ending*

la travée *aisle*

s'égrener *to range from*

la viande Halal *Halal meat*

le/la responsable *manager, person in charge*

le BTS Brevet de technicien supérieur *2-year degree*

le chef de rayon *department supervisor*

le CDD: contrat à durée déterminée *fixed-term contract*

le CDI: contrat à durée indéterminée *permanent contract*

2 a Reliez les mots et sigles à leur définition.

i	un CDD	a	le salaire minimum
ii	une licence	b	un engagement pour un travail sans limite dans le temps
iii	le Smic	c	diplôme obtenu après deux ans d'études après le bac
iv	un BTS	d	un emploi pour une période précise
v	un CDI	e	diplôme obtenu après trois ans d'études après le bac

b En utilisant le vocabulaire du texte, traduisez les phrases suivantes.

i He learnt how to deal with difficult customers.

ii More than twenty nationalities are represented.

iii The never-ending hours are hardly enticing.

iv Some people cannot believe I am in charge.

v Considering the unemployment rate, recruiting should be easy.

c En consultant le texte, écrivez le plus de détails possibles sur Dieynaba Diouf et Henri Lolonga (responsabilités, âge, origine, niveau d'étude).

d Expliquez la dernière phrase du texte:

« Travailler avec différentes cultures apporte un plus. »

3 a 🎧 Ecoutez l'extrait du journal. Quel est son sujet? Choisissez la bonne réponse.

- Les acteurs de la réforme de la justice en France
- Les grandes figures du féminisme
- La politique d'immigration en France
- Les membres du nouveau gouvernement français

b 🎧 Réécoutez et donnez un nom à chaque photo.

Rama Yade   Rachida Dati   Fadéla Amara

c Recopiez et complétez le tableau.

Nom	Age	Nombre de frères et sœurs	Pays d'origine
Fadéla Amara			
Rachida Dati			
Rama Yade			

d 🎧 Réécoutez et puis dites tout ce que vous avez appris sur Fadéla, Rachida et Rama.

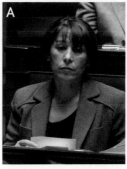

A

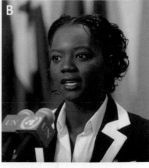

B

Secrétaire d'Etat chargée de la politique de la ville

Secrétaire d'Etat chargée des droits de l'homme

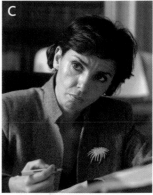

C

Ministre de la Justice

4 💡🎧 Ecoutez le témoignage d'une Chinoise en France et faites les activités interactives.

5 💡 Travail de groupe. Lisez les deux déclarations suivantes. Le premier groupe va développer et défendre les arguments de A, le deuxième groupe ceux de B. (Feuille)

A
> Pour bien s'intégrer, il faut parler la langue du pays et vivre comme les Français, c'est-à-dire adopter leur façon de vivre et leur culture. Je suis d'ailleurs pour la loi contre le port de signes religieux dans les écoles.

B
> Apprendre la langue, c'est essentiel, mais il est important de garder son identité culturelle. Ce mélange de coutumes, de religions rend notre pays plus intéressant, plus riche culturellement.

6 💡 A l'écrit: en vous inspirant de l'exercice précédant, donnez votre point de vue personnel sur l'intégration des immigrés. (Feuille)

Expressions clés

Pour que l'intégration se fasse / soit possible, il faudrait que…

Il faut apprendre à vivre ensemble.

une diversité ethnique / religieuse

une société multiculturelle

le droit à la différence

le modèle français républicain

les différences de culture et de modes de vie

l'école laïque / la laïcité

C'est une chance pour la culture / l'économie du pays.

L'interdiction des signes religieux à l'école…

Le port du foulard est interdit.

L'intégrisme religieux / musulman fait peur.

être frappé par des attentats terroristes

avoir des difficultés d'intégration

ne pas se donner les moyens de s'intégrer

🔖 Compétences

Express well-informed and sophisticated opinions in a debate

Prepare your arguments: use research to support ideas and opinions.

Introduce your topic: *Tout d'abord, En premier lieu…*

Set out arguments: *D'autre part, Par ailleurs, De plus…*

Link sentences: *parce que, puisque, car, mais, cependant, donc, alors…* (See conjunctions, page 120)

Give your opinion: *Personnellement, je pense que…,
A mon avis…,
Je ne suis pas d'accord parce que…*

B   La désintégration de la France

1 Quelles sont les raisons qui freinent l'intégration des immigrés? Mettez-les en ordre d'importance selon vous. Ensuite, écrivez les raisons de votre choix. Discutez-en avec le reste de la classe.

a   **ne pas être intéressé par la scolarité**

b   **vivre dans des quartiers difficiles**

c   **ne pas parler la langue du pays**

d   **s'habiller en costume traditionnel**

e   **avoir une religion différente**

f   **être au chômage**

g   **avoir des habitudes alimentaires différentes**

h   **continuer à suivre les coutumes de son pays d'origine**

Les racines du malaise

Les cités de banlieues apparaissent comme de véritables ghettos où de nombreux jeunes se sentent exclus, se voient de plus en plus enfermés dans les murs de leur cité. Ces jeunes sont pauvres, presque souvent d'origine étrangère et pourtant la majorité d'entre eux sont de nationalité française.

Ils n'occupent aucune place reconnue dans la société et n'ont plus cette insertion par le travail qu'avaient leurs parents. Le taux de chômage parmi ces jeunes est très élevé, même pour le petit nombre d'entre eux qui ont fait des études supérieures et qui se heurtent à des discriminations à l'embauche.

Les émeutes qui surgissent dans ces quartiers difficiles depuis quelques années sont des révoltes du désespoir et surgissent de manière récurrente. Elles sont souvent déclenchées après des interventions policières telles que des arrestations, des poursuites de jeunes qui dégénèrent parfois en accidents qui peuvent être mortels.

Les cibles visées ne sont plus seulement les forces de l'ordre, mais d'autres personnels de la fonction publique comme les pompiers et les chauffeurs d'autobus, ainsi que des biens privés. Les jeunes s'en prennent aux voitures du quartier, c'est-à-dire à celles qui sont possédées par leurs voisins. Ils mettent le feu aux écoles où les gens du quartier souvent issus de l'immigration comme eux envoient leurs enfants.

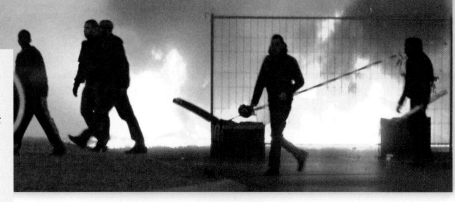

Vocabulaire

la racine *root*

la banlieue *suburb*

le taux de chômage *unemployment rate*

se heurter à *to bump into, to come up against*

une embauche *employment*

une émeute *riot*

surgir *to arise*

le quartier *area, neighbourhood*

être déclenché *to be triggered off*

la cible *target*

la fonction publique *public service*

s'en prendre à *to take it out on, to attack*

2 a Retrouvez les expressions suivantes dans le texte. (Attention: elles ne sont pas dans l'ordre du texte.)

i   many young people feel excluded

ii   accidents which can be fatal

iii they have no place in society

iv   the ones owned by their neighbours

v   the unemployment rate is very high

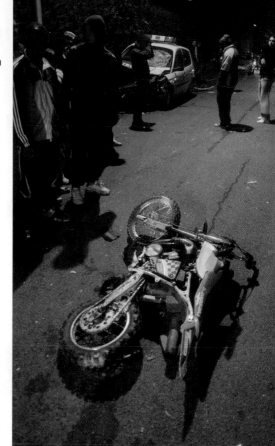

2 b Notez ce que vous avez appris sur:

- la situation des jeunes dans les cités de banlieues (travail, situation économique, origines ethniques, ce qu'ils ressentent)
- les émeutes (quand, où, facteurs déclencheurs, ce qui se passe).

3 Relisez le texte et faites les activités interactives.

4 a Ecoutez ce reportage sur les émeutes qui ont eu lieu à Villiers-le-bel. Notez les détails suivants:

- date, heure, moment de la journée
- nombre de morts
- durée des émeutes
- deux moyens de transport impliqués
- où se trouve Villiers-le-bel

b Vous allez maintenant entendre une déclaration du maire de Villiers-le-bel. Ecoutez sans regarder le texte ci-dessous. Ensuite complétez le résumé avec les mots qui se trouvent dans la case.

> Depuis deux nuits, des ...... sévissent à Villiers-le-bel. Celles-ci ne sont pas .... On ne peut pas comprendre ce qui .... On a brûlé des .... , on a détruit des ...... , on a blessé des ...... et des ....
>
> Je lance un appel au ...... pour que Villiers-le-bel retrouve sa sérénité. La ville est .... J'invite les ...... à demander à leurs ...... de rester à la maison.

traumatisée   acceptables   commerces   pompiers
violences   bâtiments   parents   s'est passé
calme   publics   enfants   policiers

c Réécoutez l'extrait et vérifiez vos réponses.

d Réécoutez et relevez quatre phrases à la forme passive (voir Grammaire, page 11).

5 Jeu de rôle: vous êtes journaliste et vous interviewez un groupe de jeunes qui ont participé aux émeutes. (Feuille)

a   Faites une liste de questions que vous pourriez leur poser.
b   Imaginez leurs réponses.
c   Préparez un dialogue et enregistrez-vous. Ensuite, changez de rôle.

6 Vous habitez Villiers-le-bel. Votre voiture a été brûlée dans la nuit lors des émeutes. Vous décidez d'écrire au maire de Villiers-le-bel pour porter plainte. (Feuille)

a   Décrivez ce qui s'est passé.
b   Exprimez ce que vous ressentez.
c   Demandez à le rencontrer pour discuter des solutions à prendre.

Grammaire

Demonstrative pronouns – *les pronoms démonstratifs*

Demonstrative pronouns **replace** nouns to say 'this one', 'those ones', etc. They always **agree** with the **noun** they refer to. See page 109.

celui – masculine sing.
celle – feminine sing.
ceux – masculine pl.
celles – feminine pl.

Ma voiture est rouge mais *celle* de Marc est grise. (*voiture* is feminine)

Expressions clés

J'habite une cité de banlieue.

Notre quartier connaît des violences...

Des émeutes ont eu lieu...

être traumatisé / choqué / en colère

Ce n'est pas acceptable.

Il faut lancer un appel au calme.

Ce n'est pas juste.

On a incendié / brûlé / mis le feu à...

Mon véhicule a été brûlé / incendié.

être assuré contre les incendies

L'intégration des jeunes

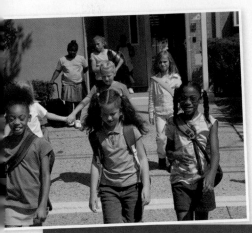

1 🎧 Ecoutez l'introduction d'une émission sur l'intégration et répondez aux questions.

a   De quelles minorités parle-t-on?

b   Dans quels domaines ne sont-elles pas représentées?

2 a Avant de lire le texte, reliez ces mots à leur définition.

i   défavorisé   a   refaire une année scolaire

ii   la scolarité   b   le fait de suivre régulièrement les cours d'un établissement d'enseignement

iii améliorer   c   privé d'un avantage

iv   redoubler   d   perfectionner

L'intégration des enfants issus de l'immigration

La discrimination commence dès l'école. Il n'y a pas vraiment de problème avec les enfants d'immigrés en France, mais un problème d'accueil des populations défavorisées dont font partie les immigrés. On sait que la réussite sociale est de plus en plus liée à la réussite scolaire. Or 'les enfants d'immigrés sont particulièrement exposés à l'échec scolaire: parmi les jeunes dont les deux parents sont immigrés, un sur trois a redoublé à l'école élémentaire, contre seulement un sur cinq quand aucun ou un seul parent est immigré. Cette plus grande difficulté se retrouve dans la suite de la scolarité, au collège et au lycée. Elle résulte directement du fait que les enfants d'immigrés vivent souvent dans un environnement familial'* dans lequel la réussite scolaire est moins favorable. Un grand nombre d'entre eux ont une mère ayant au plus terminé l'école primaire et grandissent dans une famille d'au moins quatre enfants.

Cependant, en quittant leur pays les émigrants ont manifesté une forte motivation pour améliorer leurs conditions d'existence, ambition qu'ils reportent sur leurs enfants. Ces parents attendent donc beaucoup du système scolaire, ce qui n'est pas toujours le cas des parents français des milieux populaires qui, par résignation, autolimitent le plus souvent leurs espoirs de réussite pour leurs enfants.

Les parents sont aussi placés devant le dilemme suivant: doivent-ils préserver et transmettre les normes et valeurs reçues dans le pays d'origine ou admettre que leurs enfants vont s'éloigner de ces valeurs? L'enfant d'immigré est contraint de découvrir et de construire son identité en évitant les déchirements familiaux.

Insee Première No. 1042, Sept. 2005

Vocabulaire

l'accueil *reception, welcome*

la réussite *success*

cependant *however*

améliorer *to improve*

reporter sur *to transfer to*

un espoir *hope*

s'éloigner *to move away*

être contraint de *to be forced to*

éviter *to avoid*

le déchirement *tear, breakdown*

b Lisez le texte et les phrases i–viii. Ecrivez V (vrai), F (faux) ou N (information non donnée).

i   La réussite sociale dépend de la réussite scolaire.

ii   Les enfants d'immigrés redoublent plus souvent que les autres enfants.

iii Les enfants d'immigrés n'ont pas de problèmes au collège ou au lycée.

iv   Les pères ont fait plus d'études que les mères.

v   Les immigrés aspirent à de meilleures conditions de vie.

vi   Les familles d'immigrés ont peu d'enfants.

vii Les parents français des milieux défavorisés attendent plus du système scolaire que les parents immigrés.

viii Il est plus complexe pour un enfant d'immigré de construire son identité.

3 a 🎧 Ecoutez la première partie de l'enregistrement et trouvez les erreurs dans les bulles.

i
> Conformément à la législation, on scolarise tous les enfants, avec papiers ou pas. Les majeurs de moins de dix-huit ans ont besoin de titre de séjour.

ii
> Oui, Paul est revenu en France il y a cinq mois quand ses parents sont partis. Il est hébergé par une amie.

iii
> Le problème de Paul, c'est qu'il va avoir dix-huit ans et il doit obtenir un titre de retour pour continuer ses voyages.

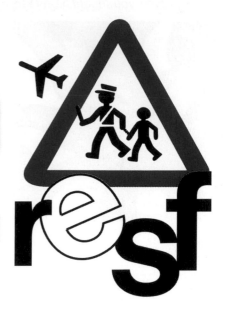

b 🎧 Ecoutez le reste de l'enregistrement et répondez aux questions.

i Qu'est-il arrivé à Paul?

ii Qui est intervenu pour l'aider?

iii En quelle classe est-il?

iv Est-ce qu'il travaille bien?

www.educationsansfrontieres.org

4 💡🎧 Réécoutez l'enregistrement et faites les activités interactives.

5 💡 A deux, à l'oral: vous avez un lycéen sans-papiers dans votre classe. (Feuille)

a Imaginez son nom, sa nationalité, date d'arrivée dans le pays, sa situation familiale. Prenez en compte les problèmes qu'il a pu rencontrer: langue, conflit de cultures, etc.

b Changez de partenaire et décrivez la personne que vous avez inventée. Prenez note des détails donnés par votre partenaire.

6 💡🖊 Ecoutez l'entretien avec le camarade imaginaire et enregistrez vos réponses.

7 💡 Ecrivez une lettre de soutien pour votre camarade qui est menacé d'expulsion, que vous envoyez à la presse locale. (Feuille)

💡 Grammaire

Relative pronouns with prepositions
– les pronoms relatifs: dans lequel, duquel, auquel, dont

In English, you can often omit the relative pronoun ('who', 'which', 'that') and a preposition can be separated from the person or thing it refers to: 'The class (that) Paul is a student **in**...'

In French, the relative pronoun cannot be omitted and the preposition must come before the relative pronoun:

*La classe **dans laquelle** Paul est étudiant...*
(See page 108.)

Expressions clés

le pays d'origine

Elle a été naturalisée.

Elle est hébergée par / logée par...

être expulsé / renvoyé dans son pays d'origine

être placé en centre de rétention

Il a besoin d'un titre de séjour.

Il faut se mobiliser / intervenir...

signer une lettre / une pétition

une demande de régularisation

poursuivre ses études

préparer son bac / un examen

C'est stupide d'interrompre la scolarité.

C'est un élève bien intégré.

Il est apprécié de...

C'est une situation incohérente.

mettre en danger

Now you should be able to:

- ■ talk about factors facilitating integration
- ■ discuss which culture immigrants should show loyalty to

- ■ consider factors making integration difficult

- ■ talk about the experiences of individual immigrants

Grammar

- ■ use conjunctions

- ■ use demonstrative pronouns: *celui, celle, ceux, celles*

- ■ use relative pronouns with prepositions: *dans lequel, auquel, duquel, dont*

Skills

- ■ express well-informed and sophisticated opinions in a debate

- ■ give precise descriptions using complex sentences

- ■ express obligation and support someone's rights

✓ Résumé

1 Comment diriez-vous en français?

The hypermarket puts its staff in the same boat.

2 Complétez la phrase:

Rachida Dati occupe le poste de...

3 Qu'est-ce que l'école laïque interdit?

4 Ecrivez une phrase, en français, qui veut dire à peu près la même chose:

Les adolescents attaquent les véhicules des forces de l'ordre.

5 Traduisez en anglais:

« Je voudrais lancer un appel au calme, de manière à ce que la ville retrouve sa sérénité. »

6 Mettez les pronoms démonstratifs qui conviennent:

« Les poubelles de mon immeuble sont intactes mais ...... de l'immeuble voisin ont été détruites. »

« L'abri bus en face est brisé et ...... de l'autre côté de la rue est couvert de graffiti. »

7 Complétez la phrase:

« Les jeunes circulaient sur une moto qui... »

8 Pourquoi les enfants d'immigrés sont-ils souvent en échec scolaire?

9 Mettez les pronoms relatifs qui conviennent:

Parmi les jeunes ...... les parents sont immigrés, un sur trois a redoublé à l'école dans ...... il est scolarisé.

10 Qu'est-ce qu'une garde à vue?

AQA Examiner's tips

Listening

Do not listen to a particular section of the recording more than three times. If you can't understand it, **come back to it later**. You will probably find it easier next time round.

Speaking

Think of **examples to explain why** you like/ think something.

Reading

If you can't find the answer to a question, **move on** and come back to it if there's time at the end.

Writing

Maintain the reader's interest by asking direct questions or using 'let's consider' statements.

La société multiculturelle
Le racisme

6

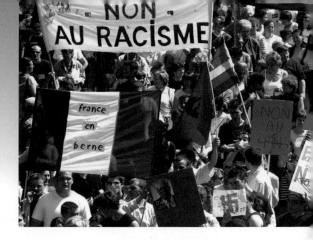

By the end of this chapter you will be able to:

	Language	Grammar	Skills
A Raciste, moi?	■ discuss the reasons for racism	■ use possessive pronouns	■ express clear ideas about important issues
B Discrimination	■ talk about discrimination in employment and education	■ revise present and past tenses of the passive voice	■ discuss anti-racism initiatives
C Victimes	■ talk about the victims of racism	■ use the perfect subjunctive	■ develop a personal explanation

Le saviez-vous?

Chaque individu sur terre partage 99,99% du même code génétique. En fait, des personnes de groupes raciaux différents peuvent présenter plus de similarités entre elles que des personnes prises au sein d'un même groupe.

Un Français sur trois se dit raciste. C'est ce qui ressort du rapport 2005 de la Commission Nationale Consultative des Droits de l'Homme.

S'informer
www.sos-racisme.org
www.mrap.asso.fr
www.afrik.com

Pour commencer

1 Un préjugé, c'est:
   a un passage devant le juge
   b la partie d'un jugement
   c un parti pris

2 Un bouc émissaire, c'est:
   a le mâle de la chèvre
   b une personne que l'on accuse
   c une personne chargée d'une mission

3 Un cliché, c'est:
   a une image négative
   b une photo
   c une idée toute faite

4 Le harcèlement, c'est:
   a tourmenter une personne
   b parler à une personne
   c se disputer avec quelqu'un

5 Une blague, c'est:
   a un mensonge
   b une histoire drôle
   c un mot raciste

A   Raciste, moi?

1 a 🎧 Ecoutez le passage. Recopiez et complétez la transcription.
Etes-vous d'accord ou pas?

> Le ...... est l'un des ...... humains les plus ...... car il ne demande aucun ....
>
> Il offre une ...... magique aux ...... comme le ...... ou la ...... , mettant la ...... sur des boucs émissaires.

b Traduisez la transcription en anglais.

Le racisme, d'où ça vient?

Etre raciste, c'est croire qu'il existe différentes races et que certaines sont supérieures aux autres. En fait, les races n'existent que chez les animaux. On ne doit pas parler de différentes races humaines mais d'un seul genre humain.

Malgré tout, des personnes affirment le contraire pour justifier une domination ou des persécutions envers certains groupes de personnes, distinguées par leur apparence physique, leurs habitudes, leurs idées, leur religion...

Globalement, nous avons souvent du mal à accepter nos différences. Nous avons peur de l'inconnu, nous cherchons à éviter ce que nous ne comprenons pas. C'est pourquoi nous avons tendance à rejeter celui qui est différent, l'étranger, car sa langue, ses coutumes sont incompréhensibles.

Personne n'est donc à l'abri de mépriser celui qui est différent. Le racisme est apparenté à la haine, la peur, le préjugé, l'ignorance, l'intolérance et l'idéologie de supériorité culturelle ou personnelle. Connaître le plus de monde possible permet de ne pas généraliser nos jugements, c'est-à-dire ne pas s'imaginer que des personnes qui ont la même apparence, la même religion, le même métier, le même âge, ont forcément les mêmes défauts. Pour lutter contre nos réflexes racistes et xénophobes, il faut aller vers les autres car les clichés parasitent notre univers.

Ce serait tellement triste si tout le monde se ressemblait!

Vocabulaire

le genre *kind*

malgré tout *in spite of everything*

avoir du mal à *to have difficulty in*

l'inconnu *the unknown*

la coutume *custom*

être à l'abri de *to be safe from*

mépriser *to despise*

le défaut *fault*

lutter *to fight*

triste *sad*

se ressembler *to resemble each other, to be the same*

2 a Lisez le texte. Reliez les mots aux définitions.

i	la persécution	a	sentiment d'antipathie
ii	une coutume	b	expression trop souvent utilisée
iii	un préjugé	c	hostilité à ce qui est étranger
iv	l'intolérance	d	manque de connaissances
v	la haine	e	opinion préconçue
vi	la xénophobie	f	manque d'indulgence et de compréhension
vii	un cliché	g	traitement injuste et cruel
viii	l'ignorance	h	habitude collective d'agir

b Vrai ou faux? Corrigez les erreurs dans les phrases suivantes:

i   Il existe différentes races chez les hommes.

ii   Pour dominer, certains affirment que les races existent.

iii   Celui qui est différent est accepté.

iv   Il faut apprendre à connaître les autres.

v   Notre univers est plein de clichés.

vi   Connaître des personnes d'origines variées nous enrichit.

vii   Si on se ressemblait tous, le monde serait plus intéressant.

3 💡 A l'oral: faites une liste des comportements quotidiens que vous considérez comme racistes. Discutez-en avec le reste de la classe. (Feuille)

> **Vidéo: un incident critique**
>
> Deux enseignants discutent dans la salle des profs. Au cours du mois dernier, plusieurs incidents de vol à la tire ont été constatés dans l'école.
>
> vol à la tire *pickpocketing*

4 a 💡 ⊒ Regardez la vidéo, faites les activités interactives et répondez aux questions suivantes:

1ère scène	Qu'auriez-vous fait à la place du principal?

2ème scène	Pensez-vous que l'affaire a été résolue de manière satisfaisante?

3ème scène	Et maintenant, que pensez-vous du fait que le garçon soit innocent?

b ⊒ Qu'auraient dû faire les enseignants, le père de Fouad et le principal pour être équitables dans cette affaire?

5 💡 En vous aidant du vocabulaire du texte à la page 50, répondez à la question suivante:
« Etre raciste », ça veut dire quoi à votre avis? (Feuille)

💡 **Grammaire**

**Possessive pronouns
– *les pronoms possessifs***

Used after verbs to express the idea of possession: 'yours', 'hers', 'mine'.

It has to agree in gender and number with the noun it replaces. (See page 109.)

*le mien   la mienne
les miens   les miennes*   (mine)

Je considérerai ton avis et je donnerai le mien.
I'll consider your opinion and I'll give mine.

■ **Expressions clés**

Le racisme, c'est la peur de l'autre.

C'est rejeter quelqu'un à cause de sa couleur, sa nationalité, son origine sociale, sa religion.

Les plaisanteries racistes sont très répandues.

Nous avons tous des clichés en tête.

On est tous un peu racistes au fond de nous.

Nous avons tous des faiblesses sur lesquelles le racisme peut s'enraciner.

le harcèlement physique / verbal

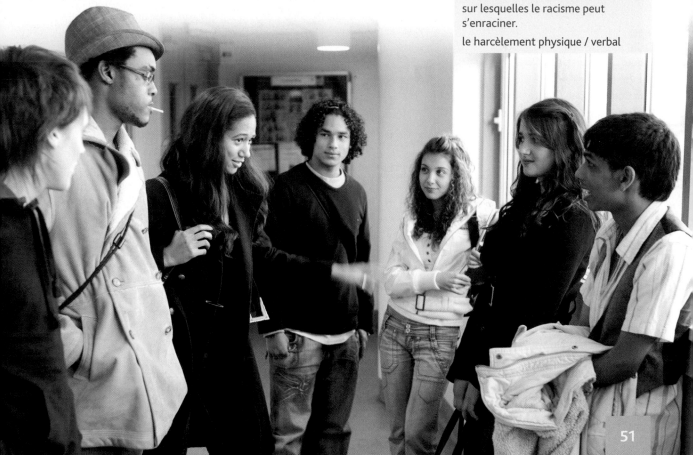

B Discrimination

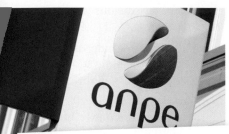

Recherche employé service entretien
Profil: race blanche, bonne tête, dynamique, esprit d'initiative.
Volonté d'apprendre et de s'intégrer.

Recherche fille ou garçon, 25 / 26 ans
Bac pro commercial ou BTS commercial
TB présentation (BCBG). Pas typé.

ANPE: Agence nationale pour l'emploi

TB: très bonne

BCBG: bon chic bon genre

typé *foreign-looking*

Vocabulaire

beur *2nd generation North African living in France*

la Cour d'appel *Court of Appeal*

le fabricant *manufacturer*

coupable *guilty*

une animatrice / un animateur *sales / promotions staff*

la grande surface *hypermarket*

une amende *fine*

prison avec sursis *suspended sentence*

les dommages et intérêts *damages*

les frais *expenses*

une agence d'intérim *temping agency*

l'inspection (f) du travail *factory inspectorate*

une équipe *team*

le fichier *file*

1 a Regardez les deux petites annonces à gauche et relevez les expressions discriminatoires.

b Pourriez-vous trouver de telles offres d'emploi dans votre pays?

Garnier, condamné pour discrimination raciale

Leurs publicités sont black, blanc, beur et même jaune. Mais pour vendre leurs produits, mieux valait être bleu blanc rouge. La Cour d'appel de Paris a condamné le fabricant de cosmétiques Garnier qui a été reconnu* coupable d'avoir demandé d'exclure les candidats d'origine arabe, africaine ou asiatique d'emplois d'animatrices en grandes surfaces, lors d'une campagne promotionnelle pour les produits Fructis Style.

Les sociétés de travail temporaire qui recrutaient pour Garnier sont également condamnées*. Chaque société devra payer 30 000 euros d'amende. Une de leurs employées est condamnée* à trois mois de prison avec sursis. Les condamnés devront également payer 35 000 euros de dommages et intérêts à SOS-Racisme, ainsi que 10 000 euros de frais de procédure.

L'accusation s'appuie sur une mention portée sur un fax, envoyé par Garnier aux agences d'intérim. Ce document précisait les exigences requises pour les animatrices commerciales: être âgée de 18 à 22 ans, faire une taille de vêtements entre 38 à 42 et avoir le type « BBR ». Trois discriminations en tout, âge, physique et ethnie. Cette mention BBR, qui signifie bleu blanc rouge, est une référence à la fête annuelle du Front national, et un code raciste connu des agences d'intérim pour exclure les candidats de couleur.

Une enquête de l'inspection du travail a montré que pour la campagne Fructis, les candidats noirs, asiatiques et arabes avaient été quasi-exclus du recrutement de l'équipe, où ils ne représentaient que 4% des employés, alors qu'ils sont environ 40% dans les fichiers sur ce type d'emplois.

the passive voice: see page 116

2 a Lisez l'article. Reliez les expressions i–vi à leur équivalent.

i la société a été reconnue coupable

ii les emplois d'animatrices en grandes surfaces

iii les sociétés de travail temporaire

iv une enquête de l'inspection du travail

v les fichiers sur ce type d'emploi

vi exclure les candidates de couleur

a une expertise faite par les autorités

b la compagnie est fautive

c évincer les postulantes non blanches

d le personnel de promotion dans les hypermarchés

e les entreprises d'emplois intérimaires

f les registres de ce genre de travail

b Relisez l'article et répondez aux questions.

i Dans l'article, à quoi correspondent ces chiffres?

35 000 euros: 3 mois de prison:
10 000 euros: 30 000 euros:

ii Quels sont les trois éléments discriminatoires chez Garnier? Donnez des détails.

iii Expliquez ce que veut dire « BBR ».

3 a 🎧 Ecoutez Abdel et Nedjma parler de leur expérience face au monde du travail. Associez un nom, Abdel ou Nedjma, à chaque information:

i 26 ans

ii BTS action commerciale

iii DEA de management

iv 25 ans

v DEUG d'allemand

vi maîtrise de droit

vii assistant du directeur d'une PME

viii travaille pour une chaîne de restauration rapide

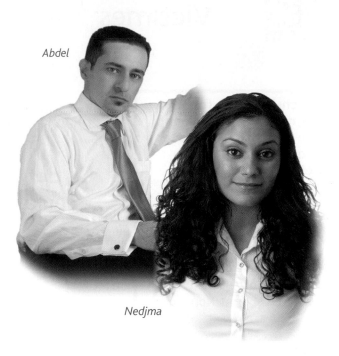

Abdel

b 🎧 Réécoutez et dites si les phrases sont vraies ou fausses. Corrigez les phrases qui sont fausses.

i Depuis qu'il a changé de nom, Thomas a moins d'entretiens d'embauche.

ii Il a envoyé de nombreuses lettres de motivation.

iii Il est fier d'avoir changé son prénom.

iv Il vient de trouver du travail.

v Cela fait trois ans que Nedjma a terminé ses études.

vi Son prénom lui déplaît.

vii Elle est immigrée de troisième génération.

viii Elle préfère contacter des organisations antiracistes en cas de discrimination.

ix Elle fait du baby-sitting.

Nedjma

4 💡🎧 Ecoutez le reportage sur SOS-Racisme et faites les activités interactives.

5 💡 Que pensez-vous de la décision d'Abdel? Et de celle de Nedjma? Discutez-en avec un(e) partenaire. (Feuille)

6 💡 Faites des recherches et résumez les mesures prises pour combattre le racisme en France. Comparez-les avec celles prises au Royaume-Uni. Sont-elles suffisantes? (Feuille)

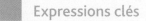

Expressions clés

Moi, je suis d'accord avec…

Je comprends la décision de…

J'aurais fait la même chose.

Je refuse / Il est hors de question que…

Ce n'est pas juste.

Je trouve ça choquant / inadmissible.

On devrait juger les gens par rapport à leurs compétences, pas par rapport à leur faciès.

Il ne fait aucun doute que…

On dirait que…

Je me demande si…

… que l'on peut comparer à…

◤ Compétences

Discuss anti-racism initiatives

In order to consider the effectiveness of measures to eliminate racism involving:

• the legal system

• anti-racist pressure groups

• the education of society as a whole

… you need to gather information and also a range of good expressions.

Introducing the subject:
Aujourd'hui, il faut dire stop à…

Reporting an event:
J'ai entendu à la radio…

Relating personal experiences:
J'en ai fait l'expérience à plusieurs reprises…

Assessing effectiveness:
Cela (n') est (pas) une bonne solution parce que…

C Victimes

Rachel s'est fait agresser en revenant de l'école. Sa faute: revenir de l'école et être juive.

Ligue internationale contre le racisme et l'antisémitisme

Tout près d'ici n'habite pas Moussa car le propriétaire n'a pas voulu louer à Moussa.

LICRA

Le videur a dit à Abdel «soirée privée». Privée d'Abdel.

Ligue internationale contre le racisme et l'antisémitisme

LICRA: Ligue internationale contre le racisme et l'antisémitisme

Vocabulaire

être le théâtre de *to be the scene of*

le répit *respite, rest*

être pris à parti *to be picked on*

le gamin *kid*

tenter *to attempt*

le domicile *home*

inscrire *to write*

la croix gammée *swastika*

faire l'objet de *to be the subject of*

taguer *to graffiti*

envahir *to invade*

déménager *to move house*

---

1 A deux, discutez du contenu des ces trois affiches de la LICRA, à gauche. Y a-t-il des campagnes similaires au Royaume-Uni?

Un petit alsacien d'origine congolaise victime d'attaques racistes

Le petit village français de Breitenbach, en Alsace, est, depuis quelques semaines, le théâtre d'attaques racistes. Les parents adoptifs de Quentin ne connaissent plus de répit. Il y a un mois, leur fils d'origine congolaise, 9 ans, est pris à parti par cinq gamins âgés de 10 à 14 ans dans une rue du village, alors qu'il joue avec trois de ses camarades de classe. L'un d'eux le menace d'un couteau et d'autres tentent ensuite de brûler ses vêtements. Trois de ses agresseurs sont aussi des camarades de classe.

Dans la nuit de jeudi à vendredi, ce sont aux murs bleus du domicile familial qu'on s'est pris en y inscrivant des croix gammées et le mot « nègres ». Malheureusement, ce n'est pas la première fois que la famille fait l'objet d'attaques racistes. Leurs murs ont déjà été tagués de croix gammées et de propos haineux puis leur boîte aux lettres a été envahie de courriers anonymes. Ils ont décidé de déménager et d'aller s'installer dans une autre région de France.

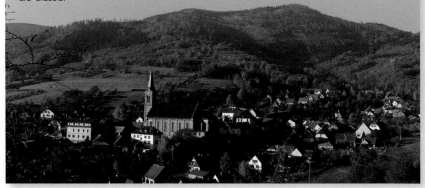

2 a Lisez l'article. Numérotez les événements suivants dans l'ordre du texte.

- On essaie de **mettre le feu** à ses habits
- Envois de **lettres** de menace
- Quentin **s'amuse** dehors
- La famille va **habiter ailleurs**
- Des propos haineux sont inscrits sur **la maison**
- Quentin est menacé **à l'arme blanche**

b Dans l'article, trouvez les synonymes des mots soulignés ci-dessus.

c Posez des questions à votre partenaire pour obtenir le plus de détails possible sur:

la victime   les coupables de l'attaque   la nature des actes racistes

3 🔆 Lisez les textes (en ligne) et faites les activités interactives.

4 a 🎧 Ecoutez ce reportage sur la profanation de tombes musulmanes et répondez aux questions.

   i   Où s'est passé l'incident?

   ii   Que représentent ces trois chiffres?
       170   40 000   52

   iii   Qu'est-il arrivé il y a presque un an?

   iv   Pour quelle raison cet incident s'est-il reproduit une deuxième fois?

b 🔆🎧 Ecoutez les réactions du président du Mrap et celles de M. Sarkozy et M. Fillon. Notez les différences entre la transcription ci-dessous et l'enregistrement.

Exemple: _____

important – urgent

_____

> Il est important que les auteurs soient vite identifiés, que des peines exemplaires soient attribuées. Il faut une mobilisation du gouvernement et des associations pour déclarer que cette sorte de racisme qu'est l'islamophobie ne doit pas avoir une possibilité de subsister sur la terre de France. Le président de la République Nicolas Sarkozy a dénoncé un acte révoltant et a souhaité que les coupables soient condamnés comme ils le méritent. Le Premier ministre François Fillon a exprimé sa colère et réprouvé ces actes racistes.

5 🔆 Que feriez-vous si vous vous trouviez face à ces situations? (Feuille)

- Vous êtes immigré(e). Dans le bus ou le métro, une personne change de place au moment où vous vous asseyez à côté d'elle.
- Vous vous faites refuser l'entrée dans une boîte de nuit parce que vous êtes noir(e).
- Votre maison a été couverte d'inscriptions antisémites sous prétexte que vous êtes juif/juive.

6 🔆 Relisez l'article à la page 54. Imaginez que votre enfant est l'un des agresseurs. Ecrivez une lettre d'excuse à la famille de Quentin. (Feuille)

7 🔆🎙 Jeu de rôle: écoutez le dialogue et enregistrez vos réponses.

💡 Grammaire

The perfect subjunctive – *le subjonctif passé*

It is used when the action happens before that of the main verb.

Present subjunctive: *Je suis content (maintenant) que la société* **perde** *le procès (maintenant).*

Perfect subjunctive: *Je suis content (maintenant) que la société* **ait perdu** *le procès (la semaine dernière).*

It is similar to the indicative perfect (the "normal" perfect tense), but uses *avoir* and *être* in the present subjunctive. See page 115.

Expressions clés

Il faut régler le problème.

Ces incidents sont inacceptables.

Un tel comportement est inadmissible.

Je trouve que...

Je ne supporte pas...

Je suis déçu par...

Je regrette que / Je suis désolé que mon fils ait agressé Quentin.

Je suis étonné que / Je suis surpris que les enfants aient eu un tel comportement.

Il faut qu'il prenne conscience de la gravité du problème.

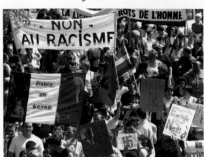

Now you should be able to:

- discuss the reasons for racism
- talk about discrimination in employment and education
- talk about the victims of racism

Grammar

- use possessive pronouns
- revise present and past tenses of the passive voice
- use the perfect subjunctive

Skills

- express clear ideas about important issues
- discuss anti-racism initiatives
- develop a personal explanation

✓ Résumé

1 Complétez la phrase:

SOS Racisme, c'est…

2 Comment diriez-vous cette phrase en français ?

He feels he has disowned his true identity.

3 Mettez les pronoms possessifs qui conviennent:

Recruteur: Ce CV est …… ?

Claire: Non, ce n'est pas ……

Recruteur: Et cette lettre, c'est bien …… ?

Claire: Oui, c'est ……

4 Qu'est-ce qu'un "beur"?

5 Remettez les mots dans l'ordre.

nos généraliser plus de jugements pas
Connaître de monde ne permet

6 Traduisez en anglais:

Personne n'est à l'abri de mépriser celui qui est différent.

7 Le "testing", c'est quoi exactement?

8 Que s'est-il passé au cimetière militaire près d'Arras?

9 Complétez avec des verbes au subjonctif passé.

Je suis désolé que cet incident …… (**se passer**). Je regrette que mon fils …… (**attaquer**) Quentin. Je suis surpris qu'il …… (**faire**) ça.

10 Quel mot décrit une attitude raciste contre l'Islam?

AQA ⁄ Examiner's tips

Listening

If numbers are needed in your answers, it is quicker to write the **number in figures**, e.g. *20* rather than *vingt*.

Speaking

If you're asked for 'reasons why', offer **several different points**.

Reading

Pay attention to the **mark scheme**: *2 marks* means that the examiner wants two details.

Writing

Build your essay up from simple sentences and use **link phrases** to connect ideas.

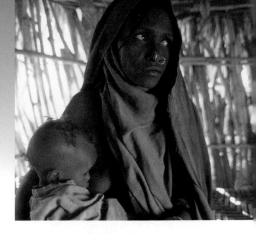

Problèmes sociaux contemporains
Richesse et pauvreté

7

By the end of this chapter you will be able to:

	Language	Grammar	Skills
A L'embarras des riches	■ talk about wealth and poverty, including links to health and social unrest	■ use the conditional perfect	■ adapt others' opinions to express your own
B Les racines de la misère	■ discuss the causes of poverty in Europe and developing countries	■ use comparative and superlative adjectives	■ construct dialogues using various sources
C Solidarité globale?	■ discuss debt and aid programmes in developing countries	■ use dependent infinitives (revisited)	■ adapt online text and data for presentations

■ Le saviez-vous?

From rags to riches?

La fabrication artisanale du papier à partir du lin continue au Musée du Papier "Le Nil", à Angoulême, où on cite le poème suivant qui raconte comment les mendiants aidaient à créer la richesse:

Les mendiants font les chiffons.
Les chiffons font le papier.
Le papier fait la monnaie.
La monnaie fait les banques.
Les banques font les emprunts
Les emprunts font les mendiants...

le lin *linen*
le chiffon *rag*

■ Pour commencer

Choisissez la bonne réponse.

1 Un chômeur est...
a actif
b fictif
c inactif
d radioactif

2 Les prestations sociales...
a aident les gens précaires
b provoquent la précarité
c s'adressent aux riches
d augmentent la pauvreté

3 Un SDF est sans...
a dettes financières
b doute familier
c devises françaises
d domicile fixe

4 Dans les pays d'Europe de l'est, combien de gens vivaient dans la pauvreté à la fin des années 90?
a 5 millions
b 50 millions
c 150 millions
d 500 millions

5 L'Unicef, c'est quoi?
a un mouvement universitaire
b une association caritative
c un pays d'Afrique
d une agence de presse

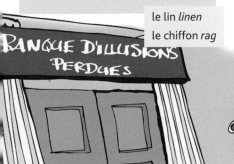

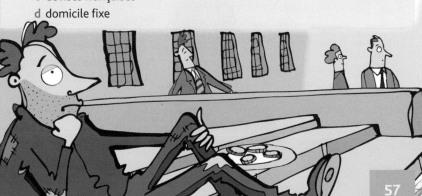

A L'embarras des riches

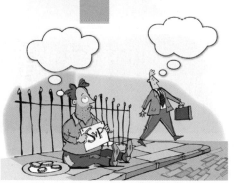

1 Choisissez les pensées de l'homme riche et du clochard.

Exemple: _____

A: L'homme riche pense: « Je mérite mieux que ça ». Il a travaillé dur et il n'apprécie pas les clochards dans la rue.

B: Mais non, le clochard pense: « Je mérite mieux que ça ». Il n'a pas eu de chance et il n'aime pas les riches sans conscience morale.

_____

> Je mérite mieux que ça.

> La richesse se donne seulement à ceux qui la méritent.

> Vous n'appréciez pas mes problèmes.

> Vous ne contribuez à rien.

> La pauvreté n'est pas ma responsabilité.

> Plus on partage, plus on est riche.

2 a Lisez le texte et reliez les termes français et anglais.

> Les Français, ayant plus de temps et plus d'argent, ont par conséquent plus de pouvoir d'achat. Le seuil de richesse correspond au double du niveau de vie médian: 2 700€ net par mois pour un individu, 4 450€ pour un couple et 5 680€ pour un couple avec deux enfants.
>
> Par contre, le seuil de pauvreté correspond à la moitié du revenu médian, moins de 700€ net par mois. Il y a donc 3,5 millions de pauvres en France ou, selon les critères européens (seuil de pauvreté = 60% du niveau de vie médian), jusqu'à sept millions, soit 12 % des ménages.

i	le pouvoir d'achat	a	*wealth threshold*
ii	le seuil de richesse	b	*average standard of living*
iii	le niveau de vie médian	c	*European criteria*
iv	le seuil de pauvreté	d	*average income*
v	le revenu médian	e	*purchasing power*
vi	les critères européens	f	*poverty threshold*

b Traduisez le texte en anglais.

c C'est comment dans votre pays? Adaptez le texte.

3 a 🔆🎧 Ecoutez deux jeunes parler de leur vie et faites les activités interactives.

b 🎧 Rédigez les textes à partir des notes, puis réécoutez pour vérifier.

Exemple: _____

J: Je me suis peu intéressé au collège...

M: J'ai été mal scolarisé, parce que...

_____

Vocabulaire

le/la SDF: sans domicile fixe *homeless person*

le chômeur *an unemployed person*

le licenciement *redundancy*

mendier *to beg*

se ficher de (fam.) *not to give a damn about*

scolariser *to educate*

bosser (fam.) *to work*

défavorisé *underprivileged*

actif *(of) working (age)*

percevoir *to earn*

traité de racaille *branded as scum*

manifester *to protest*

précaire *precarious, unsound*

Jérôme, 27 ans, SDF et chômeur
peu intéressé collège, emploi: pas de diplôme, usine
se droguer, copains: disputé avec parents
licenciements usine, logement: clochards, rues, mendier
voler de l'argent, malade: tout perdu
attitude des riches: se fichent

Mathieu, 27 ans, footballeur au PSG
mal scolarisé, sportif: contrat PSG
entraînement, matches: dur, salaire
voitures, vacances, copine: chance, bosse dur, mérite
pauvres: son affaire? auraient pu trouver emploi
services de santé

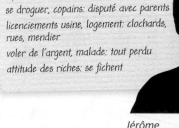

Jérôme

Mathieu

4 a 🎧 Deux étudiantes parlent de Mathieu et de Jérôme. Ecoutez: vous êtes d'accord avec qui? Ecrivez vos opinions.

b 💡 A deux. Echangez vos opinions. (Feuille)

« *Société malade?* »

En France on meurt plus tôt et les problèmes de santé surviennent plus précocement chez les défavorisés. En 2006, 9,2 millions de Français actifs avaient un problème durable de santé ou un handicap. Le taux d'emploi de cette population n'était que de 44 %, contre 65 % pour la population dont la capacité de travail restait intacte. En classe de troisième, 7,4 % des enfants d'ouvriers non qualifiés étaient obèses contre moins de 0,7 % des enfants de cadres.

Les inégalités monétaires apparaissent donc à beaucoup de Français comme des injustices. On se demande s'il est normal qu'un grand patron gagne autant que plusieurs centaines de ses salariés mal payés, ou que des stars et des grands sportifs perçoivent des millions d'euros pour quelques semaines de travail.

Quant aux milliers de jeunes chômeurs, l'avenir reste incertain sur tous les plans: souvent malades car mal nourris et mal logés, mal scolarisés et traités de "racaille" par Nicolas Sarkozy, dès qu'ils manifestent dans les rues, ils n'ont aucune possibilité d'échapper à la pauvreté ni à la violence et la délinquance qui en résultent. Ainsi tourne la roue de la pauvreté: aucune réussite scolaire, aucun diplôme, la santé précaire, le chômage et la vie en marge.

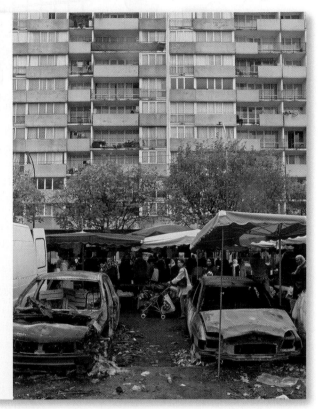

5 Lisez le texte, trouvez les quatre phrases vraies et corrigez les erreurs.

a L'espérance de vie des défavorisés est plus courte que celle des gens bien payés.

b Le taux d'obésité des enfants de cadres est nettement supérieur à celui des enfants d'ouvriers.

c Beaucoup de Français se fichent des inégalités monétaires de la société.

d Ils trouvent anormal l'écart entre le salaire des grands patrons et celui de leurs employés.

e Certaines vedettes travaillent peu pour gagner beaucoup.

f Des centaines de jeunes sont au chômage.

g Les chômeurs qui manifestent ont mauvaise réputation chez le président de la République.

h L'inclusion sociale les attend.

6 💡 Ecrivez quelques phrases sur chaque aspect de la richesse et la pauvreté dans votre pays. (Feuille)

- le chômage
- le logement
- la scolarisation
- les maladies
- la violence

Expressions clés

L'attitude des riches me dégoûte.

Ils sont chanceux / touchent des salaires fabuleux sans contribuer à la société.

Ils auraient pu partager leur fortune avec les défavorisés.

La pauvreté entraîne souvent des conséquences terribles.

C'est déprimant / honteux / inadmissible / scandaleux!

Les pauvres auraient pu s'intéresser plus au collège.

Les riches ne sont pas responsables des gens en situation précaire.

Si on a aidé à créer la richesse on a le droit de la partager.

On ne devient pas riche si on ne le mérite pas.

💡 Grammaire

The conditional perfect – *le conditionnel antérieur*

Use the **conditional** of the auxiliary (*avoir/être*) and add the **past participle** of the main verb, to say what would/should/could have happened. See page 114.

*Il **aurait dû** travailler un peu plus.*

*Il ne **serait** pas **devenu** footballeur professionnel s'il n'avait pas eu la chance d'être sportif.*

Les racines de la misère

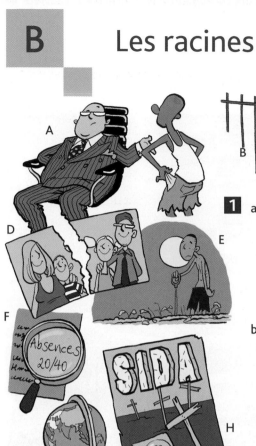

USINE FERMÉE

1 a Reliez les titres (i–viii) et les images (A–H).

i le chômage

ii la scolarité de courte durée et un faible niveau de qualification

iii les ruptures familiales

iv la famine

v les catastrophes naturelles

vi l'endettement

vii les problèmes de santé

viii la mondialisation

b Classez par ordre d'importance les causes de la pauvreté selon vous. (1 = la cause la plus profonde, 8 = la moins profonde)

Exemple: _____

A: La scolarité de courte durée: si on n'est pas bien scolarisé, on ne trouve pas de travail.

B: Le chômage: même avec peu de qualifications, on peut travailler, mais s'il n'y a pas de travail…

2 a Lisez le texte sur l'emploi en France. Reliez les expressions aux synonymes.

Les taux de chômage en Europe en 2007 (en % de la population active)	
Allemagne 8,4	Luxembourg 4,7
Autriche 4,4	Norvège 2,6
Belgique 7,5	Pays-Bas 3,2
Danemark 3,8	Pologne 9,6
Espagne 8,3	Portugal 8,0
Finlande 6,9	Royaume-Uni 5,3
France 8,3	Rép. tchèque 5,3
Grèce 8,3	Slovaquie 11,1
Hongrie 7,4	Suède 6,1
Irlande 4,5	Suisse 3,6
Italie 6,1	OCDE Europe 7,1

© OECD 2008

Sept millions d'actifs en France sont en situation de précarité, dont 2,7 millions de chômeurs. Un tiers des nouvelles embauches dans les entreprises de plus de 50 salariés fait l'objet de contrats à durée déterminée, un tiers concerne un emploi à temps partiel. Les jeunes sont les plus touchés, le taux des 15 à 29 ans remontant à 17% en situation de précarité. Le taux de chômage des personnes sans diplôme a atteint 15%. Une part importante des jeunes chômeurs ont eu une scolarité courte et une qualification faible, ce qui explique leur difficulté à trouver un emploi.

Selon les comparaisons internationales, la France a moins bien réussi à préserver l'emploi que ses partenaires de l'Union européenne. Trois pays seulement ont des taux de chômage plus élevés: l'Allemagne, la Pologne et la Slovaquie.

D'après G. Mermet, Francoscopie 2007 © Larousse 2006

i sont en situation de précarité

ii chômeurs

iii un tiers des nouvelles embauches

iv à durée déterminée

v les plus touchés

vi ont eu une scolarité de courte durée

vii un faible niveau de qualification

viii a réussi

a inactifs

b à temps fixe

c peu de ou aucun diplôme

d ont été peu scolarisés

e a eu du succès

f risquent de ne pas travailler

g trente-trois pour cent des postes créés

h ceux qui sont les plus concernés

Vocabulaire

une embauche *start, job*

la durée déterminée *fixed term*

à temps partiel *part-time*

remonter à *to reach*

atteindre *to reach*

important *significant*

plus élevé *higher*

2 b A deux: relisez le texte (page 60) et posez des questions.

Exemple: _____

A: Combien de Français sont au chômage?

B: Sept millions. Combien de nouveaux postes sont à temps partiel?

_____

c A deux: formulez des questions "vrai ou faux?" sur les pourcentages de la page 60.

Exemple: _____

A: Le Royaume-Uni a un taux de chômage plus élevé que l'Allemagne.

B: Faux. La France a un taux de chômage plus bas que...

_____

3 a 💡 Lisez le texte sur l'Europe de l'Est et faites les activités interactives.

b 🎧 Lisez les extraits du dialogue et notez F (fait) ou O (opinion), puis écoutez Elona et Antonin pour vérifier.

Exemple: _____

i – O

_____

i	Au début du deuxième millénaire, beaucoup plus de gens des pays d'Europe de l'Est vivaient dans la pauvreté que sous les régimes communistes.
ii	Plus de 30% des habitants de Hongrie vivaient sous le revenu minimum.
iii	Le taux de pauvreté était cinq fois plus élevé que celui de la France.
iv	Avant la chute du communisme, les gens n'avaient pas de liberté civile mais ils bénéficiaient de plus de protection sociale.
v	En Hongrie, 1,5 million d'emplois ont été supprimés à cause des privatisations.
vi	La privatisation détruit tous les services publics.
vii	Les salaires ont chuté, et la pauvreté et le chômage ont augmenté.
viii	On est mieux éduqué sous un système d'enseignement public.
ix	Les inégalités dans la société sont devenues de plus en plus évidentes.
x	Les problèmes de nutrition, de santé et de logement des gens pauvres sont entièrement dus au marché du travail flexible.
xi	Si les gens pauvres ont aujourd'hui plus de libertés civiles, ils n'ont pourtant pas les moyens d'en profiter.

4 a 💡 A deux: utilisez les faits et opinions ci-dessus pour faire un dialogue. Réécoutez Elona et Antonin et comparez. (Feuille)

b 💡 A l'écrit: « Les causes de la pauvreté en Europe de l'Est et en France ». (Feuille)

💡 **Grammaire**

Comparative and superlative adjectives

Add the definite article to turn **comparative** adjectives into **superlatives**. See page 105.

*Le taux de chômage est **plus élevé qu**'en France.*

*C'est le taux de chômage **le plus élevé** d'Europe.*

*Les jeunes sont **les plus concernés**.*

Elona

Antonin

■ **Expressions clés**

C'est ton opinion, et peut-être la mienne aussi, mais...

On n'en a pas la preuve.

On ne peut pas dire qu'ils n'avaient pas de libertés civiles du tout.

Il me semble bien que plus de gens vivaient dans la pauvreté / qu'ils bénéficiaient de beaucoup plus de protection sociale.

C'est sûr qu'ils avaient le plein emploi / que les inégalités sont devenues plus évidentes.

Il est indéniable que les salaires ont chuté.

C Solidarité globale?

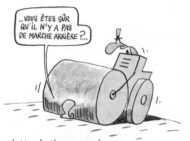

... VOUS ÊTES SÛR QU'IL N'Y A PAS DE MARCHE ARRIÈRE ?...

La dette du tiers-monde –
un frein au développement?

1 Traduisez en anglais et expliquez la signification du dessin, puis choisissez ou écrivez une légende.

L'Ouest avance, le Tiers-Monde s'incline

Les pays de l'Ouest rencontrent les pays en développement

Sommet des pays riches et des pays en développement

Les pays riches font disparaître les problèmes du Tiers-Monde

Dette, aide et autonomie

La véritable leçon des événements de la fin du premier millénaire s'impose: l'issue à la dette n'est pas la dette elle-même. En régénérant l'Europe de l'ouest après la Seconde Guerre mondiale, le "Marshall Plan" a aussi condamné une large partie du Tiers-Monde à la dépendance commerciale, technologique et financière. Après la crise du pétrole pendant les années 70, les pays riches ont imposé des intérêts variables sur les prêts aux tiers nations, qui par conséquent n'auraient pas pu s'en sortir sans changement de politique de croissance, de développement et de dette.

La dette n'est qu'un simple révélateur. En définitive, il faut permettre aux pays du Tiers-Monde de profiter eux aussi de la croissance et du développement, en leur accordant une plus grande autonomie.

En attendant, les pays en développement continuent à bénéficier de programmes d'aide et de développement essentiels, grâce à de nombreuses associations caritatives internationales, y compris:

L'Unicef France qui a pour mission d'informer le public français sur les problèmes des enfants dans les pays en développement, et plus particulièrement dans les situations de détresse.

MÉDECINS SANS FRONTIÈRES **Médecins Sans Frontières** qui, depuis plus de trente ans, apporte une assistance médicale à des populations aux prises avec des crises menaçant leur survie: principalement en cas de conflits armés, mais aussi d'épidémies, de pandémies, de catastrophes naturelles ou encore d'exclusion des soins.

Oxfam

Oxfam: grâce à ses campagnes internationales, chaque jour des enseignants, des médecins et des infirmières changent la vie des gens. Refusant la fatalité, ils s'efforcent d'apporter un enseignement et des soins de santé de qualité.

2 a 🎧 Lisez le texte et répondez aux questions, puis écoutez et vérifiez.

i Qu'est-ce que les dernières années du 20ème siècle nous ont fait comprendre*?

ii Qu'est-ce qui a régénéré les pays d'Europe de l'ouest en période d'après-guerre?

iii Quels pays n'ont pas pu en profiter?

iv Comment pourrait-on y encourager la croissance et le développement?

v Quelle association se soucie en particulier des victimes de guerres et de luttes violentes?

vi Elle intervient aussi dans quels cas?

vii L'Unicef se spécialise dans quoi?

viii Oxfam fait penser* à quelle catastrophe naturelle? Quels sont ses autres domaines d'intervention?

*faire comprendre, faire penser: *see dependent infinitives, page 118*

b 🎧 A deux: réécoutez puis répondez de mémoire aux questions.

Exemple: _____

A: Que se passerait-il si on changeait...?

B: Les pays en développement auraient... Ils pourraient exporter leurs produits et...

Vocabulaire

la marche arrière *reverse (gear)*

véritable *real*

s'imposer *to be assertive / convincing*

l'issue (à la dette) *the solution (to debt)*

le révélateur *indicator*

accorder *to grant, allow*

une association caritative *charitable foundation, charity*

aux prises avec *struggling against*

s'efforcer d'apporter *to strive to provide*

3 a 💡 Lisez les textes (en ligne) sur les Objectifs du Millénaire pour le Développement (OMD) et faites les activités interactives.

b Mettez les objectifs A–H dans l'ordre du rapport OMD.

A   la promotion d'un environnement durable

B   la réduction de la mortalité infantile

C   la réduction de la pauvreté et de la faim

D   la lutte contre le sida, le paludisme et autres maladies

E   la mise en place d'un partenariat mondial pour le développement

F   l'enseignement primaire pour tous

G   l'égalité entre hommes et femmes

H   l'amélioration de la santé maternelle

c 🎧 Lisez les phrases i–x. Ecoutez l'interview et notez le numéro des phrases que vous entendez.

i   On a fait des progrès mais beaucoup reste à faire.

ii   D'abord parce que la réussite est mal répartie.

iii   En Asie, la pauvreté baisse lentement, grâce à la croissance économique.

iv   En Afrique subsaharienne, le nombre de personnes très pauvres s'est stabilisé.

v   Il est probable qu'on atteigne la cible fixée.

vi   Je suis plus pessimiste en ce qui concerne l'enseignement primaire.

vii   L'Afrique subsaharienne est en avance sur d'autres régions, avec 30% des enfants non scolarisés.

viii   Seul un des huit groupes régionaux risque d'atteindre tous les objectifs.

ix   Toutes les régions rencontrent des difficultés dans les domaines de la santé et de l'environnement.

x   Au minimum, les pays développés doivent tenir entièrement leur promesse.

d 🎧 Corrigez les erreurs dans les phrases qui restent (ci-dessus), puis réécoutez et vérifiez.

e 💡 A deux: rejouez l'interview. (Feuille)

4 💡🖎 Ecoutez la conversation puis enregistrez vos réponses.

5 💡 A l'écrit: « La solidarité globale: seule solution ou rêve impossible à réaliser? » (Feuille)

Objectifs du Millénaire pour le développement

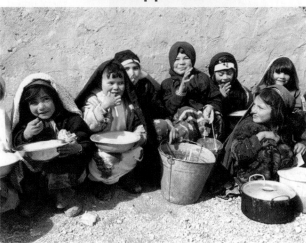

■ **Expressions clés**

La réussite du projet est encore possible / inégalement répartie.

(En Asie) la pauvreté baisse rapidement.

Il se peut qu'on n'atteigne pas la cible fixée.

Je suis optimiste en ce qui concerne l'éducation / la scolarisation / la réduction de la faim.

(L'Afrique subsaharienne) reste à la traîne derrière d'autres régions.

Le problème du chômage des jeunes me semble insurmontable, ainsi que les inégalités entre les sexes / la déforestation / la pénurie d'eau / la forte prévalence du VIH

Il faut doubler l'aide accordée à l'Afrique.

L'accès libre au marché global sans condition pour tous les pays en développement est absolument essentiel.

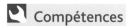 Compétences

Adapting online text and data for presentations

Enhance presentations by:

• highlighting key phrases for bullet points

• simplifying or adapting data electronically

• combining statements with questions to involve listeners.

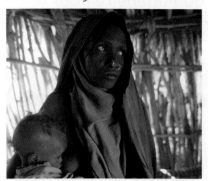

Now you should be able to:

■ talk about wealth and poverty, including links to health and social unrest

■ discuss the causes of poverty in Europe and developing countries

■ discuss debt and aid programmes in developing countries

Grammar

■ use the conditional perfect

■ use comparative and superlative adjectives

■ use dependent infinitives (revisited)

Skills

■ adapt others' opinions to express your own

■ construct dialogues using various sources

■ adapt online text and data for presentations

✓ Résumé

1 A quoi correspond le seuil de richesse?

2 Mettez les verbes au conditionnel antérieur:

Mathieu ...... (**pouvoir**) s'intéresser un peu plus au collège, comme ça il ...... (**avoir**) plus de diplômes et peut-être qu'il ...... (**ne pas devenir**) footballeur.

3 Complétez la phrase:

« Si on a aidé à créer la richesse... »

4 Traduisez en français:

The unemployment rate for people without qualifications has reached 15%.

5 Complétez les phrases avec le comparatif ou superlatif des adjectifs entre parenthèses:

Les jeunes sont ...... (**concerné**) ...... les adultes, mais les mal scolarisés sont ...... (**touché**).

6 Traduisez en anglais:

Sept millions d'actifs en France sont en situation de précarité, dont 2,7 millions de chômeurs.

7 Complétez la phrase:

Les pays en développement bénéficient de programmes d'aide et de développement grâce aux...

8 Ecrivez une phrase qui veut dire:

MSF se soucie en particulier des victimes de guerre et de luttes violentes.

9 Que se passerait-il pour les pays en développement si on changeait les mécanismes et les politiques de croissance?

10 Qu'est-ce qu'il faut faire pour assurer en partie le succès des Objectifs du Millénaire pour le Développement? (2 détails)

AQA Examiner's tips

Listening

Write down any numbers or percentages **as soon as you hear them**. You will then be prepared for questions that might need them as an answer.

Speaking

Choose vocabulary that allows you to **demonstrate your ability** at this level of study.

Reading

In **matching exercises**, watch out for 'extra' options. Don't be led away from the correct answer.

Writing

Simplify ideas if it helps you to **express yourself accurately**.

8

Problèmes sociaux contemporains
L'ordre public

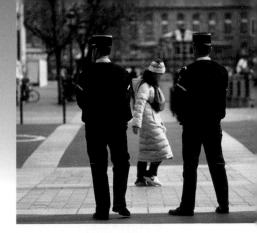

By the end of this chapter you will be able to:

	Language	Grammar	Skills
A **La délinquance: causes et effets**	▦ discuss crime, especially among young people ▦ talk about reasons for criminal and antisocial behaviour	▦ use the perfect tense	▦ structure a coherent analysis of causes and effects
B **La criminalité en baisse**	▦ discuss the effectiveness of measures to reduce crime	▦ use infinitive constructions (revisited)	▦ combine data with opinions in debates and presentations
C **Crime et châtiment**	▦ consider alternatives to imprisonment	▦ use the future tense of the passive voice	▦ consider the values society holds on major issues

Le saviez-vous?

Ma parole!

A la suite de la Bataille d'Hastings (1066) et du couronnement de Guillaume duc de Normandie, la langue anglaise ou anglo-saxonne a absorbé de la langue française plusieurs termes légaux dont on se sert toujours. Quant aux termes suivants, à vous de juger: français ou anglais d'origine?

action, appeal, assises, complaint, counsel, court, defendant, evidence, jury, justice, parole, plaintiff, sentence, sue, summon, trespass

Pour commencer

1 Trouvez l'intrus:
- a précarité
- b pauvreté
- c inclusion
- d chômage

2 Quel est le contraire du terme "en hausse"?
- a en marge
- b en baisse
- c en général
- d en fait

3 Complétez la phrase:
"...... entraîne souvent la criminalité".
- a l'échec scolaire
- b la richesse
- c la stabilité familiale
- d la réussite scolaire

4 "Taux de criminalité" veut dire:
- a nombre total de prisonniers
- b total global de délinquants
- c nombre de crimes commis
- d méthodes criminelles

5 Classez (1–6) les aspects de la criminalité par ordre personnel (1 = l'aspect le plus inquiétant pour vous).
- a le trafic de drogue
- b le cybercrime
- c les jeunes délinquants violents
- d le terrorisme
- e les crimes financiers
- f autres crimes

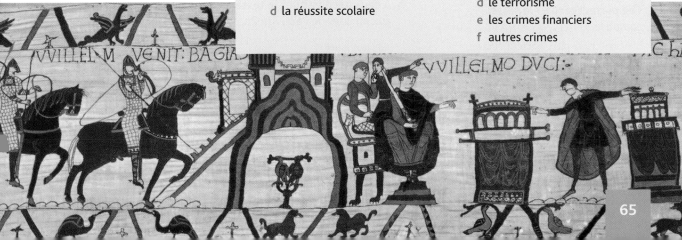

1 Discutez des causes de la délinquance.

> C'est la faute des ruptures familiales. Il y a trop de divorces et donc trop d'enfants avec des problèmes sociaux.

> Pour moi, c'est à cause de l'exclusion sociale qu'on a tous ces délinquants. Ils n'ont pas le choix...

FRANCE DÉLINQUANCE

ruptures familiales

exclusion sociale

chômage, précarité et personnes défavorisées

écart entre les riches et les pauvres

enfants mal scolarisés sans diplômes

culte de l'individu

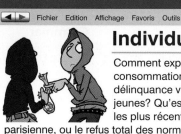

Fichier Edition Affichage Favoris Outils

Individualisme ou société?

Comment expliquer la hausse de la consommation de drogues et des actes de délinquance violents, notamment chez les jeunes? Qu'est-ce qui a incité les émeutes les plus récentes dans la banlieue parisienne, ou le refus total des normes et des valeurs collectives de la société traditionnelle?

La société, ou plus précisément le système économique, constitué par les entreprises, les médias et la publicité, nous a fait croire que chacun a par principe le droit de tout obtenir de la vie, car "il le vaut bien". Malheureusement, comme la vie ne fournit pas en même temps les clés permettant à tout le monde d'y parvenir, ce culte de l'individu entraîne une "difficulté d'être soi", qui peut aboutir au suicide. Les membres de cette non-société ne peuvent "survivre" qu'en développant des stratégies d'adaptation individuelles, y compris délits, infractions, délinquance, vols et meurtres, au détriment de la cohésion sociale et de la solidarité.

D'après Gérard Mermet, Francoscopie 2007 © Larousse 2006

Vocabulaire

la délinquance *crime, criminality*
il le vaut bien *he/they deserve(s) it*
fournir *to provide*
parvenir *to succeed*
entraîner *to entail, to lead to*
soi *oneself*
aboutir *to end up*
le délit *offence*
une infraction *breach, infringement*

Grammaire

The perfect tense – *le passé composé*

Use the two-part perfect tense (**auxiliary** + **past participle**) to talk and write about completed events in the past. See pages 110–1.

*Qu'est-ce qui **a incité** les émeutes?* What caused the riots?

2 **a** Lisez le texte et reliez les deux parties des phrases.

i	Les jeunes consomment...	a	que tout est à obtenir dans la vie.
ii	Beaucoup de gens s'opposent...	b	crée des frustrations et même le désespoir.
iii	On a accepté l'idée...	c	d'amener une crise sociale par la criminalité.
iv	Cette notion fausse...	d	de plus en plus de drogues.
v	L'individualisme risque...	e	aux règles de la société.

b A deux: reconstituez le texte en ajoutant les expressions suivantes aux phrases de l'activité 2a.

de nos jours	aujourd'hui	en même temps
à la fois	en plus	il paraît que
ce qui est étonnant, c'est que	sans aucun doute	évidemment
il est indéniable que	par conséquent	en conclusion

Exemple: _____

A: De nos jours, les jeunes consomment de plus en plus de drogues.

B: En même temps, il paraît que beaucoup de gens s'opposent...

3 a 💡🎧 Ecoutez la discussion et faites les activités interactives.

b 🎧 Complétez les réponses ci-dessous, puis réécoutez pour vérifier.

i On a le choix d'...... ou de rejeter ...... Mais je n'accepte pas que ...... aient le droit de ...... des crimes parce qu'ils se sentent frustrés ou ...... Ce n'est pas la faute de la société, après tout!

ii Moi aussi, je trouve déraisonnable ...... les jeunes désaffectés se permettent de ...... , de s'...... aux gens et de se ...... et se ...... dans les rues. C'est inadmissible!

iii Certes, notre société est ...... Si on refuse de reconnaître ...... des jeunes et des ...... en situation précaire, c'est l'ordre ...... qui en souffrira.

iv Le ...... public est impensable. Il ...... réorienter la société avant qu'il ne soit ...... Il faut abolir ...... , assurer ...... pour tous et ...... les gens en situation précaire.

v D'accord, ... , l'amour de ...... est bien, mais où reste le ...... d'autrui?

vi Ce sont les ...... et les ...... qui ont déformé la société par la ...... Le bonheur individuel est ...... , mais pas au coût de ...... et des ...... collectives. Sinon, qui va s'...... des personnes ...... et en marge?

4 💡 A l'oral: adaptez les réponses de l'exercice 3b pour en faire un mini-débat. (Feuille)

Exemple: _____

A: La délinquance est due au rejet de la société, surtout par les jeunes.

B: C'est possible, on peut accepter ou rejeter la société, mais je n'accepte pas que....

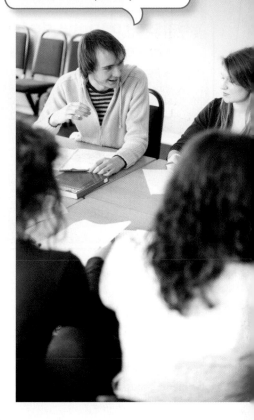

Vous êtes d'accord que la délinquance est due au rejet de la société, surtout par les jeunes?

La société n'existe pas?

Faut-il que l'individualisme et la disparition des valeurs collectives de la société entraînent une hausse du taux de criminalité et un climat généralisé de peur et de haine même d'autrui? Les gens, sont-ils vraiment convaincus que les groupes minoritaires, comme les immigrés, les mal scolarisés, les précaires et les fragiles, représentent une menace quelconque au bonheur individuel et méritent donc d'être punis, non seulement par la loi mais aussi par leurs concitoyens?

Il faut rejeter d'urgence l'image fausse de la vie représentée par les médias et la publicité et accepter son rôle d'individu dans un cadre social collectif, avant qu'il ne soit trop tard.

Expressions clés

C'est possible / inadmissible.

Ce n'est pas la faute de la société.

Le désordre public est impensable / affreux / à éviter à tout prix.

Je n'accepte pas / Je trouve déraisonnable que + subj.

... que les jeunes se permettent / aient le droit de commettre des crimes.

Que reste-t-il de la solidarité / du respect d'autrui?

Il faut protéger les gens en situation précaire / réorienter la société / reconnaître les problèmes / abolir la pauvreté / assurer la scolarité.

5 a Lisez l'article ci-dessus et traduisez-le en anglais.

b 💡 Rédigez un article (250 mots) au sujet des causes et effets de la délinquance. (Feuille)

B La criminalité en baisse?

Baisse continue de la délinquance enregistrée depuis cinq ans

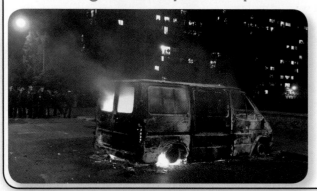

Comme au Royaume–Uni et dans l'Union européenne en général, selon les chiffres publiés par l'Office national de la délinquance, la délinquance générale a diminué de 3,66 % par rapport à l'année dernière. La délinquance de voie publique recule encore plus nettement de 7,29 %. Parallèlement, le taux d'élucidation a atteint 36,11%, soit une progression de deux points. En plus, les violences contre les personnes, connaissant pour la première fois depuis 12 ans un recul, ont diminué de 3,16 % au second semestre.

Le nombre de violences "crapuleuses", ayant le vol pour objet, a baissé de 11,26 % mais elles ne représentent qu'environ le quart des atteintes à l'intégrité physique. Par contre, les violences "gratuites" ou "non crapuleuses", qui ont augmenté de 6,07 %, en représentent près de la moitié.

C'est la cinquième année consécutive à voir une baisse du nombre d'atteintes aux biens, qu'il s'agisse des cambriolages, des vols violents ou de ceux liés aux véhicules à moteur.

Vocabulaire

enregistré *recorded*
la voie publique *public highway*
le taux d'élucidation *clear-up rate*
le semestre *term (of six months)*
une atteinte *attempt, attack*
les biens *goods, property*
le cambriolage *burglary*

la récidive *reoffending*
dissuader *to deter*
à peine *hardly*
engorgé *overcrowded*
obsédé *obsessed*

1 Lisez le texte ci-dessus puis jouez au baseball verbal. A dit une expression des cases ci-dessous (en anglais ou en français), B répond sans hésiter avec l'équivalent dans l'autre langue.

Exemple: _____

A: Gratuitous violence?   B: Violence gratuite.

_____

street crime	gratuitous violence
a reduction	more clearly
crimes against property	compared with
general crime	physical assault

atteinte à l'intégrité physique	un recul
plus nettement	atteintes aux biens
délinquance générale	violence gratuite
	délinquance de voie publique
	par rapport à

2 Relisez le texte, puis corrigez une erreur par phrase.

a La baisse générale concerne tous les actes de délinquance commis en France.

b L'Office nationale de la délinquance a refusé les chiffres.

c Le taux de délinquance générale a reculé de moins de trois pour cent.

d Les actes délinquants dans les rues sont en hausse.

e Pendant les six premiers mois de l'année, les violences contre les personnes ont baissé de plus de 3%.

f Les violences "non crapuleuses" ne représentent que 25% environ du nombre total des atteintes à l'intégrité physique.

g Les actes de violence gratuite ont diminué d'au moins six pour cent.

h Depuis plus de quatre ans les cas d'atteintes aux biens enregistrés sont en hausse.

3 a 🎧 A qui donnez-vous raison? Choisissez des réponses (dans les bulles à gauche), puis écoutez pour comparer.

b 💡 A deux, discutez-en, en recyclant et adaptant les opinions de Charlotte et Natacha. (Feuille)

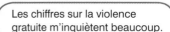

Les chiffres sur la violence gratuite m'inquiètent beaucoup.

Je me sens rassurée par tous ces chiffres.

Charlotte

Je n'ai pas l'impression que la délinquance soit en baisse.

La délinquance enregistrée ne donne pas forcément les chiffres réels.

La hausse du taux d'élucidation est encourageante.

Ce n'est pas tout à fait rassurant.

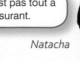

Natacha

4 💡 Les prisons: lisez le texte (en ligne) et faites les activités interactives.

5 🎧 Ecoutez et mettez les extraits (A–J) dans l'ordre de la conversation. Commencez par G.

A Il ne faut pas emprisonner le problème, il faut le résoudre.

B Le taux de récidive suggère que l'emprisonnement, avec ses conditions inhumaines, dissuade à peine les futurs délinquants.

D Au contraire, les prisons sont engorgées et le taux de récidive est beaucoup trop élevé.

E D'accord, la violence s'excuse mal dans tous les cas, mais l'incarcération des mineurs et des jeunes n'est pas la bonne solution.

I Si on veut désengorger les prisons, on n'a qu'à respecter autrui et ne pas commettre de crimes.

F Mais il faut absolument protéger les citoyens innocents contre toute forme de violence.

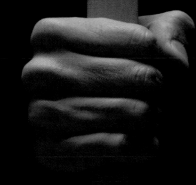

C Tout à fait, mais il ne s'agit pas uniquement d'atteintes violentes. Notre société est obsédée par la notion du "risque zéro" en tout, ce qui est impossible à achever.

G Les statistiques montrent qu'on est en train de briser le cycle infernal de la criminalité.

H Il faut comprendre que l'emprisonnement devrait servir à la fois à punir et à dissuader.

J Et le respect de la dignité humaine des victimes innocentes des délinquants?

to revise infinitive constructions, see pages 117–8

6 💡 A deux: préparez un petit dossier (300 mots) sur:
« La criminalité est-elle vraiment en baisse? »
Ajoutez des statistiques actuelles d'Internet, des opinions et des raisonnements sur les dispositifs. (Feuille)

Expressions clés

Le taux de violence gratuite / récidive est en hausse / affreux / trop élevé.

Où reste le respect de la dignité humaine de ces prisonniers / des victimes innocentes de la délinquance?

Cela ne m'étonne pas, vu les conditions de détention inhumaines.

Je ne dis pas le contraire, mais il ne s'agit pas uniquement de…

L'emprisonnement devrait servir à la fois à punir et à dissuader.

Il (ne) faut (pas) emprisonner / résoudre le problème.

Traitons les causes fondamentales et pas les symptômes de la maladie.

Tu n'es pas / Vous n'êtes pas un peu trop laxiste / punitif/ve?

🖋 Compétences

Combining data with opinions in debates and presentations

With careful use of reasons and data such as pie charts, graphs and results of surveys, you can enhance significantly the impact of your arguments and conclusions in presentations and in controversial debates.

C Crime et châtiment

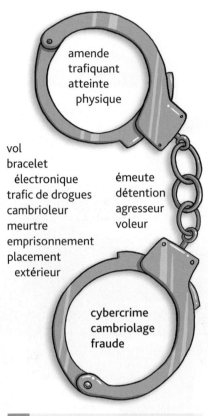

amende
trafiquant
atteinte
physique

vol
bracelet
électronique
trafic de drogues
cambrioleur
meurtre
emprisonnement
placement
extérieur

émeute
détention
agresseur
voleur

cybercrime
cambriolage
fraude

Vocabulaire

apaiser *to quell, to appease*

une échelle *scale*

le dispositif *measure, arrangement*

mettre en place *to set up, to put in place*

le milieu *environment, setting*

périscolaire *outside school*

le brevet *certificate, diploma*

Grammaire

The future tense of the passive voice

This describes a future event without explaining who is responsible for the action.

It is formed using the **future tense** of *être* and a **past participle**. See page 116.

*4 000 policiers **seront déployés**.*
4 000 police officers will be deployed.

---

1 Classez les termes à gauche sous les catégories relatives à la délinquance.

Crime/Infraction	Accusé/Coupable	Punition
vol		

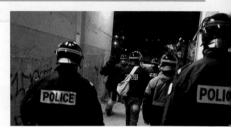

Plus ça change...?

La lutte contre toutes les formes de criminalité se poursuivra sans cesse à partir de 2008. Afin d'apaiser les banlieues, environ 200 unités territoriales de quartier viendront renforcer la sécurité des banlieues les plus marquées par les violences, alors 4 000 policiers supplémentaires en trois ans seront déployés. Pour faire échec à la criminalité organisée et au trafic de drogue, des coopérations seront organisées à l'échelle européenne. La France se placera au premier rang de la lutte contre la cybercriminalité. Finalement, afin de s'opposer au terrorisme, en développant un dispositif national de vidéosurveillance, le nombre de caméras sera augmenté jusqu'à un million en 2009.

Ces mesures, risquent-elles de réussir? Pas évident! Sans compter le coût social des prisons engorgées et de la récidive, au début du troisième millénaire, le coût global de la délinquance au lieu de diminuer s'élevait à 20 milliards d'euros, une augmentation significative depuis 1981. Ceci démontre une bien faible productivité des moyens de lutte contre la délinquance. Les dispositifs mis en place par l'Etat n'ont pas été efficaces. Parallèlement, les dépenses en sécurité privée n'ont cessé aussi de progresser. De quelques milliers dans les années 1980, les agents de sécurité privée seraient aujourd'hui environ 180 000.

Que faire donc pour combattre la criminalité? On peut être pour ou contre la vidéosurveillance, le fait est qu'elle est efficace dans la lutte contre la délinquance. Il est nécessaire de concentrer aussi les efforts sur la prévention. On ne naît pas délinquant. Il est donc important de mettre en place des programmes de prévention couvrant le milieu scolaire, périscolaire et même familial. Au niveau scolaire, on pourrait développer la formation à la citoyenneté, et faire passer à tous les enfants un "brevet citoyen".

2 a Lisez l'article. Ecrivez un résumé en anglais (120 mots) des paragraphes 1 et 2, sous ces catégories:

street violence   organised crime   internet fraud   terrorism   costs of crime

b 🎧 Ecoutez quatre suggestions et trouvez dans l'article les détails qui correspondent.

Exemple: _____

1 – 4 000 policiers supplémentaires seront déployés

_____

c 🎧 Réécoutez et répétez en incorporant vos réponses à 2b.

2 d A deux: servez-vous du texte de la page 70 pour répondre aux questions. (Feuille)

> Alors, les mesures proposées risquent-elles d'avoir du succès?

> Ce n'est pas évident!

i Les mesures proposées risquent-elles d'avoir du succès?

ii Pourquoi pas?

iii Les dépenses en sécurité privée ont-elles diminué sur la même période?

iv Comment peut-on combattre la criminalité, alors?

v C'est la seule solution?

vi Qu'est-ce qu'on pourrait faire vis-à-vis de la citoyenneté?

3 a Ecoutez l'interview et faites les activités interactives.

b Remplissez les blancs dans les trois extraits ci-dessous, pour faire un résumé de l'interview.

La justice

La justice ne consiste pas uniquement en (1) ...... légitime en (2) ...... d'individus délinquants. Peu importe le rôle (3) ...... des Etablissements Pénitentiaires pour Mineurs et Centres éducatifs fermés, qui eux aussi impliquent l'incarcération et tous les problèmes de (4) ...... qui y sont associés.
   Il faut reconnaître les (5) ...... et les effets de la délinquance. Notre société individualiste (6) ...... les gens en situation précaire: c'est déjà une grosse (7) .... S'ils répondent à l'(8) ...... de la société envers eux-mêmes par la violence ou la délinquance, ils en seront (9) ...... pour une deuxième fois, d'habitude par l'incarcération.

> réinsertion   injustice   éducatif   punis   vengeance   rejette   causes   indifférence   punition

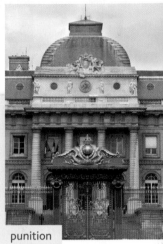

Le rôle de la prison

La prison doit punir, mais aussi rééduquer ou (10) ...... La prison doit rester un lieu (11) ...... , intégré à la ville, et (12) ...... , donc, dans la ville. En ville, la prison peut (13) ...... les familles plus facilement et facilite le travail des (14) ...... en milieu carcéral.

> bénévoles   social   accueillir   situé   resocialiser

Les alternatives à l'incarcération

Des (15) ...... alternatives existent, par exemple le (16) ...... avec mise à l'épreuve, le travail d'intérêt général qui connaît une forte (17) ...... , ou encore la semi-liberté avec l'usage du (18) ...... électronique. Ces peines évitent l'(19) .... de l'individu par la loi et la prison, et relancent dès le départ le projet de (20) ......

> écrasement   sursis   resocialisation   progression   bracelet   peines

4 Ecoutez la conversation, puis enregistrez vos propres réponses.

5 En groupes: faites une présentation écrite (jusqu'à 500 mots) sur la criminalité: causes et effets, dispositifs ratés et réussis, attitudes de la société individualiste et solutions proposées. (Feuille)

Expressions clés

La justice consiste en vengeance légitime / rééducation / resocialisation.

L'exclusion sociale est aussi une injustice.

Il faut protéger toutes les victimes / traiter les causes de la criminalité.

Sinon les gens en situation précaire continueront à être incarcérés / les prisons seront même plus engorgées / la récidive ne s'arrêtera pas.

Le rôle de la prison est de punir / rééduquer / resocialiser.

Les peines alternatives évitent l'écrasement de l'individu / relancent la resocialisation.

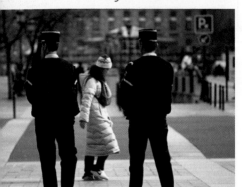

Now you should be able to:

- ■ discuss crime, especially among young people
- ■ talk about reasons for criminal and antisocial behaviour
- ■ discuss the effectiveness of measures to reduce crime
- ■ consider alternatives to imprisonment

Grammar

- ■ use the perfect tense
- ■ use infinitive constructions
- ■ use the future tense of the passive voice

Skills

- ■ structure a coherent analysis of causes and effects
- ■ combine data with opinions in debates and presentations
- ■ consider the values society holds on major issues

✓ Résumé

1 Nommez trois causes de la délinquance.

2 Traduisez en anglais:

« Cette notion fausse que tout est à obtenir dans la vie crée des frustrations et même le désespoir. »

3 Mettez les verbes au passé composé:

Qui (**inciter**) les émeutes de Paris? Comment les policiers (**réagir**) quand les jeunes (**s'attaquer**) à eux? La délinquance générale enregistrée (**diminuer**) peut-être et le taux d'élucidation (**progresser**), mais le problème de la criminalité (**ne pas disparaître**) encore.

4 Ecrivez une phrase qui veut dire la même chose que cette phrase:

Les violences contre les personnes connaissent un recul, mais les violences "non crapuleuses" sont en hausse.

5 Traduisez en français:

« I find unreasonable the notion that criminality is down to young people rejecting society. »

6 Complétez la phrase:

La délinquance enregistrée ne donne pas...

7 A quoi la prison devrait-elle servir? (3 détails)

8 Mettez les mots dans le bon ordre.

beaucoup trop le récidive Les engorgées et taux de sont est prisons élevé

9 Mettez les verbes à la forme passive et au futur:

Des mesures supplémentaires (**prendre**), la sécurité des banlieues (**renforcer**) et le nombre de caméras de vidéosurveillance (**augmenter**).

10 Remplissez les blancs:

Comme alternatives à l'incarcération, il y a le ...... avec mise à l'épreuve, le travail .... et la semi-liberté avec l'usage du ....

AQA Examiner's tips

Listening

Use a **separate piece of paper for rough work**. Make sure that any notes made on the paper to be handed to the examiner are crossed out before you hand it over.

Speaking

Speak confidently towards the microphone.

Reading

If you have to fill in **boxes with letters**, double-check that you've answered every one.

Writing

Dedicate the **conclusion of an essay** to a summary of what you've written and confirm your opinion.

Problèmes sociaux contemporains

9 Sciences et technologie: avances ou régression?

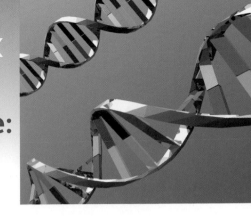

By the end of this chapter you will be able to:

	Language	Grammar	Skills
A Diagnostic: informatique	■ discuss advantages and drawbacks of ICT at home and at work	■ use present participles	■ summarise opposing views and draw balanced conclusions
B On va où exactement?	■ consider pros and cons of space and satellite technology	■ use interrogative pronouns (revisited)	■ make and counter controversial statements about contentious issues
C Science ne rime pas toujours avec conscience	■ discuss ethical issues relating to scientific, technological and medical progress and research	■ invert verb and subject after direct speech and adverbs	■ use anticipation and nuance to advance debates

---

■ Le saviez-vous?

La déchetterie du Monde

Selon l'Agence Spatiale Européenne (ESA) quelques 12 000 engins sont toujours en orbite autour de la Terre, dont seulement 700 satellites en service. Parmi les restes figurent 2 000 carcasses de fusées, toujours chargées de carburant et dont cinq par an explosent, projetant davantage de débris à l'encontre des satellites en service.

> **une déchetterie** *rubbish tip*
> **un engin** *man-made device*
> **à l'encontre de** *in the path of*

■ Pour commencer

Choisissez a, b, c ou d.

1 Pour accéder à votre compte e-mail, il vous faut votre ...... et votre code secret.
  a clé USB   c identifiant
  b portable   d ordinateur

2 ...... d'internautes travaillent depuis chez eux.
  a De moins en moins
  b De temps en temps
  c De nos jours
  d De plus en plus

3 La navigation par satellite ...... la surveillance du trafic.
  a facilite   c contredit
  b empêche   d amoindrit

4 La gestion du trafic ferroviaire concerne .....
  a les avions   c les trains
  b les voitures   d les bateaux

5 Le décryptage du génome est ...... scientifique le/la plus extraordinaire.
  a l'avancée   c le résultat
  b la reculée   d le problème

visiter   accéder à   vendre

perdre   manipuler   organiser

contacter   copier   embêter

recevoir   diffuser   répandre

envoyer   faire

1 Servez-vous des notes à gauche pour faire des phrases sur les avantages et les désavantages de l'informatique.

Exemple: _____

Avantages: Grâce à l'informatique, on peut vendre ses produits et envoyer des reportages électroniques.

Désavantages: A cause de l'informatique, il est possible de manipuler les informations et les gens.

---

produits   copains
photos numériques
reportages électroniques
études à la maison
infos et gens   virus   avec publicité
rencontres violentes
propagande   sans autorisation
sites interdits   argent et identité

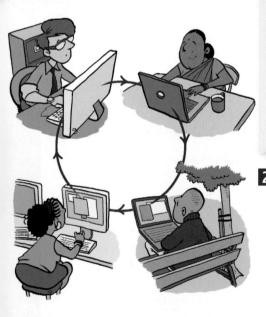

Solidarité virtuelle?

'En matière de communication, la diffusion du téléphone portable, l'accès à Internet et au multimédia ont transformé le rapport au temps, en imposant le "temps réel", qui est celui de l'immédiateté. Ils ont modifié aussi le rapport à l'espace en satisfaisant le vieux rêve d'ubiquité, en faisant éclater les frontières géographiques, politiques, linguistiques ou culturelles dans un contexte de mondialisation.'*

On est de moins en moins obligés de se déplacer afin de travailler, puisque le domicile connecté s'est vite transformé en lieu de travail et centre de communications personnel. C'en est de même pour les informations, les loisirs et la consommation: on peut gérer ses affaires financières depuis chez soi, en faisant des achats électroniques, en réglant ses comptes et en accédant à tout moment à son compte bancaire.

'Pour la première fois, tout habitant d'un pays développé peut être connecté par le son et par l'image à tous les autres.'*

L'individualisme étant sûrement en train de remplacer la collectivité et la solidarité sociale, peut-on aussi espérer que la génération techno établira une solidarité d'abord virtuelle puis, par la suite, réelle en se servant d'outils technologiques?

Quant à la France, même si plus d'un Français sur deux surfe le Web et 93% des utilisateurs disposent d'une connexion ADSL, la pénétration d'Internet a pris du retard en comparaison à ses voisins européens.

* G. Mermet, Francoscopie 2007 © Larousse 2006

2 Lisez le texte et les phrases a–h. Ecrivez V (vrai), F (faux) ou N (information non donnée), puis corrigez les erreurs.

a   La téléphonie et Internet ont bouleversé les attitudes envers le temps et l'espace.

b   La mondialisation impose des barrières à la communication.

c   En se connectant, on n'est plus obligé de travailler aussi dur qu'auparavant.

d   Un nombre croissant d'internautes profitent d'Internet pour travailler depuis chez eux.

e   Si on a une connexion Internet, on doit régler ses affaires en ligne.

f   La technologie électronique facilite la vie active, la recherche de renseignements, les loisirs et les contacts sociaux à distance.

g   En se servant trop d'Internet, on risque de perdre contact avec la société réelle.

h   Les pays européens voisins de la France sont en avance vis-à-vis de la pénétration d'Internet.

Vocabulaire

le rapport *relationship*
l'immédiateté *immediacy*
l'ubiquité *being/going everywhere*
le lieu de travail *workplace*

3 A deux: discutez des avantages de la technologie électronique.

Exemple: _____

A: Pour ma part, je profite d'Internet en faisant des achats en ligne et en... Mais je ne...

B: Moi, j'en profite en téléchargeant des fichiers et en...

4 a 💡🎞 Regardez la vidéo et faites les activités interactives.

b 🎞 A trois. Rédigez le texte de la discussion, en vous servant des termes ci-dessous. Regardez la vidéo à nouveau pour vérifier.

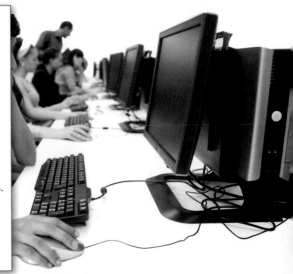

> ### 💡 Grammaire
>
> **Present participles**
> *– les participes présents*
>
> Use *en* + a present participle to talk about concurrent events or to give reasons (see page 116):
>
> *En me **connectant**, je peux prendre contact avec qui je veux.* By going on line, I can contact anyone I like.

Tolérance zéro, risque zéro, progrès zéro?

Nathalie: On ne peut pas nier que...

Marcus: Tu veux dire que...?

Nathalie: Tout à fait, oui.

Alima: Mais tu ne vas pas me dire que...?

N: Bien sûr que non, mais...

A: Par exemple?

N: De nos jours, chaque individu...

M: Evidemment, pour...

N: En principe, oui, mais...

A: Ah oui, je vois... Dès qu'on est connecté...

N: Exactement. C'est comme...

M: Et j'imagine que...

N: Et des...

A: Et des...

M: Et d'autres individus, comme...

A: Quelle horreur!... Et toi, tu ne crains pas...?

N: Si, ce sont là...

M: Et qu'il faut accepter, d'ailleurs. Après tout,...

A: En effet. Moi, je me sers de...

M: Justement. Acceptons...

---

5 💡 A deux: nommez à tour de rôle les avantages ou les désavantages de la technologie informatique. (Feuille)

> Grâce à l'informatique, je peux garder le contact avec mes copains en envoyant des SMS et en...

> Oui, mais à cause de l'informatique, on risque de laisser des empreintes électroniques, en se connectant, et on peut être surveillé et manipulé.

6 💡 Ecrivez un article (250 mots) sur « Diagnostic: informatique – avenir positif ou menaçant? » Ajoutez-y vos opinions. (Feuille)

Expressions clés

La technologie tend à renforcer le phénomène de l'individualisme.

A cause d'Internet, on se retire de la société / ne prend plus conscience d'autrui.

Toutes les avances comportent aussi des risques et des menaces.

Chaque individu est associé à des mots de passe / codes.

En utilisant les codes, on laisse des empreintes électroniques / on peut être surveillé et manipulé.

Les traces / empreintes électroniques peuvent être appropriées par des entreprises commerciales / administrations / terroristes / trafiquants / opérateurs de sites porno / pédophiles.

On risque de ne plus avoir de vie privée.

Il existe aussi des instruments de contrôle / régulation pour combattre les risques et les menaces.

Grâce à la technologie moderne, on peut travailler chez soi / gérer ses affaires en ligne / être connecté par le son et par l'image à tous les autres.

Acceptons les progrès et profitons-en, sans prendre trop de risques.

Si on insiste sur la tolérance zéro et le risque zéro dans la vie, il faudra accepter en même temps les progrès zéro.

On va où exactement?

A la surveillance de voitures volées

E la navigation par satellite en voiture

B la gestion du trafic maritime par satellite

C la gestion du trafic aérien par satellite

D la surveillance du système bancaire par satellite

F la gestion du trafic ferroviaire par satellite

1 a 🎧 Ecoutez et identifiez le bon contexte (A–F).

b Expliquez à votre partenaire les autres usages de la technologie par satellite.

Exemples: _____

La technologie par satellite facilite la surveillance de voitures volées.

En se servant de… / Si on se sert de… / A force d'utiliser…

… on peut gérer / surveiller…

Points de repère?

Malgré l'incontestable amélioration spectaculaire de la sécurité routière constatée depuis plusieurs années, due sans doute aux mesures de prévention et de répression technologiques, notamment la "peur des radars", l'utilisation de la technologie en voiture pose à la fois des problèmes considérables de sécurité.

Qui ne reconnaît pas l'image de l'automobiliste insouciant, roulant à 130 km/h dans la voie de dépassement, le portable à la main, en pleine conversation avec n'importe qui? Même les portables à mains libres ne résolvent pas les problèmes fondamentaux de la distraction du conducteur et du manque d'attention critique, qui risquent d'enchaîner des accidents mortels autrement bien évitables.

C'en est de même pour les systèmes de navigation par satellite en voiture: dès qu'on prête attention à la voix disloquée émanant de l'écran de l'appareil de navigation, on court le risque de déclencher une catastrophe routière. Quant aux conducteurs de poids lourds qui perdent la raison en croyant tout ce que l'appareil de navigation leur propose comme directions logiques, et qui finissent par se coincer dans une voie sans issue impossible ou bien par plonger dans une rivière ou même la mer, un bon conseil: ne permettez pas à la technologie de maîtriser votre technique de conduite.

Vocabulaire

la gestion *management*

ferroviaire *railway (adj.)*

gérer *to manage, to conduct*

le point de repère *landmark*

la répression *punishment*

la voie de dépassement *overtaking lane*

c'en est de même pour *the same applies to*

disloqué *disembodied*

émanant *emanating*

déclencher *to trigger*

se coincer *to get stuck*

la conduite *driving*

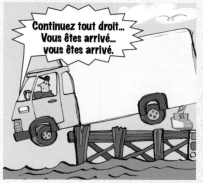

Continuez tout droit… Vous êtes arrivé… vous êtes arrivé.

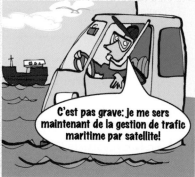

C'est pas grave: je me sers maintenant de la gestion de trafic maritime par satellite!

2 a Lisez le texte et trouvez l'équivalent des expressions suivantes:

i en dépit de

ii punition

iii en particulier

iv en même temps

v négligent

vi inattention

vii peuvent provoquer

viii immobiliser

ix un cul-de-sac

x dominer

2 b Relisez le texte et reliez les débuts et fins de phrases.

i   Il est indéniable que…

ii Il faut…

iii Certains aspects de la technologie…

iv L'utilisation inadmissible du portable…

v   Les portables à mains libres ne…

vi La navigation par satellite en voiture…

vii Trop de conducteurs sont prêts à…

viii La technologie devrait améliorer mais…

a   en voiture sont problématiques.

b   font pas disparaître les problèmes de base.

c   faire des bêtises en suivant toutes les directions de la navigation par satellite.

d   jamais remplacer une bonne technique.

e   la sécurité des routes s'est améliorée spectaculairement.

f   accepter le rôle positif de la technologie dans la prévention routière.

g   au volant continue à causer des accidents.

h   provoque l'inattention et potentiellement des accidents graves.

3 🗣 A deux: partenaire A accepte les opinions ci-dessus (2b), mais partenaire B n'accepte pas tout. Ensuite, écoutez pour comparer.

Exemple: _____

A: Il est indéniable que…. et il faut accepter que…

B: Pas d'accord! La police se sert des radars rien que pour obtenir des sommes d'argent excessives des automobilistes.

4 💡 Lisez le texte (en ligne) et faites les activités interactives.

5 🎧 Ecoutez et mettez les extraits dans le bon ordre.

a   Et la liberté de mouvement des particuliers ne sera pas restreinte?

b   Cela peut vite devenir un affront à la vie privée de tout individu.

c   Sous ce système on pourra positionner n'importe qui n'importe quand, selon son empreinte électronique, à son insu.

d   Tu n'en vois que les grands avantages. Fais bien attention!

e   Il ne faut pas exagérer. C'est un système à buts positifs pour la société.

f   Le système Galileo de navigation par satellite nous fournira toutes les informations possibles.

g   On pourra aider les personnes âgées, secourir les gens en détresse, contrôler les frontières…

h   On pourra guider le trafic aérien, maritime, ferroviaire et routier, faciliter l'utilisation des transports en commun, aider les voyageurs à trouver leur chemin, contrôler la vitesse…

6 💡 Travail de groupe: discutez des pour et des contre de la navigation par satellite. (Feuille)

7 💡 A l'écrit: présentez les bienfaits et les dangers de la technologie par satellite. (250 mots). (Feuille)

Compétences

Making and countering controversial statements about contentious issues

Technological advances that have social and political implications generate discussion. Engage in debate by drawing on several sources – factual, speculative, partisan – and by adding personal opinions.

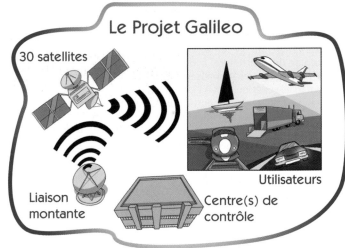

Le Projet Galileo

30 satellites

Liaison montante

Centre(s) de contrôle

Utilisateurs

Expressions clés

Grâce à la navigation par satellite on peut:
trouver son chemin / guider le trafic / secourir les gens en détresse / surveiller les délinquants portant un bracelet électronique / découvrir les terroristes / contrôler les frontières / faciliter l'utilisation des transports en commun.

C'est extraordinaire / fantastique / rassurant.

Par contre, on peut aussi surveiller / positionner n'importe qui à son insu.

C'est affreux / inadmissible / déprimant / un affront à la vie privée.

C Science ne rime pas toujours avec conscience

la surveillance – la navigation par satellite

la richesse – la pauvreté

la mondialisation – la dette du Tiers-Monde

le chômage – la violence

l'informatique – le Projet Galileo

1 Jeu de mémoire. Nommez à tour de rôle un aspect positif ou négatif des thèmes dans les bulles.

Exemple: _____

A: L'informatique facilite l'obtention de renseignements, les loisirs et les contacts.

B: Oui, mais en se servant trop d'Internet on perd contact avec la société réelle.

Les bénéfices de l'innovation?

La science a permis depuis des siècles de lutter contre l'ignorance, de soigner les maladies, d'allonger la durée de vie. Il en est de même des possibilités offertes en matière d'information, de communication, de transport, de travail ou de loisir. Alors que la révolution de la communication se poursuit, celle des biotechnologies ouvre la voie à des progrès considérables dans la lutte contre certaines maladies. Grâce au décryptage du génome, on peut dès aujourd'hui s'attendre à des soins et des guérisons personnalisés contre les maladies génétiques et à l'identification précise de régimes nutritionnels et corporels adaptés à l'individu.

D'après G. Mermet, Francoscopie 2007
© *Larousse 2006*

2 a Lisez le texte à gauche. Reliez les titres A–D aux phrases i–iv pour expliquer les "bénéfices de l'innovation".

A Le développement personnel de l'individu

B Les déplacements

C Le travail et les loisirs

D Le décryptage du génome

i On peut profiter d'une bonne santé et de l'accroissement de la longévité.

ii On a plus de temps, plus d'argent et plus de possibilités de détente.

iii On est mieux éduqué et mieux formé.

iv On profite de transports mieux adaptés et plus efficaces.

b A deux: échangez vos opinions sur les bénéfices de la liste.

Exemple: _____

A: Le développement de l'individu.

B: Eh bien, on est mieux éduqué et mieux formé. Tu es d'accord?

Vocabulaire

lutter *to struggle*

le décryptage du génome *decoding of the human genome*

la guérison *cure*

le régime nutritionnel *diet*

3 a 🎧 Ecoutez et trouvez l'équivalent français des termes i–x.

i *don't make me laugh!*

ii *widespread*

iii *the gap*

iv *from bad to worse*

v *our carbon footprints*

vi *frowned upon*

vii *sedentary lifestyle*

viii *to threaten stability*

ix *biofuel production*

x *the cost of food*

💡 Grammaire

Inversion of subject and verb

Some <u>adverbs at the beginning of clauses</u>, like statements in **direct speech**, cause the subject and the verb to switch places. See page 121.

« <u>Rarement</u> les automobilistes **peuvent-ils** profiter de leur liberté, » **dit-il**.

3 b 🎧 **Lisez les phrases, réécoutez et corrigez l'erreur dans chaque phrase.**

i On peut être mieux éduqué, si on habite le Tiers-Monde.

ii La scolarisation de courte durée est bien rare dans les pays développés.

iii L'écart entre les riches et les pauvres, les actifs et les chômeurs diminue.

iv Pourquoi insiste-t-on toujours pour rouler en ville, malgré le réchauffement de la terre et nos empreintes carboniques inadmissibles?

v Rarement, à cause de la surveillance par satellite, les automobilistes veulent-ils profiter de leur liberté individuelle.

vi Rien n'est surveillé, noté et désapprouvé.

vii Les sociétés d'assurance feront beaucoup moins attention à notre histoire génétique.

viii La vie sédentaire d'un nombre croissant de jeunes internautes, qui mangent mal aussi, entraîne un taux d'obésité en baisse.

ix La biotechnologie risque aussi d'améliorer la stabilité sociale et politique dans les pays aux populations pauvres.

x A cause de la déforestation pour la production de biocarburants, le prix de l'alimentation ne cesse de monter et va encore provoquer des centaines de personnes affamées dans le Tiers-Monde.

c 💡 **A deux: servez-vous des phrases de 3b pour contredire votre partenaire. (Feuille)**

Exemple: _____

A: L'écart entre les actifs et les chômeurs <u>diminue</u>.

B: Au contraire, ça <u>augmente</u>.

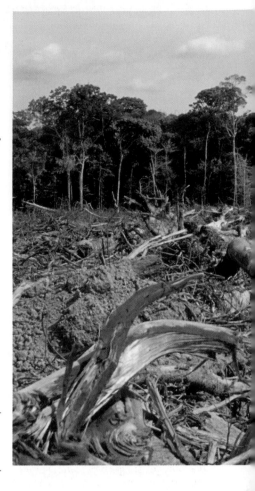

4 a 💡 **Lisez le texte (en ligne) et faites les activités interactives.**

b 🎧 **Ecoutez et remplissez les blancs. Réécoutez pour vérifier.**

i Tu trouves les perspectives de la science aussi …… qu'effrayantes?

ii La confiance dans la science est …… forte, car l'émotion est …… forte que la raison.

iii Les manipulations génétiques …… peur.

iv C'est le rôle des scientifiques d'améliorer notre …… , même si cela comporte ……

v Je ne cherche pas à …… les scientifiques de tous les maux du ……

vi « Science rime avec …… »

vii Le progrès technique engendre la croissance …… et le bien-être …… et individuel?

viii L'avidité et la folie ont révélé les …… liés à l'industrialisation de l'…… , comme la crise de la "vache folle", le …… à la dioxine et la …… aviaire.

ix Cela renforce le …… commun que le rapport bénéfice–risques de l'innovation est de moins en moins favorable.

x Il ne manque que la …… volonté des …… pour …… une nouvelle ……

5 💡🎤 **Ecoutez le dialogue et enregistrez vos réponses.**

6 💡 **A deux: écrivez les deux parties du débat, pour et contre: « Science et technologie, victoire de la raison sur l'émotion et l'incompréhension ». 250 mots par personne. (Feuille)**

Expressions clés

La biotechnologie menace la stabilité globale / risque d'augmenter la faim.

L'industrialisation de l'alimentation est / Le réchauffement de la terre est / Nos empreintes carboniques sont inadmissible(s).

Rarement peut-on profiter de sa liberté personnelle.

L'innovation est de moins en moins favorable.

Grâce à la science et la technologie, on peut guérir les maladies graves / soigner les problèmes psychologiques / combattre le chômage et la faim dans le monde.

C'est le rôle des scientifiques d'améliorer notre qualité de vie.

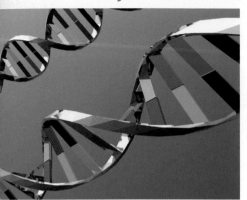

Now you should be able to:

- ■ discuss advantages and drawbacks of ICT at home and at work
- ■ consider pros and cons of space and satellite technology
- ■ discuss ethical issues relating to scientific, technological and medical progress and research

Grammar

- ■ use present participles
- ■ use interrogative pronouns (revisited)
- ■ invert verb and subject after direct speech and adverbs

Skills

- ■ summarise opposing views and draw balanced conclusions
- ■ make and counter controversial statements about contentious issues
- ■ use anticipation and nuance to advance debates

✓ Résumé

1 Traduisez en anglais:

La téléphonie et Internet ont bouleversé les attitudes envers l'espace et le temps.

2 Complétez la phrase avec les bons participes présents:

Tu profites d'Internet en (**faire**) des achats, en (**télécharger**) des fichiers et en (**écrire**) ton blog?

3 Ecrivez une phrase qui veut dire à peu près la même chose:

Chaque individu est associé à des codes personnels.

4 Complétez la phrase:

A cause d'Internet, on risque...

5 Mettez les mots dans le bon ordre:

satellite de La voiture en navigation risques beaucoup comporte par accidents peut spectaculaires. et des déclencher

6 Traduisez en français:

"Technology should improve but never replace good technique."

7 Complétez la phrase avec trois avantages du système Galileo de navigation:

On pourra...

8 L'innovation est-elle bénéfique pour le développement de l'individu? Ecrivez votre opinion.

8 Comment dit-on cette phrase en français?

Therefore (*Aussi*) the gap is going from bad to worse.

10 Expliquez pourquoi vous êtes pour ou contre les avancées scientifiques les plus récentes.

AQA Examiner's tips

Listening	Speaking	Reading	Writing
Always go back and **check your work.**	You are **not expected to ask questions** of the examiner.	Allow time at the end to **check your answers.**	Remember that you will be **graded on your use of the French language.** Check your grammar, spelling and vocabulary.

10 Dossier culturel

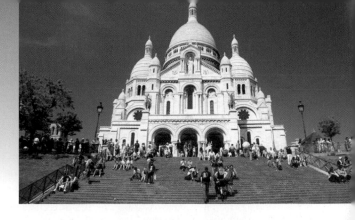

To help you speak and write effectively about the culture of France, we will consider the following areas:

- how to talk and write about the geography of a French region, a period of French 20th-century history, or the work of French authors, dramatists, poets, musicians, film directors, artists and architects

- how to evaluate the influence these aspects have had on the country's development

- how to talk and write about a range of characteristics and features of the chosen cultural topic

- how to give a personal perspective on a topic

- how to develop the scope of your vocabulary, including appropriate specialist terms

- how to speak and write about the topic in an accurate and precise manner.

France is one of the largest countries in Europe, about double the size of the UK, with roughly the same population. It is the world's most popular tourist destination; not surprising when you consider the geographical and cultural diversity that make up the country. France is divided into 22 regions, including the Mediterranean island of Corsica.

As a result of its imperial past, France includes islands scattered around the world (in the Atlantic Ocean, the Caribbean, Indian Ocean and South Pacific) as well as part of South America. The term *France métropolitaine* is used to specify the European parts of France. The *République française* denotes all of France, in Europe and overseas. The *départements d'outre-mer* are four overseas departments: Guadeloupe, Martinique, French Guiana and the island of Réunion. These together with other French territories are known as *les DOM-TOM*.

The country has had a turbulent history, experiencing successive revolutions and wars, but now has a vital role in the construction of the European Union. The French are rightly proud of their rich historical, cultural and political heritage.

France is well known throughout the world as a leader in the fields of literature, the arts, science and industry. French literature is very rich and wide-ranging, from novelists such as Balzac, Flaubert and Camus, to poets such as Verlaine, Rimbaud and Prévert. French drama is equally rewarding, from the classical dramatists Racine and Molière to modern writers such as Anouilh and Ionesco. The most famous French artists are probably the 19th-century Impressionist painters, Renoir and Monet, whose work remains popular to this day. Composers and musicians include Bizet (who wrote the opera *Carmen*), Chopin and Ravel; this tradition is maintained today by such figures as Jean-Michel Jarre. The work of the Lumière brothers led to the invention of the modern cinema, an influence further developed by directors such as Truffaut, Chabrol and Besson.

At the same time, France has been a leader in technology. The tremendously efficient high-speed train network (TGV) now runs throughout the country and is the envy of other nations. Many modern scientific advances were the result of the work of French scientists such as Louis Pasteur, Henri Becquerel and Marie Curie.

This chapter will introduce you to geographical, historical and cultural aspects of France as well as the skills you need to carry out research on an aspect of your choice.

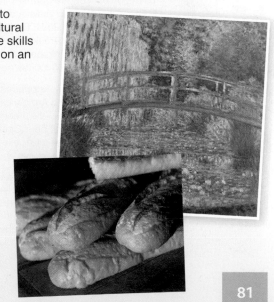

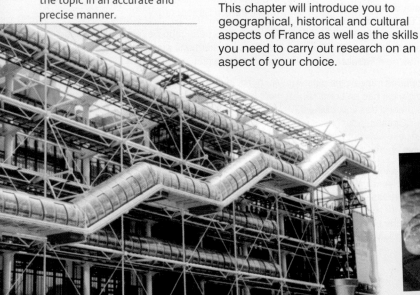

Une région française

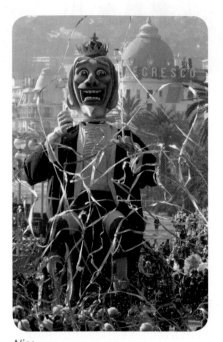

Dans cette section, on va vous présenter des régions de France métropolitaine et un département d'outre-mer. Vous allez apprendre des renseignements sur la géographie, l'histoire, la population et les activités économiques de la région. On va considérer aussi les avantages et les inconvénients d'habiter une telle région.

Selon vos intérêts, vous pourrez étudier une région de France riche en histoire, comme l'Alsace, ou vous pourrez peut-être étudier une région que vous avez déjà visitée, comme la Bretagne. Vous pourrez choisir un grand centre urbain comme Paris ou peut-être une région rurale, comme le Limousin. La littérature ou le cinéma pourraient vous donner envie d'en savoir plus sur une région, par exemple les romans de Marcel Pagnol et les films Jean de Florette et Manon des Sources vous encourageront à étudier la Provence. Vous pouvez aussi, bien sûr, étudier un département d'outre-mer, comme la Martinique.

Nice

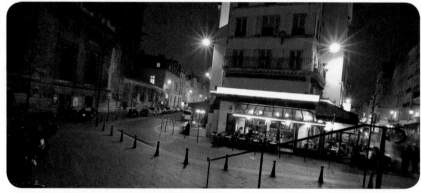

Paris

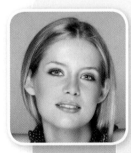

Patricia Giardi, 17 ans, habite à Nancy

La Lorraine

Je vais vous présenter ma région, la Lorraine, qui a une population de plus de deux millions d'habitants. La région est connue pour ses industries lourdes comme la sidérurgie, mais la dernière mine de charbon a fermé en 2004. Comme ressources agricoles, il y a les céréales et les vergers de pruniers comme la mirabelle. La Lorraine produit chaque année 40 000 tonnes de mirabelles.

Un des personnages historiques français les plus célèbres est Jeanne d'Arc qui est née en Lorraine, à Domrémy. A 13 ans, elle entend des voix divines lui ordonnant de partir pour Orléans, pour chasser les Anglais. En janvier 1431, elle est capturée par les Anglais et elle est brûlée vive en mai 1431.

La Première Guerre mondiale a touché durement la Lorraine. En 1916 autour de Verdun, plusieurs villages ont été entièrement détruits et jamais reconstruits. Pendant la Seconde Guerre mondiale, la Lorraine a été annexée par les Allemands en 1940 jusqu'à sa libération en 1944–45.

Après la guerre, de nombreux immigrants, principalement d'Italie, sont venus s'y installer, dont mon père qui est maçon.

Actuellement, les transports sont en pleine expansion avec notamment la nouvelle ligne TGV reliant Paris à Strasbourg.

Comme dans beaucoup de régions de France, la gastronomie tient une place importante. La quiche lorraine est le plat le plus connu.

Au nord, le plateau lorrain est assez uniforme mais vers le sud s'élève le massif des Vosges. Ici, on fait des sports d'hiver.

Je suis fière de ma ville. La place Stanislas à Nancy est une des plus belles places d'Europe.

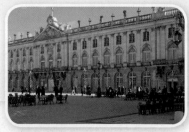

Place Stanislas, Nancy

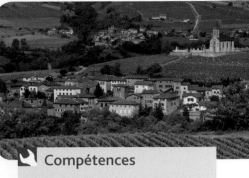

1 Lisez le texte sur la Lorraine, page 82, et les phrases a–j et écrivez vrai ou faux.

a   Il n'y a plus de mines de charbon en Lorraine.

b   La mirabelle est une petite prune, cultivée en Lorraine.

c   Jeanne d'Arc est née à Orléans.

d   On a reconstruit tous les villages détruits pendant la Première Guerre mondiale.

e   Le père de Patricia est né en France.

f   La nouvelle ligne TGV passe par la Lorraine.

g   Il y a des montagnes dans le nord de la région.

h   On peut faire du ski dans la région.

i   Patricia aime habiter à Nancy.

j   La place Stanislas n'est pas très jolie.

2 💡 Choisissez une région française et faites des recherches sur les aspects suivants. Ecrivez un exposé de 200 mots. (Feuille)

- la population
- la géographie et l'histoire de la région
- un personnage célèbre qui est né dans la région
- les industries de la région, y compris le tourisme
- la culture et la gastronomie
- l'avenir de la région

3 🎧 Ecoutez l'entretien et faites-en un résumé en anglais. Donnez les informations suivantes:

- les avantages et inconvénients de la vie en ville
- les avantages et les inconvénients de la vie rurale

4 💡 Choisissez une région rurale en France. Faites des recherches sur les aspects suivants pour faire une présentation orale. (Feuille)

- les jeunes et les études
- le chômage et l'emploi
- l'exode rural et les résidences secondaires
- l'avenir de la région
- les avantages d'habiter une région rurale pour les jeunes
- les inconvénients d'habiter une région rurale pour les jeunes

5 Pour connaître une région de France, posez ces questions à votre partenaire qui va parler d'une région qu'il/elle a étudiée.

a   Où se trouve la région exactement?

b   Pourquoi as-tu choisi cette région?

c   Que sais-tu de la géographie de la région?

d   Quelles sont les industries principales de la région?

e   Est-ce que l'économie locale est dynamique?

f   Quels sont les avantages d'habiter cette région?

g   Et quels en sont les inconvénients?

h   Est-ce que tu aimerais habiter dans cette région?

Compétences

Structuring a written response

Your written presentation can be enhanced by the use of link phrases:

… est une superbe région avec une belle campagne.

En plus, il y a l'océan…

Quant au climat, il est…

D'ailleurs, la gastronomie est riche: huîtres…

Il faut dire aussi que le… est splendide, particulièrement à…

En ce qui concerne l'économie…

Il y a vingt ans, il y avait peu de… Cependant de nos jours, il y a un…

Actuellement… est en pleine expansion.

Pour conclure…

ℹ️ Vos enquêtes

When you have chosen a region to study, you may wish to gain a broader knowledge of the area by researching novels, stories or films set in the vicinity. For example, the films *Le Fabuleux Destin d'Amélie Poulain* and *La Haine* give two very different and contrasting views of life in Paris. Alternatively, find out about a famous person who came from the area and see if he/she wrote about their childhood experiences in the region.

L'île de la Réunion

La Réunion est une île volcanique de l'océan Indien, située à environ 700 km à l'est de Madagascar et à 200 km au sud-ouest de l'île Maurice. Certainement déjà connue des navigateurs arabes, l'île de la Réunion a été découverte par des marins portugais au seizième siècle. Ils la décrivent comme « un véritable paradis terrestre ».

La Réunion offre des paysages naturels impressionnants et une diversité culturelle, qui constituent ses principaux avantages touristiques. Les Français ont pris possession de l'île au nom du roi en 1649, principalement pour chasser les pirates qui y habitaient, et l'ont baptisée « île Bourbon », du nom de la famille royale.

La dernière éruption d'un volcan remonte à 2007. L'érosion a donné aux paysages volcaniques des reliefs abrupts, des canyons, de multiples cascades, qui rendent l'île très belle.

La diversité des végétations est aussi impressionnante avec des fleurs et des arbres exotiques. Il y a plus de mille espèces de plantes sur l'île.

Le climat est tropical, avec des températures de 30°C en janvier et de 20°C en hiver (juillet).

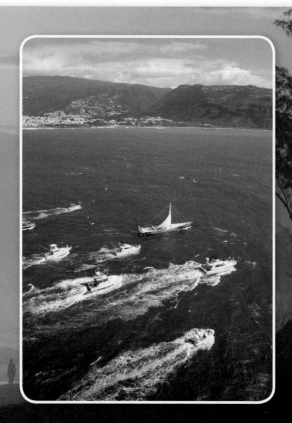

Depuis la Seconde Guerre mondiale, la Réunion connaît une croissance économique dynamique, à cause de la modernisation, l'introduction de l'électricité, l'éradication du paludisme et la construction d'une université. Cependant, malgré ces progrès, le taux de chômage est toujours supérieur à 30%.

Naturellement, le tourisme constitue la première ressource économique de l'île mais il y a aussi la production de canne à sucre et la pêche. Les fruits de mer sont une spécialité de la cuisine locale.

En 2005, le tourisme était sérieusement menacé par l'épidémie du chikungunya, qui a touché 157 000 personnes donc plus de 20 pour cent de la population avec 77 morts. Cette maladie est transmise par un moustique et se traduit par une forte poussée de fièvre accompagnée de douleurs causant même des paralysies d'où le nom chikungunya « celui qui marche courbé » en swahili.

1 Lisez le texte et corrigez le détail incorrect dans chaque phrase.

a   La Reunion a été découverte par des navigateurs français au 16ème siècle.

b   Les Français ont baptisé l'île « l'île des pirates ».

c   Les volcans ne sont plus actifs.

d   Il fait moins chaud au mois de janvier.

e   Le risque de paludisme est grave.

f   L'université date du 19ème siècle.

g   Le taux de chômage est en baisse.

h   On ne mange pas de fruits de mer.

i   La plupart des habitants sont tombés malades à cause du chikungunya.

j   Cette maladie est provoquée par une mauvaise alimentation.

2 L'île de la Réunion a trois ressources économiques principales: le tourisme, la canne à sucre et la pêche. Faites des recherches et décrivez les ressources économiques des régions suivantes:

- la Bretagne
- l'Auvergne
- l'Alsace
- la Guadeloupe
- la Corse

3 🎧 Ecoutez l'entretien et notez les quatre phrases qui sont vraies.

a Isabelle a réussi au bac.

b Elle n'a jamais visité la France.

c Elle n'aime pas beaucoup voyager.

d Selon Isabelle, il n'y a pas assez d'emplois à la Réunion.

e Elle trouve les Canadiens très sympas.

f Elle va avoir sa licence cette année.

g Elle va retourner à la Réunion à la fin de ses études.

h La cuisine réunionnaise lui manque.

i Il neige beaucoup à la Réunion.

4 💡 Imaginez que vous avez quitté votre ville natale pour étudier dans un autre pays francophone. Faites une présentation orale en répondant aux questions suivantes. (Feuille)

- Qu'est ce qui vous a décidé à partir?
- Que pensez-vous de votre ville natale?
- Comment trouvez-vous la ville où vous étudiez?
- Comment s'est passée votre arrivée?
- Quels sont vos projets pour l'avenir?
- Qu'est-ce qui vous manque de votre ville natale?

5 💡 Posez ces questions à un/une partenaire qui va parler d'un pays francophone. (Feuille)

a Où se trouve la région que tu as étudiée?

b Que sais-tu de son histoire?

c Combien d'habitants y a-t-il?

d Est-ce que la population est en hausse ou en baisse?

e Que sais-tu de la géographie de la région et de son influence sur le progrès régional?

f Quelles sont les principales industries?

g Comment est-ce que ces industries ont changé ces dernières années?

h Qu'est-ce qui va se passer à l'avenir?

i Qu'est-ce qui favorise ou freine le développement économique de la région?

j Est-ce que tu aimerais habiter dans cette région? Pourquoi/Pourquoi pas?

Compétences

Structuring a spoken response

Use link phrases to develop your presentation:

Pour moi, l'aspect le plus attrayant de cette région, c'est sans doute...

Ce qui me plaît aussi, c'est...

En ce me qui concerne, c'est...

Ce que j'aime le plus, c'est...

Ce qui me manque, c'est...

En fin de compte, je dois avouer que...

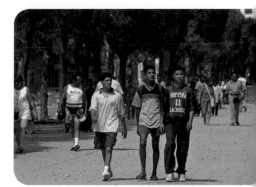

Vos enquêtes

You should now have an idea of which region you would like to study further. Consider historical, geographic and economic influences and how the region is likely to change over the coming years. Finally, decide what you find attractive about the area and be prepared to say whether you would like to live there.

WebQuest

Paris et l'Ile-de-France, est-ce qu'il fait bon vivre dans cette région?

Faites des recherches sur Paris et sa région pour participer à un débat qui essaie de répondre à la question: « Fait-il bon vivre à Paris? »

La France au vingtième siècle

1981

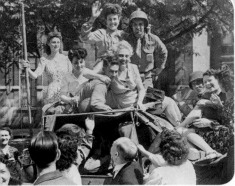

Dans cette section, on va vous présenter des événements importants dans l'histoire de la France du vingtième siècle. Vous allez apprendre des renseignements sur les causes et les conséquences de ces événements et on va considérer le rôle joué par des personnages importants pendant cette période.

Selon vos intérêts, vous pouvez étudier les guerres qui ont eu lieu au siècle dernier, comme la Première et la Seconde Guerre mondiales, ou vous pourrez peut-être étudier les effets des événements de mai 1968. Vous pourrez choisir d'analyser les conséquences de l'élection du président socialiste François Mitterrand en 1981.

Charles de Gaulle

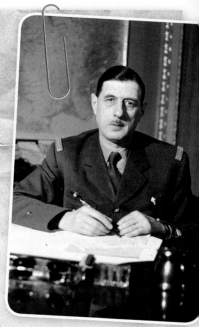

Charles de Gaulle est né le 22 novembre 1890 à Lille. C'était un général français qui est devenu, après son exil à Londres, le chef de la résistance à l'occupation allemande de la France pendant la Seconde Guerre mondiale. Après la Libération en 1944 il est devenu brièvement président de la France, puis le fondateur de la Ve République en 1958, dont il a été le premier président de 1959 à 1969. Il est mort le 9 novembre 1970 à Colombey-les-Deux-Eglises, en Haute-Marne.

La France a déclaré la guerre à l'Allemagne nazie en septembre 1939, mais c'est seulement en mai 1940 que l'armée allemande attaque la France. Les Français sont vite battus.

En juin 1940, le gouvernement de la France, confié au maréchal Pétain, signe un armistice avec Hitler. Une grande partie de la France est occupée par les Allemands. La partie sud du pays devient la zone libre sous le contrôle du gouvernement établi par Pétain à Vichy. En exil à Londres, où il a trouvé asile après la défaite, de Gaulle trouve cet accord inacceptable et lance un appel à la Résistance dans un célèbre discours diffusé par la BBC le 18 juin 1940... Sa tâche est difficile, mais une armée de résistance extérieure est créée.

Le général de Gaulle, à la tête de la France libre, voulait unifier la Résistance extérieure et la Résistance intérieure. Il a donc envoyé Jean Moulin en France en 1942.

La Résistance participe à la libération de la France. Après le débarquement en Normandie du 6 juin 1944 (le jour J), Paris est libéré le 25 août 1944. De Gaulle est salué comme un héros sur les Champs-Elysées. Beaucoup de Français le considèrent toujours comme un grand homme.

1 Lisez le texte et mettez ces événements dans le bon ordre.

- a   Les Alliés envahissent la France.
- b   Les Allemands envahissent la France.
- c   Charles de Gaulle s'échappe à Londres.
- d   Pétain devient chef de l'Etat de la zone libre.
- e   La Seconde Guerre mondiale commence.
- f   De Gaulle est acclamé par des foules à Paris.
- g   Les groupes de résistants sont réunis.
- h   De Gaulle prononce un discours important à la radio.

1944

2 💡 Choisissez un personnage qui a joué un rôle important dans l'histoire de la France du 20ème siècle. Faites des recherches pour écrire un article sur les aspects suivants. (Feuille)

- sa naissance et son enfance
- son éducation
- les événements qui ont influencé le personnage
- les actions du personnage
- son importance
- sa réputation

Pour vous aider, utilisez ces phrases:

Il/Elle a passé son enfance…

Il/Elle a reçu une éducation à…

En… un événement s'est passé qui a beaucoup influencé…

En conséquence, … a décidé de…

Selon ses proches, c'était un homme/une femme qui…

Il/Elle voulait… / avait pour but…

3 🎧 Ecoutez un professeur d'histore-géo parler de Jean Moulin et répondez aux questions en anglais.

a What do we know about Jean Moulin's father?

b What were the three essential values which Jean Moulin learnt from his father?

c What significant event happened in 1937?

d Why, according to Christian, is Moulin such a good role model?

e How did Moulin succeed in uniting the French Resistance?

f What has never been proved?

g What happened to Moulin after his arrest?

h How is he often remembered today?

4 💡 Faites des recherches sur les aspects suivants de l'Occupation pour faire une présentation orale. (Feuille)

- les raisons de la défaite de la France en 1940
- le rôle du maréchal Pétain
- le traitement des Juifs (par exemple la rafle du Vélodrome d'hiver)
- les succès de la Résistance française
- la collaboration (par exemple le rôle de René Bousquet)
- Pour vous, quelle est l'importance de la Résistance française?

5 Posez ces questions à votre partenaire qui va parler d'un événement historique qu'il/elle a étudié.

a Quand est-ce que l'événement s'est passé?

b Pourquoi as-tu choisi d'étudier cet événement?

c Parle-moi de ce qui s'est passé exactement.

d Quelles ont été les conséquences de cet événement?

e A ton avis, quelle est l'importance de cet événement?

🧭 **Compétences**

Narrating events in the past

The following expressions can be used to help:

Il y a quatre jours
Par cette belle journée

En début de
Tout d'abord
Puis
Ensuite

En quelques secondes
Peu de temps après
Le lendemain

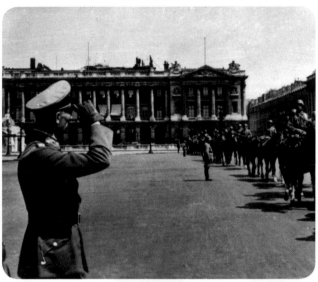

L'Occupation de Paris, 14 juin 1940

i **Vos enquêtes**

If you have chosen to study France during the Second World War, you may wish to gain a broader knowledge of the subject by researching novels, stories or films set at the time. For example, the film *Au revoir, les enfants* deals with the treatment of the Jews during the Occupation, as does the novel *Un Sac de billes*. The short novel by Vercors, *Le Silence de la mer,* deals with the effect of war and resistance on ordinary people. Alternatively, such films as *Lacombe Lucien* and *L'Armée des ombres* deal with collaboration and resistance. Marcel Ophul's controversial documentary *Le Chagrin et la pitié* examines these issues in great depth.

La guerre d'Algérie 1954–1962
« La sale guerre »

A la fin de la Seconde Guerre mondiale, de violentes manifestations eurent lieu en Algérie contre l'occupation française. Les manifestants demandaient l'indépendance. En Algérie, environ un million de pieds-noirs (des Français d'Algérie) possédaient les meilleures terres agricoles et ne voulaient pas partager le pouvoir avec les huit millions de musulmans qui avaient un niveau de vie très bas.

Le Front de libération nationale (FLN) soutint la lutte armée pour l'indépendance nationale de l'Etat algérien. En novembre 1954, une vague d'attentats contre les Français en Algérie signala le début de la guerre et le gouvernement français envoya des renforts militaires. En 1955, le FLN organisa un soulèvement de musulmans qui attaquèrent les quartiers européens des villes et tuèrent les habitants des fermes isolées, faisant une centaine de morts. Les forces françaises répondirent par une dure répression. On compta un millier de victimes.

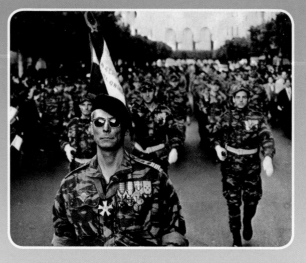

Militairement, la France avait des forces supérieures mais elle ne put empêcher la guérilla et le terrorisme. La population musulmane soutenait le FLN, par conviction ou par crainte des représailles.

La réputation de la France souffrit dans le monde entier à cause des histoires de torture en Algérie et l'économie de la France fut menacée par l'inflation provoquée par la guerre. En même temps, le conflit algérien provoqua une crise morale: des intellectuels, des étudiants et des représentants des Eglises exigeaient la fin de la guerre et protestaient contre l'utilisation de la torture.

En 1958, de Gaulle retourna au pouvoir et il imposa à l'armée et aux Européens l'indépendance de l'Algérie. En 1960, il commença des pourparlers avec le FLN qui aboutirent en 1962 aux accords d'Evian, reconnaissant l'indépendance de l'Algérie.

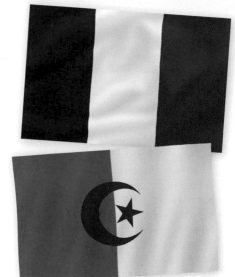

1 Lisez le texte et les phrases suivantes et écrivez vrai ou faux.

a La guerre d'Algérie a commencé avant la Seconde Guerre mondiale.

b Les pieds-noirs sont des musulmans.

c Les musulmans algériens n'avaient pas une très bonne qualité de vie.

d Le FLN était opposé à la violence.

e Les Français ont réagi d'une façon violente aux massacres dans les quartiers européens.

f La France avait du mal à combattre le terrorisme malgré sa supériorité militaire.

g D'autres pays ont condamné les actions des Français en Algérie.

h Tous les Français ont soutenu la politique du gouvernement.

i De Gaulle n'était pas en faveur de l'indépendance de l'Algérie.

j L'Algérie est devenue indépendante en 1962.

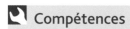 Compétences

Understanding the past historic

When reading about historical events, you are likely to come across the *passé simple* or past historic tense. You do not need to use this tense yourself, but it is helpful to recognise key verb forms. See page 114.

Find the verb in the past historic in the following sentences. Which verb do you think they are from?

A la fin de la Seconde Guerre mondiale, de violentes manifestations eurent lieu en Algérie.

L'économie de la France fut menacée par l'inflation.

En 1958, de Gaulle retourna au pouvoir.

En 1960, il commença des pourparlers avec le FLN.

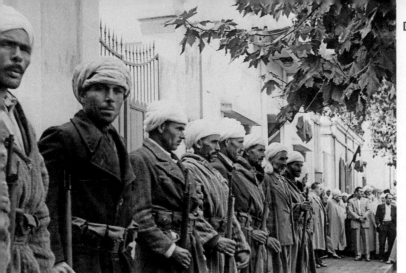

2 Faites des recherches et décrivez le rôle joué par les personnages ci-dessous pendant la guerre d'Algérie. A votre avis, quelle a été l'importance des actions de chaque personnage? (Feuille)

- Guy Mollet
- François Mitterrand
- Ben Bella
- Mohamed Khider
- le général Massu
- Charles de Gaulle

3 Ecoutez l'entretien avec Fatima, la fille d'un harki, c'est-à-dire un musulman qui était engagé dans l'armée française pendant la guerre d'Algérie.

Complétez les phrases.

a Pour Fatima, un harki est un …… qui ne voulait pas l'indépendance de l'Algérie.

b Le père de Fatima a décidé de quitter l'Algérie à cause des ……

c En arrivant en France, la famille de Fatima habitait dans un ……

d L'attitude des Français envers les harkis a rendu le père de Fatima très ……

e Fatima se sent …… par ses expériences en France.

4 Imaginez que vous avez quitté l'Algérie pour venir en France à la fin de la guerre. Faites une présentation orale en répondant aux questions suivantes. (Feuille)

a Pourquoi avez-vous quitté l'Algérie?

b Quels étaient vos espoirs en arrivant en France?

c Comment a été votre accueil en France?

d Où avez-vous logé après votre arrivée?

e Quels sont vos projets pour l'avenir?

f Qu'est-ce que vous pensez de l'attitude du gouvernement français envers les harkis?

5 Posez ces questions à votre partenaire qui va parler des expériences d'un pied-noir.

a Que sais-tu de l'origine du terme "pied-noir"?

b Parle-moi des caractéristiques d'un pied-noir.

c Qu'est-ce qui s'est passé pendant la guerre d'Algérie?

d Quelles ont été les conséquences de la guerre pour les pieds-noirs?

e Que penses-tu de leur accueil en France?

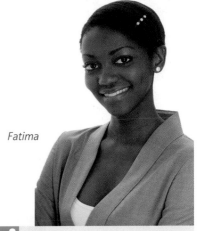

Fatima

i WebQuest

Mai 68: comment l'avez-vous vécu?

Faites des recherches sur les événements de mai 68 pour faire une présentation sur ce qui s'est passé et les conséquences de cette période, du point de vue d'un étudiant/une étudiante qui a participé aux manifestations.

i Vos enquêtes

You will by now have studied some significant events of the history of 20th-century France and should have an idea of which period you would like to study in more depth. Examine the causes behind the key events of your chosen period and consider the lasting importance of these events. Look closely at the specific actions of at least two important individuals who were influential at the time. Finally, be prepared to give a personal perspective on the period of history and say whether you would have liked to have lived then.

C. L'œuvre d'un auteur français

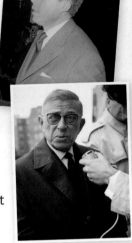

Albert Camus

Dans cette section vous allez trouver des renseignements sur plusieurs auteurs et leur œuvre. On va considérer les thèmes majeurs de leurs livres et les influences qui les ont poussés à les écrire. Les Français sont fiers de leur longue tradition littéraire.

Selon vos intérêts, vous pourrez étudier des livres classiques du 19ème siècle par des auteurs comme Flaubert, Zola ou Balzac ou vous pourrez choisir un livre que l'on a adapté pour le cinéma. Les romans de Jean-Paul Sartre, André Gide, Albert Camus ou François Mauriac restent toujours très populaires en France, mais vous pourrez étudier un auteur plus récent comme Tahar Ben Jalloun (*L'enfant de sable*) ou Faïza Guène (*Kiffe kiffe demain*).

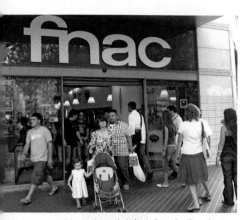

Magasin spécialisé dans la distribution de produits culturels: musique, littérature, cinéma

Jean-Paul Sartre

Faïza Guène

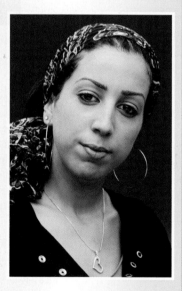

Kiffe kiffe demain est le premier roman de Faïza Guène. Elle avait 20 ans quand le roman est sorti en 2004. Elle a écrit le roman qui est en partie autobiographique pour parler de la vie dans les banlieues parisiennes. Elle n'essaie pas de cacher les problèmes des cités, mais elle nous donne en même temps une galerie de portraits pleine d'humour.

Doria, quinze ans, vit avec sa mère dans un appartement de la banlieue parisienne. Elle raconte les événements de sa vie et elle nous présente sa mère, qui est femme de ménage dans un hôtel. Elle nous parle aussi de son père, qui est parti pour trouver une nouvelle femme au Maroc. Elle nous décrit enfin son monde, ses rêves, la réalité de sa vie.

Doria a des problèmes à l'école, une psychologue pour l'aider et une assistante sociale qu'elle surnomme Barbie. A travers les yeux de Doria, Faïza Guène jette un regard vif, amusant et parfois moqueur sur la vie d'une adolescente qui habite un quartier difficile.

Appréciations des lecteurs

Karine, 16 ans
Je trouve ce livre très rafraîchissant, c'est drôle et bien écrit. Malheureusement, l'histoire m'a un peu déçue parce qu'entre le début et la fin, il ne se passe pas grand-chose.

Georges, 17 ans
J'ai trouvé ce livre impressionnant et je le recommande à tous mes copains.

Audrey, 15 ans
La cité de Doria n'a pas bonne réputation. Tout y est: le racisme, l'ennui et le pessimisme. Faïza Guène examine la société française d'un œil tendre et marrant. Le langage est réel et direct. Les émotions sont vraisemblables.

Salma, 18 ans
Encore un livre qui parle de la banlieue. J'en ai marre. J'ai envie de lire des livres qui présentent un point de vue plus optimiste du monde.

Isabelle, 16 ans
Le personnage de Doria est intéressant et évolue pendant le livre. Pour moi, pourtant, le roman dans l'ensemble est un peu artificiel puisque l'auteur mélange le langage des quartiers avec un style assez littéraire qui sonne un peu faux.

Olivier, 15 ans
Je ne peux pas supporter ce livre. Les personnages ne m'intéressent pas et les situations ne me semblent pas réelles.

1 Lisez (à la page 90) les appréciations des lecteurs de *Kiffe kiffe demain*. Décidez si chaque personne a une opinion positive, négative ou une opinion partagée du livre.

> Karine   Georges   Audrey   Salma   Isabelle   Olivier

2 💡 Choisissez un auteur français et faites des recherches pour écrire un article sur les aspects suivants. (Feuille)

- son enfance, son éducation et les événements qui l'ont influencé(e)
- son premier livre et la réaction des critiques
- ses autres livres et son plus grand succès
- sa réputation

3 🎧 Ecoutez un reportage sur Faïza Guène. Répondez aux questions en anglais.

a   What was Faïza's original intention?

b   What was her main influence when she was younger?

c   What do we know about the plot of the short film *Rien que des mots*?

d   Why did Faïza decide to write *Kiffe kiffe demain*?

e   How does the reporter illustrate the success of the novel?

4 💡 Faites des recherches sur le deuxième roman de Faïza Guène, *Du rêve pour les oufs*. Faites une présentation orale. (Feuille)

a   De quoi s'agit-il?

b   Que savez-vous du personnage principal?

c   Où habite-t-elle?

d   Quelle est sa personnalité?

e   Que savez-vous de sa famille?

f   Quelles sont les différences entre ce livre et *Kiffe kiffe demain*?

g   Comment a-t-on accueilli le livre à sa sortie?

5 Posez ces questions à un/une partenaire qui va parler de *Du rêve pour les oufs*.

a   On a publié le livre en quelle année?

b   C'est quel genre de livre?

c   Quand est-ce que l'action se passe?

d   Où se passe le roman?

e   Est-ce que l'auteur nous donne explicitement la caractérisation ou est-ce que le lecteur doit se servir de son imagination?

f   Décris un événement important dans la vie d'un de ces personnages et les conséquences de cet événement.

g   Quelle vue du monde nous présente l'auteur?

h   Est-ce que tu recommanderais ce livre? Pourquoi/Pourquoi pas?

🔖 Compétences

Talking or writing about a book

1   *L'auteur, le titre du roman et la date de publication*

2   *Un résumé de l'histoire*

3   *Le rôle du narrateur*

4   *Les personnages*

5   *La structure (le temps et l'espace)*

6   *Les thèmes*

7   *Votre opinion*

Un long dimanche de fiançailles

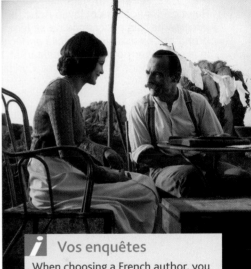

ℹ Vos enquêtes

When choosing a French author, you may wish to select a book that has been made into a film.

Marcel Pagnol's novels *Jean de Florette* and *Manon des Sources* were successfully adapted by Claude Berri. There are also film versions of the same author's autobiographical works, *La Gloire de mon père* and *Le château de ma mère*.

More recently, Sébastien Japrisot novel *Un long dimanche de fiançailles*, set during and just after the First World War, has been filmed by Jean-Pierre Jeunet.

Claude Chabrol has filmed Flaubert's masterpiece, *Madame Bovary*, and the same author's story, *Un Cœur simple,* has been adapted by Marion Laine.

Novels by Balzac adapted for the big screen include *Le Colonel Chabert* and *La Cousine Bette*.

Bonjour tristesse par Françoise Sagan

Ce roman a été publié en 1954, quand Françoise Sagan avait seulement 19 ans. Le roman a connu un succès immédiat. Elle était la fille d'industriels aisés, et elle a passé une enfance heureuse mais elle n'était pas une brillante élève: elle préfère lire Sartre et Camus tout en fréquentant les clubs de jazz du quartier latin. Elle rate ses examens universitaires.

Dans le roman, Cécile, 17 ans, a passé son enfance en pension. Après la mort de sa mère, elle vit depuis deux ans avec son père Raymond. Elle mène une existence paresseuse et Raymond lui accorde une grande liberté. Son père a de nombreuses liaisons amoureuses.

Cet été, Cécile, son père Raymond, et Elsa, sa maîtresse, partent en vacances sur la Côte d'Azur. Raymond a également invité Anne, une femme intelligente, qui était l'amie de sa femme. Très vite Anne prend en main la vie de Cécile et décide notamment de la faire réviser pour son baccalauréat. Anne n'approuve pas les rapports de Cécile avec Cyril, un jeune étudiant.

Raymond abandonne Elsa et devient l'amant d'Anne. Il pense même l'épouser. Cécile a peur de perdre sa liberté. Furieuse, elle réussit à persuader son petit ami Cyril de faire semblant de tomber amoureuse d'Elsa. Raymond ne peut pas supporter de voir Elsa avec un adolescent à peine plus âgé que sa fille, et il se retrouve bientôt dans les bras de son ancienne maîtresse.

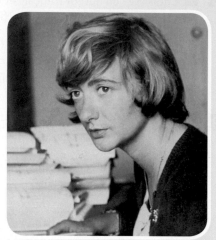

Anne les surprend. Désespérée, elle part tout de suite mais elle est tuée dans un accident de voiture. Pour Cécile, la vie ne sera jamais la même car elle connaît maintenant un sentiment nouveau: la tristesse.

---

1 Trouvez l'équivalent de ces expressions dans le texte.

a on a fait paraître ce roman

b une réussite

c elle vit d'une façon indolente

d lui donne beaucoup d'indépendance

e se charge de

f se marier avec elle

g craint

h convaincre

i feindre

j tolérer

k effondrée

l une nouvelle émotion

2 Faites des recherches sur trois des livres suivants pour en faire un résumé écrit. Mentionnez les aspects suivants:

- l'auteur
- le contexte du livre
- les personnages principaux
- les thèmes du livre
- avez-vous envie de lire le livre?

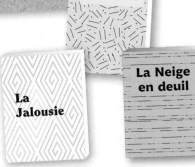

Thérèse Desqueyroux

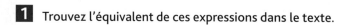
La Peste

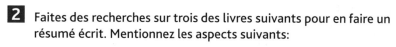
La Jalousie

La Neige en deuil

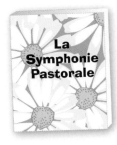
La Symphonie Pastorale

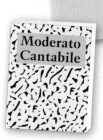
Moderato Cantabile

Les Particules Elémentaires

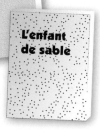
L'enfant de sable

3 🔊 Ecoutez une discussion sur le roman *Le Petit Prince* d'Antoine de Saint-Exupéry. Lisez les phrases a–h; c'est Lorie, Thierry, Karine ou Ludovic?

a   Who thinks that the book is suitable for people of all ages?

b   Who has read aloud an extract from the book?

c   Who has had the book read aloud to them?

d   Who believes one reading is not enough?

e   Who thinks everyone likes the book?

f   Who finds the style childish?

g   Who claims the book has influenced them greatly?

h   Who could not put the book down?

4 💡 Choisissez un livre que vous avez lu. Faites une présentation orale en considérant les aspects suivants. (Feuille)

a   Le titre et la date de publication.

b   Au début du livre, qu'est-ce que nous apprenons du cadre de l'intrigue: le lieu, l'époque, les personnages…?

c   Parlez d'un événement important qui fait avancer l'intrigue: par exemple, une rencontre, une découverte ou un événement inattendu…

d   Parlez d'une suite d'événements de résolution qui se passent à la fin de l'intrigue.

e   Décrivez la conclusion.

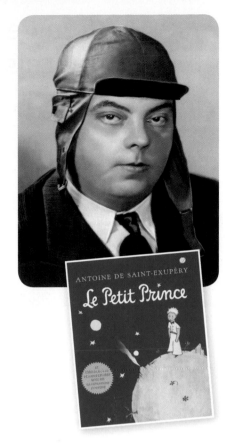

5 💡 Posez ces questions à un/une partenaire qui va parler d'un livre qu'il/elle a lu. (Feuille)

a   Le récit est-il facile ou difficile à lire?

b   Le roman est-il vraisemblable ou invraisemblable?

c   Les thèmes du roman t'intéressent?

d   Les personnages principaux t'intéressent?

e   As-tu apprécié le style?

f   Le roman te paraît-il bien ou pas bien construit?

g   Le récit semble original?

h   Quelle est ta réaction émotionnelle au livre?

🔖 **Compétences**

Giving a personal evaluation of a book

Le livre est accessible et facile à lire / compliqué et difficile à lire.

L'intrigue est vraisemblable / n'est pas tout à fait convaincante.

Les thèmes du roman m'intéressent / ne m'intéressent pas du tout.

Les personnages m'intéressent / ne m'intéressent pas du tout.

Le style est direct et simple / trop poétique pour moi.

Le livre est bien construit / n'est pas bien construit.

Le livre est tout à fait original / est plein de clichés.

Je me passionne pour ce livre / Ce livre ne me dit rien.

---

i WebQuest

L'Etranger de Camus: un point de vue personnel

Faites des recherches sur *L'Etranger* d'Albert Camus pour écrire une composition dans laquelle vous donnez votre point de vue personnel sur le roman.

i Vos enquêtes

You will by now have studied a variety of French novels and stories and should have an idea of which author you would like to study in more depth. You need to consider the context and background of the author's work. You will have to identify the main themes, ideas and messages of the author and what techniques the author uses to convey these. Include some research into what influenced the author and how successfully their work was received. Finally, do not forget to give your own personal appraisal and evaluation of the author's work.

D. L'œuvre d'un dramaturge ou d'un poète français

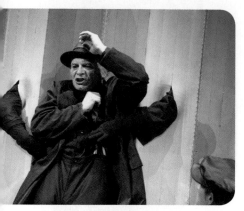

L'Avare, par Molière

Dans cette section, on va vous présenter des informations sur des dramaturges et des poètes français. On va considérer les thèmes majeurs de leurs œuvres et les techniques que ces auteurs utilisent pour créer l'impact de leurs pièces et leurs poèmes. Selon vos intérêts, vous pouvez étudier des dramaturges et des poètes classiques ou plus récents; le théâtre français est riche en textes anciens, modernes ou contemporains. Vous pourrez étudier les comédies de Molière, les tragédies de Racine ou le théâtre français du 20ème siècle, avec des dramaturges comme Jean Anouilh ou Jean-Paul Sartre. Les plus beaux fleurons de la poésie française comprennent des poètes comme Baudelaire, Verlaine et Rimbaud. Vous avez aussi la possibilité d'étudier différents genres de poésie, par exemple la poésie de guerre ou la poésie romantique.

Molière

Molière n'était pas seulement acteur et dramaturge mais aussi metteur en scène et directeur de troupe. C'était un des plus grands écrivains français, pas seulement à cause de la façon dont il manipulait la langue française, mais surtout parce qu'il faisait rire. Dans ses pièces, il a attaqué des défauts comme l'hypocrisie, l'avarice et l'amour propre.

Dans *Le Misanthrope*, Alceste déteste l'amabilité artificielle. Il préfère une sincérité absolue et critique sévèrement l'hypocrisie. *Le Tartuffe* aussi traite le thème de l'hypocrisie. Orgon est tombé sous l'influence de Tartuffe, hypocrite et faux dévot. Tartuffe réussit à manipuler facilement Orgon. Cet hypocrite essaie de séduire Elmire, la femme de son bienfaiteur.

Dans *Dom Juan,* Molière a créé un personnage plein de vices qui sait expliquer clairement ses buts et ses convictions. *L'Avare* est une comédie qui traite de sujets sérieux: l'avarice, bien sûr, mais aussi la tyrannie domestique et l'égoïsme. Dans *Le Bourgeois Gentilhomme*, Monsieur Jourdain veut devenir gentilhomme en apprenant la danse ou la musique, des choses qui lui semblent indispensables pour se transformer en gentilhomme. Naturellement, il est ridicule et sa famille se moque de lui.

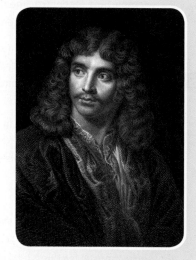

Dans la dernière comédie de Molière, *Le Malade imaginaire,* Argan se croit toujours malade et les médecins en profitent pour lui prendre son argent. Son obsession est telle qu'il veut marier sa fille à un médecin.

Selon Molière, le but de ses pièces était « d'attaquer par des peintures ridicules les vices du siècle » et pour lui « le devoir de la comédie est de corriger les hommes en les divertissant. »

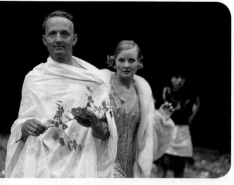

Tartuffe, par Molière

1 Lisez le texte. Identifiez la pièce:

a In which play is the main character obsessed with social standing?

b What play shows how money leads to selfishness and threatens domestic harmony?

c Which play deals with hypochondria?

d In which play does the main character believe in total frankness and honesty?

e In which play does the main character speak coherently about his vices and motivation?

f In which play does religious hypocrisy almost destroy a family?

2 💡 Faites des recherches pour identifier les thèmes d'une des pièces suivantes et écrire des détails sur le personnage principal. (Feuille)

L'Avare

Dom Juan

Le Bourgeois Gentilhomme

Le Malade imaginaire

Le Misanthrope

3 🎧 Ecoutez l'entretien avec des spectateurs qui ont assisté à des représentations théâtrales. C'est qui: Lucie, Thomas, Angélique, Faroud ou Cécile?

a   Qui n'a pas aimé les vêtements des comédiens?

b   Qui n'a pas aimé les acteurs?

c   Qui voudrait devenir actrice?

d   Qui a trouvé la pièce très sombre?

e   Qui a aimé le rythme rapide de la pièce?

f   Qui a vu une pièce sur la politique?

g   Qui a apprécié l'interprétation mais n'a pas aimé la pièce?

h   Qui a aimé la pièce mais n'a pas aimé l'interprétation?

4 💡 Présentez une critique orale d'une pièce que vous avez vue. Parlez des aspects suivants. (Feuille)

- l'intrigue
- les personnages
- les acteurs
- la mise en scène
- la musique
- l'éclairage
- le rythme de la représentation
- votre avis personnel

5 Posez ces questions à un/une partenaire qui va parler d'une pièce qu'il/elle a vue.

a   C'est quel genre de pièce?

b   De quoi s'agit-il?

c   Comment est le personnage principal?

d   Quels sont les thèmes de cette pièce?

e   Quel est le message principal du dramaturge?

f   Est-ce que tu as apprécié l'interprétation des acteurs?

g   Comment as-tu trouvé le dénouement de la pièce?

h   Est-ce que tu as apprécié la pièce?

Compétences

Describing the work of a dramatist

When talking about the work of a dramatist, examine the following aspects:

- *l'exposition*
- *l'intrigue*
- *les personnages*
- *la langue*
- *les thèmes abordés*
- *le dénouement*

When talking about a performance of a play, you could consider the following:

- *le décor*
- *les costumes*
- *la mise en scène*
- *l'interprétation des acteurs*
- *le rythme de la représentation*
- *la musique*
- *l'éclairage*

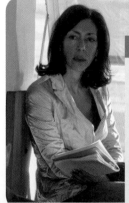

Yasmina Reza

i Vos enquêtes

Many classic French plays are available on DVD. La Comédie Française has recorded many of its plays by Molière, Racine, Corneille, Marivaux and Beaumarchais. More recent dramatists of note include Eugène Ionesco, Jean Cocteau and Jean Anouilh. The contemporary playwright, Yasmina Reza, is well regarded and has had her plays translated into English and performed throughout the world.

If you want to find out more about Molière, films such as Laurent Tirard's *Molière* could be a good starting point. Eugène Ionesco's *La Cantatrice chauve* is a modern play that may appeal to you; this is an example of the 'Theatre of the absurd'. Writers of this style of drama demonstrate the originality and vitality of French theatre.

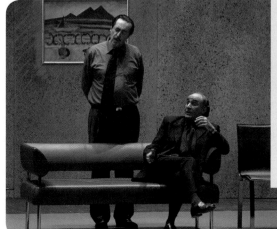

Art, par Yasmina Reza

Jacques Prévert

Jacques Prévert est né en 1900 à Neuilly-sur-Seine, dans une famille bourgeoise. Dans ses poèmes, il ne cessera de se moquer des obsessions et des convenances de la bourgeoisie. Ses études lui donneront une antipathie envers la religion.

En 1920, il a fait son service militaire à Saint-Nicolas-de-Port, près de Lunéville. Ici, il rencontre le peintre Yves Tanguy. Peu de temps après, Jacques est envoyé en Turquie. A la suite de son service militaire, il devient un pacifiste convaincu.

De retour à Paris en 1922, Jacques fait partie du mouvement surréaliste auquel participent Louis Aragon et André Breton. Prévert prendra ses distances avec le parti communiste malgré l'influence du communisme dans sa défense des faibles et des opprimés.

Pendant la guerre, il quitte Paris et habite dans le sud à la Tourette-sur-Loup. Ici il tombe amoureux de Janine Loris, dont il s'inspire pour écrire des poèmes romantiques. Sa collection *Paroles* est publiée pour la première fois en 1945.

L'ouvrage est accueilli avec enthousiasme et est réédité à 5000 exemplaires dans la semaine suivant le jour de sa publication.

La Seconde Guerre mondiale finie, Prévert revient à Paris. Mais la guerre lui donne une haine du militarisme qui restera avec lui toute sa vie. Jacques Prévert est mort auprès de sa femme Janine en 1977 à Omonville.

Dans ses poèmes, il parle de la religion, de la guerre et de la violence, de l'amour et de la tristesse.

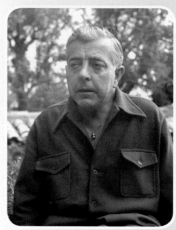

1 Lisez le texte. Reliez les étapes de la vie de Prévert (a–g) aux sujets que l'on trouve dans son œuvre (i–vii).

a   son milieu familial
b   l'école
c   son service militaire
d   Paris dans les années 20
e   le communisme
f   son séjour à la Tourette-sur-Loup
g   la guerre

i   la défense des victimes
ii   le pacifisme
ii   l'amour
iv   l'antimilitarisme
v   la religion
vi   la bourgeoisie
vii le surréalisme

2 a Lisez ces extraits de l'œuvre de Prévert et identifiez le sujet du poème.

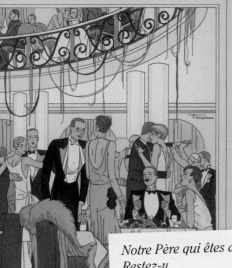

Notre Père qui êtes aux cieux
Restez-y
Et nous nous resterons sur la terre
Qui est quelquefois si jolie...

A

Ils m'ont tiré au mauvais sort
par les pieds
et m'ont jeté dans la charrette des morts
des morts tirés des rangs

C

Des milliers et des milliers d'années
Ne sauraient suffire
Pour dire
La petite seconde d'éternité
Où tu m'as embrassé
Où je t'ai embrassée

B

Et il est parti
Sous la pluie
Sans une parole
Sans me regarder
Et moi j'ai pris
Ma tête dans ma main
Et j'ai pleuré.

D

2 b 💡 Faites des recherches sur un poète de votre choix. Faites un résumé des thèmes d'inspiration du poète et de ce qui l'a influencé. Donnez des citations de ses poèmes pour illustrer votre réponse. (Feuille)

3 🎧 Ecoutez le poème d'Arthur Rimbaud et répondez aux questions.

a   Où se passe la scène décrite dans le poème?

b   Quel temps fait-il?

c   Trouvez quatre couleurs mentionnées dans le poème.

d   A première vue, que fait le jeune soldat?

e   Qu'est-ce qui s'est passé en réalité?

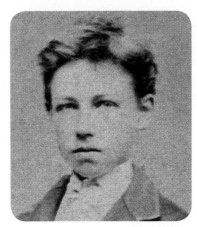

Arthur Rimbaud

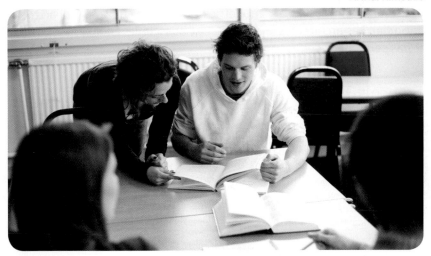

4 💡 Faites une analyse d'un poème de votre choix et faites une présentation orale sur les aspects suivants. (Feuille)

• le contexte

• le sujet

• type de poème / vers / rime

• assonances, allitérations

• personnifications

• comparaison et métaphore

• la conclusion: est-ce que le poème est réussi?

5 Posez ces questions à un/une partenaire qui va parler d'un poème qu'il/elle a étudié.

a   Quel est le contexte du poème que tu as choisi?

b   Donne quelques renseignements sur le poète – sa vie, ses influences.

c   Quel est le sujet du poème?

d   Quelles sont les techniques utilisées par le poète?

e   Parle-moi de ta réaction personnelle au poème.

🔲 Compétences

Widening vocabulary to give personal reaction

Positive

bon, agréable, amusant, approprié, beau, convaincant, efficace, excellent, exemplaire, habile, intéressant, juste, remarquable, sensible, sentimental, sérieux, simple, supérieur, vrai

Negative

mauvais, abominable, affreux, atroce, catastrophique, débile, déplorable, désastreux, épouvantable, exécrable, incompétent, inefficace, inférieur, insuffisant, insupportable, lamentable, pénible

i Vos enquêtes

You will by now have studied poems by several poets, including Jacques Prévert and Arthur Rimbaud. There are a huge number of poets for you to choose, ranging from the Renaissance (Du Bellay) to the modern poems of Aimé Césaire from Martinique. The best-known poet of the 18th century is André Chénier, but the 19th century is particularly rich, starting with the romanticism of Victor Hugo and Alfred de Vigny, moving on to the naturalist movement of Charles Baudelaire, ending with the symbolism of Stéphane Mallarmé or Paul Verlaine. French poets of the 20th century include Paul Eluard, André Breton, Louis Aragon and Robert Desnos.

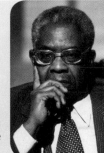

Aimé Césaire

i WebQuest

La poésie de la Résistance

Faites des recherches sur la poésie de la Résistance. Ecrivez une composition dans laquelle vous donnez votre point de vue personnel après avoir étudié en profondeur un poème.

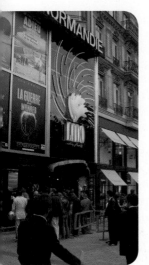

E

L'œuvre d'un artiste français
(réalisateur, architecte, musicien ou peintre)

Dans cette section, vous allez étudier les thèmes et les techniques d'un artiste français et le contexte dans lequel il a évolué. Il y a quatre domaines possibles: le cinéma, l'architecture, la musique ou la peinture.

En France, **le cinéma** est souvent désigné comme le septième art. Une étude approfondie d'un film est utile pour l'apprentissage d'une langue: il y a l'aspect linguistique mais aussi le décor, les attitudes, l'ambiance du film.

Le prestige de **l'architecture** française se porte bien au rang mondial. Les architectes français ne réalisent pas seulement des "grands travaux" en France mais partout dans le monde.

En ce qui concerne **la musique**, vous pouvez étudier un compositeur de musique classique ou un musicien contemporain; il existe beaucoup de genres musicaux à travers le monde francophone.

La peinture française est variée. Le mouvement impressionniste du dix-neuvième siècle est toujours populaire, mais les mouvements artistiques plus modernes, comme le cubisme ou l'art abstrait, ont aussi leurs adeptes.

François Truffaut

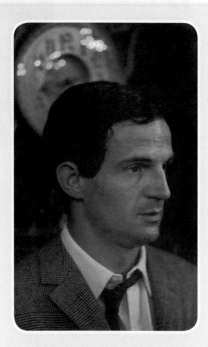

François Truffaut naît le 6 février 1932 à Paris. Il connaît une enfance solitaire et donc il trouve refuge dans le cinéma. Il manque les cours pour passer ses journées dans les cinémas de Paris.

En 1953, Truffaut fait son entrée aux Cahiers du cinéma. Dans ses articles, il attaque "le cinéma de Papa", cinéma traditionnel français. Il est un des fondateurs de la nouvelle vague. C'est un mouvement qui rompt avec le cinéma classique.

C'est avec *Les Quatre cents coups* en 1958 que Truffaut fait sa marque. L'histoire est autobiographique. Elle raconte la vie d'un jeune adolescent parisien, Antoine Doinel, interprété par Jean-Pierre Léaud. Avec *Fahrenheit 451* (1966), Truffaut fait une incursion dans le monde de la science-fiction. Truffaut y décrit un monde du futur où les livres sont interdits.

Jusqu'en 1982, Truffaut tourne pratiquement un film par année. On peut citer en particulier *L'Enfant sauvage* (1969), dans lequel il joue un rôle principal; *La nuit américaine* (1973), un film sur le cinéma qui a gagné l'Oscar du meilleur film étranger; *L'Histoire d'Adèle H.* (1975) avec Isabelle Adjani dans le rôle de l'une des filles de Victor Hugo; *Le Dernier métro* (1980) avec Catherine Deneuve et Gérard Depardieu et *Vivement dimanche!* (1982), son dernier film.

François Truffaut meurt le 21 octobre 1984. Il laisse une œuvre importante: 21 films en tout. La variété des sujets traités par Truffaut est importante: polar noir, comédie romantique, science-fiction et film historique. Cette diversité thématique est mélangée de deux éléments: une humanité sincère et des sujets autobiographiques.

1 Lisez le texte. Vrai, faux, ou information non donnée?

a   Truffaut avait beaucoup d'amis quand il était jeune.

b   Il aimait beaucoup l'école.

c   Dans ses articles, il critiquait le cinéma classique français.

d   Jean-Pierre Léaud avait le même âge que Truffaut.

e   Dans *Fahrenheit 451*, on supprime la littérature.

f   On ne voit jamais Truffaut dans ses films.

g   Il n'a jamais tourné un film historique.

h   Son œuvre est très variée.

2 💡 Faites des recherches pour écrire un paragraphe sur un des films suivants. Parlez du contexte, du metteur en scène, des thèmes du film et de la réaction des critiques. Donnez votre avis personnel. (Feuille)

- *Jean de Florette* de Claude Berri
- *Le Boucher* de Claude Chabrol
- *Le Fabuleux Destin d'Amélie Poulain* de Jean-Pierre Jeunet
- *La Haine* de Mathieu Kassovitz
- *Au revoir, les enfants* de Louis Malle

3 🎧 Ecoutez ce reportage sur l'architecte Jean Nouvel. Choisissez les quatre phrases vraies.

a Jean Nouvel a toujours voulu devenir architecte.
b Au début de sa carrière, il a tout de suite travaillé sur de grands projets.
c La façade de l'Institut du monde arabe est bien connue.
d Jean Nouvel a un style qui est typique de lui.
e Dans ses bâtiments, il essaie de créer autant d'espace que possible.
f Il ne s'intéresse pas aux effets de lumière.
g Il travaille souvent sur la rénovation de vieux bâtiments.
h Il ne travaille jamais à l'étranger.
i C'est un architecte dont le travail est souvent original.

4 💡 Faites une description orale d'un bâtiment qui est l'œuvre d'un architecte français que vous avez étudié. Parlez des aspects suivants. (Feuille)

- quelques renseignements sur l'architecte
- l'environnement
- la fonction de la construction
- le style
- le matériel
- la façade
- l'intérieur
- votre avis personnel

5 Posez ces questions à un/une partenaire qui va parler d'un bâtiment qu'il/elle a étudié.

a C'est quel genre de construction?
b Qui en est l'architecte et quand est-ce qu'on l'a construite?
c Quels sont les caractéristiques de cette construction?
d Que penses-tu de l'extérieur?
e Décris l'architecture intérieure et la décoration.
f Quelle a été la réaction initiale des critiques envers la construction?
g Pourquoi est-ce que tu apprécies la construction?
h Quelle a été l'influence de cette construction sur d'autres architectes?

Institut du monde arabe, Paris

🔍 **Compétences**

Widening vocabulary: using alternatives

Use alternatives to avoid repetition of words in your written work.
The following are very common:
*beaucoup de   des gens
il y a   intéressant
un problème   un avantage
un inconvénient*

Match up these alternative expressions to the ones above:
*un atout
un grand nombre de
un obstacle   une difficulté
il existe   remarquable
certaines personnes*

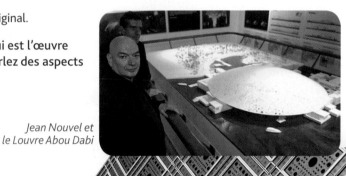
Jean Nouvel et le Louvre Abou Dabi

ℹ️ **Vos enquêtes**

DVD box sets of French films are a good way to explore an overview of the work of a director. If you are interested in the work of film-makers of the *Nouvelle Vague,* the works of Jean-Luc Godard, Claude Chabrol and Louis Malle are readily available. Recent directors of note include Claude Berri, Luc Besson, Jean-Pierre Jeunet and Jean-Hugues Anglade.

If you want to find out more about French architecture, a good place to start is the construction of some recent *grands travaux* in Paris. Architects such as Jean Nouvel, Dominique Perrault and François Grether have all been involved in changing the urban landscape. If you wish to examine architecture from an earlier era, the work of Auguste Perret, Claude Parent or Le Corbusier may be of interest.

Jean-Michel Jarre

Fils de Maurice Jarre, un compositeur de musiques de film (*Lawrence d'Arabie* et *Docteur Jivago*), Jean-Michel Jarre apprend le piano depuis l'âge de cinq ans et reçoit une formation classique au Conservatoire. Il quitte le Conservatoire pour le Groupe de recherches musicales, un groupe créé par Pierre Schaeffer pour des musiciens étudiant les musiques contemporaines et expérimentales. Passionné par la musique électroacoustique, Jean-Michel veut explorer de nouvelles voies et montre beaucoup de talent à la manipulation de magnétophones et de bandes magnétiques.

Jean-Michel Jarre commence à composer pour le cinéma, l'opéra et les variétés sans vraiment attirer beaucoup d'attention. Mais sa carrière commence réellement en 1976 lorsqu'il sort son album *Oxygène*. Les sonorités évoquent des bruits de navettes spatiales et des vagues. Jarre a du succès deux ans plus tard avec *Equinoxe*, un hommage symphonico-électronique aux créatures marines: méduses, dauphins, algues. Juste après, il commence à donner ses

premiers concerts monstres dans la planète entière: Pékin, Houston, Lyon, Londres, Moscou.

Jean-Michel Jarre continue à sortir des albums comme *Les Chants magnétiques*, *Révolution*, *Chronologie*, *Métamorphose* et *Aero*. Il a une réputation mondiale et ses spectacles, des concerts multimédias, sont des rendez-vous magiques. Il donne à la musique électronique une dimension populaire depuis plus de 30 ans.

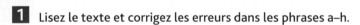

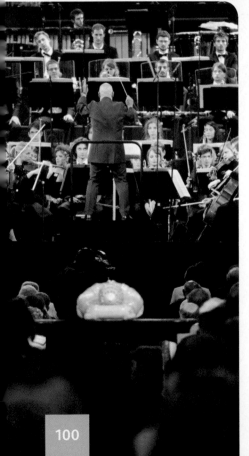

1 Lisez le texte et corrigez les erreurs dans les phrases a–h.

a Le père de Jean-Michel Jarre composait des opéras.

b Jean-Michel a quitté le Conservatoire pour faire des recherches sur la musique classique.

c La musique électroacoustique ne l'intéressait pas tellement.

d Ses premières compositions ont eu beaucoup de succès.

e La musique de son premier album évoque la mer.

f Ses concerts ont lieu devant peu de spectateurs.

g Ses concerts ont lieu en France.

h Il est maintenant moins populaire qu'il y a trente ans.

2 a Classez ces musiciens par ordre chronologique.

- Charles Trenet
- Claude Debussy
- Jean-Philippe Rameau
- Jean-Jacques Goldman
- Georges Bizet
- Jean-Baptiste Lully

b 💡 Choisissez un musicien de la liste et faites des recherches pour écrire sur les aspects suivants. (Feuille)

- l'époque où il a vécu
- le genre de musique qu'il a composée
- son importance et son influence
- son chef-d'œuvre

Orchestre français des jeunes

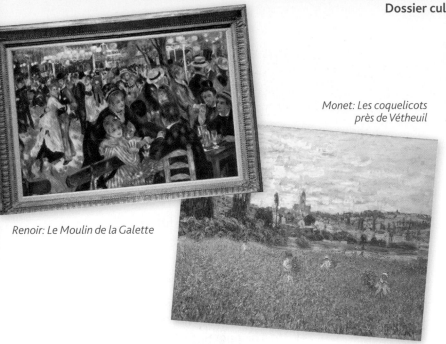

Monet: Les coquelicots près de Vétheuil

Renoir: Le Moulin de la Galette

3 🎧 Ecoutez trois commentaires sur les impressionnistes. Qui parle? Franck, Morgane ou Sylvie?

a   Mon artiste favori a peint beaucoup de figures féminines.

b   J'aime les peintures qui représentent des hommes et des femmes.

c   Ces peintres ont travaillé surtout à l'extérieur.

d   J'aime beaucoup les paysages.

e   J'aime les représentations des lacs et des fleuves.

f   J'aime les impressionnistes, mais Renoir ne me plaît pas beaucoup.

g   Avant les impressionnistes, on a encouragé les peintres à imiter les artistes du passé.

h   Ce peintre a influencé d'autres mouvements artistiques.

4 💡 Faites une analyse de plusieurs mouvements artistiques français pour en faire une présentation orale. Parlez des styles suivants en considérant: l'époque, les peintres français, les techniques et votre opinion sur ce mouvement artistique. (Feuille)

le pointillisme   **le surréalisme**   **le fauvisme**

le romantisme   **le cubisme**   **le baroque**

5 Posez ces questions à un/une partenaire qui va parler d'un mouvement artistique qu'il/elle a étudié.

a   Pourquoi as-tu choisi d'étudier ce mouvement?

b   Que sais-tu de l'origine du mouvement?

c   Parle-moi des techniques caractéristiques du mouvement.

d   Quels peintres sont associés à ce style?

e   Décris une œuvre bien connue qui représente ce style.

f   A ton avis, quelle est l'importance de ce mouvement?

g   Est-ce que tu recommanderais ce style? Pourquoi?

🔲 Compétences

Making a personal analysis of a work of art

Premier constat: ce qui me saute aux yeux et pourquoi j'ai choisi cette œuvre.

Inventaire: ce que je remarque et ce que j'en comprends.

Mise en perspective: ce que je sais de l'œuvre – mes connaissances culturelles et le contexte historique.

Mise en forme: une présentation raisonnée des éléments de l'œuvre qui me semblent importants.

Conclusion: pourquoi je recommanderais cette œuvre aux autres.

ℹ Vos enquêtes

You have now studied the work of French artists in a variety of fields and although the focus has been very much on metropolitan France, it is equally valid to study the work of Francophone artists in other parts of the French-speaking world.

The French architect Roland Simounet was born in Algeria and this country greatly influenced his subsequent work. Férid Boughedir is Tunisia's best known film director. The band Kassav' from Guadeloupe and Martinique invented a pan-Caribbean sound by taking elements from reggae and salsa, and became the most famous musicians of *le zouk*. Painters from Ivory Coast (known as *peintres naïfs*) such as Korhogo are said to have greatly influenced Pablo Picasso in the 1930s.

ℹ WebQuest

Les artistes des années 30

Faites des recherches sur des artistes des années trente pour écrire une composition dans laquelle vous donnez votre point de vue personnel sur cette époque.

Grammaire

1 Nouns and articles

1.1 Gender of nouns

Knowing the gender of a French noun is largely a question of careful learning, but there are guidelines to help you. The following general rules apply, but be careful as there are exceptions.

Masculine nouns

Nouns ending in the letter groups listed below are masculine – but note the exceptions.

ending	example	exceptions
-acle	un obstacle	
-age	le courage	la cage, une image, la page, la plage
-al	le total	
-ail	le portail	
-amme	le programme	la gamme
-eau	un oiseau	
-ème	le problème	
-er	le fer	la mer
-et	le billet	
-isme	le tabagisme	
-ment	le commencement	la jument
-oir	le miroir	

Feminine nouns

Nouns ending in the letter groups listed below are feminine – but note the exceptions.

ending	example	exceptions
-ance	la tendance	
-anse	la danse	
-ée	la journée	le lycée, le musée
-ence	la prudence	le silence
-ense	la défense	
-esse	la jeunesse	
-eur	la douceur	le bonheur, le malheur
-ie	la vie	le génie
-ière	la matière	le cimetière
-ise	la valise	
-sion	une expression	
-tié	une amitié	
-té	la santé	le côté, le pâté, le traité, le comité
-tion	la natation	le bastion
-ure	la nature	

Masculine nouns with modified feminine form

The feminine equivalent of many masculine nouns is formed by adding -e:

un commerçant – une commerçante
un Américain – une Américaine

Other patterns for masculine and feminine nouns are listed below.

masc. ending	fem. ending	masculine noun	feminine noun
-eur	-euse	le chanteur	la chanteuse
-eur	-rice	un instituteur	une institutrice
-eau	-elle	le jumeau	la jumelle
-er	-ère	le boulanger	la boulangère
-ien	-ienne	un Italien	une Italienne
-on	-onne	le Breton	la Bretonne
-f	-ve	le veuf	la veuve
-x	-se	un époux	une épouse

Single gender nouns

Some nouns retain the same gender, irrespective of the person described.

Always masculine:

un amateur, un auteur, un bébé, un écrivain,
un ingénieur, un médecin, un peintre,
un professeur (but un/une prof), un témoin

Always feminine:

une connaissance, une personne, une recrue,
une sentinelle, une star, une vedette, une victime

1.2 Plural forms of nouns

The plural of a noun is normally formed by adding -s:

un livre – des livres

Other patterns for singular/plural forms are listed below.

sing. ending	pl. ending	example (sing./pl.)
-al	-aux *or* -als	animal/animaux bal/bals, festival/festivals
-ail	-aux *or* -ails	travail/travaux détail/détails
-au, -eau, -eu	*add* -x	bateau/bateaux, jeu/jeux
-ou	-ous *or* -oux	trou/trous bijou/bijoux, genou/genoux
-s, -x, -z	*no change*	fils/fils, voix/voix, gaz/gaz

Learn these special cases:

le ciel – les cieux
un œil – les yeux
le grand-parent – les grands-parents
madame – mesdames
mademoiselle – mesdemoiselles
monsieur – messieurs

1.3 Definite articles: *le, la, l', les* – 'the'

The definite article is usually used in the same way as 'the' in English. However, in French it is often required where 'the' is omitted. Learn these in particular:

1 Before abstract nouns or nouns used to generalise:

L'argent donne la liberté. Money gives freedom.

2 Before names of continents, countries, regions and languages:

La France est le pays d'Europe le plus visité. France is the most visited country in Europe.

Le français n'est pas trop difficile.
French is not too difficult.

But the definite article is not required after *en* and *de*, with feminine place names only:

Cette année, nous allons en Normandie.
Elle revient de Norvège.

It is also not required with languages placed immediately after the verb *parler*:

Ici, on parle japonais.

3 Before arts, sciences, school subjects, sports, illnesses:

La physique nous permet de mieux comprendre l'univers. Le sida nous fait bien peur.

4 Before parts of the body:

Pliez les genoux. Il s'est cassé la jambe.

5 Before meals and drinks:

Le petit déjeuner est servi à partir de sept heures.

6 Before fractions:

Les trois quarts de l'électorat sont indifférents.

7 Before titles:

Le président Sarkozy.

1.4 Indefinite articles: *un*, *une*, *des* – 'a', 'an', 'some', 'any'

Note that *un/une* is not needed in the following situations:

1 When stating a person's occupation:

Mon père est médecin. My father is **a** doctor.

2 After *quel, comme, en, en tant que, sans, ni*:

Quel frimeur! What a show off!

Je vous parle en tant que professeur.
I'm speaking to you as a teacher.

Tu n'as ni crayon ni stylo?
Haven't you got either a pencil or a pen?

3 In a list:

Etudiants, ouvriers, cadres: tous étaient là.
Students, workers, managers: they were all there.

1.5 Partitive articles: *du, de la, de l', des* – 'some', 'any'

The partitive article means 'some' or 'any' and describes an unspecified quantity.

*Je voudrais **du** beurre, s'il vous plaît.*
I'd like **some** butter, please.

	singular	plural
masculine	du / de l'	des
feminine	de la / de l'	des

All the forms change to *de* in the following situations:

1 After a negative verb (this also applies to the indefinite article *un* and *une*):

*Je joue **du** violon, je ne joue pas **de** piano.*
I play the violin, I don't play the piano.

(But note there is no change after *ne… que*:

*Il ne mange que **du** poisson.* He only eats fish.)

2 In expressions of quantity such as *assez de*, *trop de*:

*Ça cause trop **de** pollution.*
It causes too much pollution.

3 With plural nouns preceded by an adjective:

*On fait **des** efforts/On fait **de** gros efforts pour…*
We're making great efforts to…

4 In expressions such as:

bordé de, couvert de, entouré de, plein de, rempli de

2 Adjectives and adverbs

2.1 Adjective agreement and position

Adjectives must agree in gender and number with their noun. Usually a masculine singular form needs to add -e for the feminine form, -s for the plural and -es for feminine plural.

masc. sing.	fem. sing.	masc. pl.	fem. pl.
vert	verte	verts	vertes

Adjectives that already end in -e do not need an extra -e in the feminine form: *jeune/jeune*. Those that end in -s or -x do not change in the masculine plural form: *dangereux/dangereux*.

Other patterns for masculine/feminine endings:

masc. sing.	fem. sing.	example
-er	-ère	mensonger/mensongère
-eur	-euse	trompeur/trompeuse
-f	-ve	informatif/informative
-x	-se	dangereux/dangereuse
-l	-lle	nul/nulle
-on	-onne	bon/bonne
-eil	-eille	pareil/pareille
-el	-elle	officiel/officielle
-en	-enne	moyen/moyenne
-et	-ète	inquiet/inquiète
-c	-che *or* que	blanc/blanche, public/publique

Invariable adjectives

Some adjectives never change; in dictionaries these are marked **inv.** for invariable. They include compounds such as *bleu foncé, bleu marine*, and colours where a noun is used as an adjective, such as *marron* ('chestnut').

Position of adjectives

Most adjectives <u>follow</u> the noun they describe: *une jupe bleue, une chemise blanche*.

However several common adjectives come <u>before</u> the noun they describe: *le mauvais temps, le premier avril*. These include:

beau	bon	gentil	joli	mauvais	méchant
vilain	grand	gros	haut	petit	vaste
jeune	nouveau	vieux	premier	deuxième	

2.2 Comparatives and superlatives

By adding *plus... que* (more... than), *moins... que* (less... than) or *aussi... que* (as... as) around adjectives, you can compare one thing to another. Each adjective still has to agree with its noun.

*Le taux de chômage est **plus élevé qu**'en Italie.*
The unemployment rate is **higher than** in Italy.

*La vie est **moins difficile qu**'en Pologne.*
Life is **less difficult than** in Poland.

To form superlatives (the most/biggest/best, etc.), use *le/la/les plus/moins* + adjective:

*C'est le problème **le plus difficile**.*
It's **the most difficult** problem.

*Les jeunes sont **les plus concernés**.*
Young people are **the most affected**.

Some useful irregular forms:

bon – meilleur(e)(s) – le/la/les meilleur(e)(s)
good – better – the best

mauvais – pire – le/la/les pire(s)
bad – worse – the worst

2.3 Adverbs and adverbial phrases

Formation

Most adverbs are formed from the feminine form of an adjective plus –*ment*:

franc/franche frank – *franchement* frankly

Adjectives ending in a vowel use the masculine form to form the adverb:

absolu – absolument

Adjectives ending in -ent or -ant use the following pattern:

évident – évidemment, constant – constamment

A number of adverbs end in -*ément*:

profond – profondément, énorme – énormément

Note two irregular forms:

bon – bien
good – well

mauvais – mal
bad – badly

Usage

Adverbs qualify verbs and once they are formed never change (unlike adjectives). Very often an adverb describes how or when an action happens.

Il chante constamment. He sings constantly.

Adverbs usually follow verbs. In a compound tense, they come between the auxiliary and the past participle:

*J'ai **poliment** demandé la permission.*
I asked permission politely.

But many adverbs of time and place follow the past participle:

*Je l'ai vu **hier**.* I saw him yesterday.

Some adverbs are words you already know but may not think of as adverbs.

- Intensifiers and quantifiers, i.e. to show how strongly an adjective applies:
  très, un peu, trop, si, seulement, beaucoup, assez, plus, moins, tellement, presque
- Adverbs of time:
  après, avant, toujours, hier, aujourd'hui, demain, d'abord, enfin, parfois, souvent, tard, tôt
- Adverbs of place:
  ici, là, ailleurs, loin, dessus, dessous, dedans, devant, derrière, partout

Comparatives and superlatives of adverbs

These are formed in the same way as for adjectives:

***moins** souvent **que**...*

***plus** vite **que**...*

***aussi** facilement **que**...*

Note two irregular forms:

bien – mieux – le mieux
well – better – the best

mal – pire / pis – le pis / le pire
badly – worse – the worst

NB. *(le) pis* is rarely used except in the expressions *tant pis* and *ça va de mal en pis*.

*Il parle **bien** allemand mais il parle **mieux** français.*
He speaks German well but French better.

3 Pronouns

3.1 Subject pronouns

	singular		plural
je	*I*	nous	*we*
tu	*you*	vous	*you (plural or polite)*
il	*he, it*	ils	*they (m. or m. & f.)*
elle	*she, it*	elles	*they (f.)*
on	*one, we*		

These are the familiar pronouns which are learned with verb forms.

Use *tu* when talking to a child, a person your own age or an adult you know very well such as a member of your family.

Use *vous* when talking to more than one person, a person you don't know or an adult you know but are not on familiar terms with.

Use *on* when talking about people in general and also, in informal speech, for 'we' (instead of *nous*).

When referring to a mixed group of people, remember to use the masculine plural *ils*.

3.2 Object pronouns

An object pronoun replaces a noun that is not the subject 'doing' the verb but is affected by that verb, i.e. is the object. Unlike in English, the pronoun goes before the verb.

A <u>direct</u> object pronoun replaces a noun linked 'directly' to the verb.

*Tu aimes **les haricots**? Je **les** adore!*
Do you like beans? I love **them**!

*S'il y a **un problème**, il faut **le** résoudre.*
If there is a problem, we must solve **it**.

An <u>indirect</u> object pronoun replaces a noun that is linked to the verb by a preposition, usually *à*.

*Je téléphone **à ma mère**. Je **lui** téléphone tous les jours.* I phone **her** every day.

*Je demande **à mes copains** de sortir. Je **leur** demande de jouer au tennis.* I ask **them** to play tennis.

- Verbs that are used with a direct object include:
  attendre to wait for, *chercher* to look for

- Verbs that are used with an indirect object include these (*qn = quelqu'un, qch = quelque chose*):
  demander à qn de faire to ask someone to do
  dire à qn to tell/say to someone
  parler à qn to speak/talk to someone
  promettre à qn de faire to promise someone to do
  téléphoner à qn to telephone someone

- Verbs that can be used with a direct and an indirect object include:
  donner qch à qn to give something to someone
  envoyer qch à qn to send something to someone

direct object pronouns		indirect object pronouns	
me (m')	*me*	**me (m')**	*(to) me*
te (t')	*you*	**te (t')**	*(to) you*
le (l')	*him, it*	**lui**	*(to) him/it*
la (l')	*her, it*	**lui**	*(to) her/it*
nous	*us*	**nous**	*(to) us*
vous	*you*	**vous**	*(to) you*
les	*them*	**leur**	*(to) them*

Note that for the first and second persons, (me, you, us, you pl.), the direct and indirect object pronouns are identical: *me, te, nous, vous*.

For the third person (him, her, it, them), the object pronouns are different: *le, la, les* for direct and *lui, leur* for indirect.

Object pronouns also precede verbs in other tenses:
*Je **lui** ai téléphoné hier.* I phoned him/her yesterday.
*Je **vous** dirai tout.* I will tell you everything.
*Elles **nous** invitaient toujours.* They always invited us.

With a negative, the negative expression goes around the pronoun as well as the verb:
*Je **ne lui** ai **pas** téléphoné.* I didn't phone him/her.

If two object pronouns occur together, this is the sequence: *me, te, nous, vous* go before *le, la, les* which go before *lui, leur*.

*Vous **me l'**avez dit.* You told me. (You told it to me.)

*Je **les lui** ai offerts.* I gave them to her.

See 3.6 for order when used with *y* and *en*.

3.3 Disjunctive (or emphatic) pronouns

	singular		plural
moi	*me*	**nous**	*us*
toi	*you (sing.)*	**vous**	*you (plural)*
lui	*him*	**eux**	*them (m. or m. & f.)*
elle	*her*	**elles**	*them (f.)*
soi	*one, oneself (used with* on*)*		

Disjunctive pronouns, which always refer to people not things, are used:

1 For emphasis:
__Moi__, je ne suis pas d'accord. **I** don't agree.

*C'est **lui** qui devrait céder, pas **elle**.* It's him who should give way, not her.

2 Before *-même(s)*, meaning '-self' or '-selves':
*Il l'a construit **lui-même**.* He built it himself.

3 After prepositions such as *chez, pour, sans, avec*:
*Tu vas rentrer directement chez **toi**?*
Are you going straight back home?

*Chacun pour **soi**!* Each one for himself!

*Ils sont partis avec/sans **nous**.*
They left with/without us.

4 After certain verbs followed by *à* or *de*:
verb + *à*, e.g. *faire attention à, penser à, s'adresser à, s'intéresser à*
*Elle pense toujours **à lui**.*
She's always thinking about him.
*Il faut faire attention **à eux**.*
You have to pay attention to them.
verb + *de*, e.g. *dépendre de, penser de, profiter de, s'approcher de*
*Qu'est-ce qu'elle pense **de moi**?*
What does she think of me?
*Elle s'est approchée **de lui**.* She approached him.

3.4 Relative pronouns

Relative pronouns are words like 'who', 'which' and 'that', used to connect two parts of a sentence.

qui	*who, which, that*
que	*who, whom, which, that*
ce qui	*what, something that*
ce que	*what, something that*
quoi	*what*
où	*where, when*
dont	*of which, whose*
lequel, laquelle,	*which*
lesquels, lesquelles	*which*

1 *Qui* is the most common of these. It represents someone or something that is the subject of the verb that follows:
*Elle s'entend bien avec sa mère, **qui** l'écoute attentivement.* She gets on well with her mother, who listens to her carefully.

2 *Que* represents someone or something that is the object of the verb that follows:
*C'est quelqu'un **que** j'écoute attentivement.*
He/She is someone (whom/that) I listen to carefully.

3 *Qui* is used for 'who' or 'whom' after a preposition:
*La tante **avec qui** il habite...*
The aunt whom/that he lives with...
The relative pronoun can be left out in English – the aunt he lives with – but not in French.

4 *Ce qui* is used for the subject of a verb:
__Ce qui__ est essentiel, c'est... What is essential is...
and *ce que* is used for the object of a verb:
__Ce que__ je préfère, c'est... What I prefer is...

5 *Quoi* is used for 'what' after a preposition such as *de*:

*Je ne sais pas de **quoi** tu parles.*
I don't know what you're talking about.

6 *Où* means 'where' or, after a noun referring to time, 'when':

*La ville **où** j'habite est...* The town where I live is...
*Le jour **où** il est né, on a dit que...*
On the day (when) he was born, they said...

7 *Dont* means 'whose' or 'of which'. It replaces *de + qui*, or *de + lequel* and can refer to people or things.

*Un étudiant **dont** je connais la tante...*
A student whose aunt I know...

*Voilà le magasin **dont** j'ai parlé.*
There's the shop (that) I spoke about.

Dont is used to connect a noun to verbs followed by *de*, such as *avoir besoin de* (to need):

*Voici le livre **dont** il a besoin.* Here's the book he needs. ('the book of which he has need')

Dont is also used with numbers and expressions of quantity:

*Trois étudiants **dont** deux Africains...*
Three students, of whom two are Africans...

8 *Lequel* agrees in gender and number with the noun it refers to. It also changes to combine with the prepositions *à* and *de*.

	à + (= to which)	de + (= of which)
lequel	auquel	duquel
laquelle	à laquelle	de laquelle
lesquels	auxquels	desquels
lesquelles	auxquelles	desquelles

*Le journal **auquel** je suis abonné coûte cher.*
The journal to which I subscribe is expensive.

*La classe **dans laquelle** elle est étudiante...*
The class that she is a student in / in which she is a student...

3.5 Pronouns *y* and *en*

The pronoun *y* has two main uses:

1 Meaning 'there' or 'to there', replacing a place already mentioned:
*On **y** va?* Shall we go (there)?

2 Replacing a noun (not a person) or a verb introduced by *à*, such as *penser à quelque chose*:
*As-tu pensé aux conséquences? Non, je n'**y** ai pas pensé.*
Have you thought of the consequences? No, I have not thought about them.

The pronoun *en* has two main uses:

1 Meaning 'from there' or 'out of there':
*Il a mis la main dans sa poche et il **en** a sorti un billet de 100 euros.*
He put his hand in his pocket and got out a 100-euro note.

2 Replacing a noun (not a person) or a verb introduced by *de*, such as *empêcher quelqu'un de faire*:
*Marie, que penses-tu de ton cadeau? J'**en** suis ravie.*
Marie, what do you think of your present? I'm delighted with it.
*Pourquoi n'a-t-il pas protesté? Parce que les autorités l'**en** ont empêché.*
Why didn't he protest? Because the authorities prevented him (from protesting).

In this case, *en* often has the sense of 'some', 'any', 'of it', 'about it', 'of them':
*Tu n'as pas de l'argent à me prêter? Si, j'**en** ai.*
Haven't you got any money to lend me? Yes, I have some.

3.6 Order of pronouns

The sequence of pronouns before a verb is as follows:

1	2	3	4	5
me te se nous vous	le la les	lui leur	y	en

*Il **m'en** a parlé. Il ne comprend pas la blague: il faut **la lui** expliquer.*
He has talked **to me about it**. He does not understand the joke: you have to explain **it to him**.

4 Demonstrative adjectives and pronouns

Demonstrative adjectives are the equivalent of 'this', 'that', 'those', 'these' used before a noun.

*Je voudrais **ces** chaussures.* I'd like **these/those** shoes.

	singular	plural
masculine	**ce** (**cet** before vowel or silent h)	ces
feminine	**cette**	ces

To be more precise you can add *-ci* or *-là* after the noun:

Je voudrais ce manteau-ci. I'd like this coat here.

Je voudrais ces bottes-là. I'd like those boots there.

Demonstrative pronouns are similar to the adjectives above but replace the noun, so are the equivalent of 'this one', 'that one', 'these ones', 'those ones'.

	singular	plural
masculine	celui	ceux
feminine	celle	celles

They are often followed by *qui*, *que* or *de*, as in the examples below.

*Il a choisi une voiture – **celle qui** est la plus chère.*
He chose a car – the one that is the most expensive.

*Regardez les modèles, prenez **ceux que** vous préférez.*
Look at the models, take the ones you prefer.

*Ma voiture est rouge mais **celle de** Marc est grise.*
My car is red but Marc's is grey.

They can be used with a preposition:

*Le quartier où je suis né est en banlieue, mais **celui où** j'habite maintenant est dans le centre.*
The area where I was born is in the suburbs, but the one where I live now is in the centre.

You can add *-ci* or *-là* to emphasise that you're referring to 'this one here' or 'those ones there'.

*Je préfère **celles-ci**.* I prefer these ones.

*Quelle voiture? **Celle-ci** ou **celle-là**?*
Which car? This one or that one?

5 Indefinite adjectives and pronouns

These are words like *autre*, *chaque/chacun*, *même*, *plusieurs*, *quelque/quelqu'un*, *tout*.

J'ai choisi l'autre film. J'ai vu les autres.
I chose the other film. I've seen the others.

Chaque semaine, je joue au badminton.
Each week, I play badminton.

Chacun choisit un sport. Each person chooses a sport.

- *Quelque* has a plural form: *quelques semaines, quelques jours*. It is used without an *-s* before numbers, to mean 'about':

  Les quelque 300 mille estivants...
  The 300,000 or so holidaymakers...

- Note the use of *de* + adjective in phrases like *quelque chose d'intéressant, quelqu'un de bien, rien de nouveau*.

6 Possessive adjectives and pronouns

A **possessive adjective** must agree with its noun.

***Mon** père m'énerve. **Ma** mère est trop stricte.*
My father annoys me. My mother is too strict.

	masculine	feminine	masc. & fem. plural
my	mon	ma	mes
your	ton	ta	tes
his, her, its, one's	son	sa	ses
our	notre	notre	nos
your	votre	votre	vos
their	leur	leur	leurs

Possessive pronouns incorporate a definite article (a word for 'the') – see table below.

	masc. sing.	fem. sing.	masc. pl.	fem. pl.
mine	le mien	la mienne	les miens	les miennes
yours	le tien	la tienne	les tiens	les tiennes
his, hers, one's	le sien	la sienne	les siens	les siennes
ours	le nôtre	la nôtre	les nôtres	les nôtres
yours	le vôtre	la vôtre	les vôtres	les vôtres
theirs	le leur	la leur	les leurs	les leurs

*C'est votre sac, madame? Oui, c'est **le mien**.*
Is this your bag, madam? Yes, it's mine.

Another way to express possession, with *être*, is to use *à* + name, *à* + disjunctive pronoun, or *à* + *qui*:

*C'est **à Patrick**?* Is this Patrick's?

*C'est **à toi**? Non, c'est **à elles**.*
Is this yours? No, it's theirs (fem.).

*C'est **à qui** ce sac?* Whose is this bag?

7 Verbs

7.1 The present tense

There is only one form of the present tense in French but it has various meanings in English:

Il cherche une émission.
He <u>is looking for</u> a programme.

Il cherche en ligne?
<u>Does he look</u> on line?

Non, il cherche dans le journal.
No, <u>he looks</u> in the newspaper.

Also (see 7.26):

Il cherche depuis une heure.
<u>He's been looking</u> for an hour.

Regular verbs

Many verbs fall into three main groups or 'conjugations' according to whether their infinitive ends in *-er*, *-ir* or *-re*. You find the present tense stem by removing the two-letter ending, and then add the regular endings shown in bold in the table below.

	-er: jouer	-ir: finir	-re: attendre
je/j'	jou**e**	fin**is**	attend**s**
tu	jou**es**	fin**is**	attend**s**
il/elle/on	jou**e**	fin**it**	attend
nous	jou**ons**	fin**issons**	attend**ons**
vous	jou**ez**	fin**issez**	attend**ez**
ils/elles	jou**ent**	fin**issent**	attend**ent**

Irregular verbs

Some key verbs are irregular in the present tense; you need to learn these patterns by heart.

avoir (*to have*)	j'ai, tu as, il a, nous avons, vous avez, ils ont
être (*to be*)	je suis, tu es, il est, nous sommes, vous êtes, ils sont
aller (*to go*)	je vais, tu vas, il va, nous allons, vous allez, ils vont
venir (*to come*)	je viens, tu viens, il vient, nous venons, vous venez, ils viennent
tenir (*to hold*)	je tiens, tu tiens, il tient, nous tenons, vous tenez, ils tiennent
faire (*to do/make*)	je fais, tu fais, il fait, nous faisons, vous faites, ils font
prendre (*to take*)	je prends, tu prends, il prend, nous prenons, vous prenez, ils prennent
dormir (*to sleep*)	je dors, tu dors, il dort, nous dormons, vous dormez, ils dorment

dire (*to say*)	je dis, tu dis, il dit, nous disons, vous dites, ils disent
écrire (*to write*)	j'écris, tu écris, il écrit, nous écrivons, vous écrivez, ils écrivent
lire (*to read*)	je lis, tu lis, il lit, nous lisons, vous lisez, ils lisent
mettre (*to put*)	je mets, tu mets, il met, nous mettons, vous mettez, ils mettent
recevoir (*to receive*)	je reçois, tu reçois, il reçoit, nous recevons, vous recevez, ils reçoivent
voir (*to see*)	je vois, tu vois, il voit, nous voyons, vous voyez, ils voient
connaître (*to know*)	je connais, tu connais, il connaît, nous connaissons, vous connaissez, ils connaissent
jeter (*to throw*)	je jette, tu jettes, il jette nous jetons, vous jetez, ils jettent

Modal verbs

	pouvoir (*can/to be able to*)	devoir (*must/to have to*)	vouloir (*to want to*)	savoir (*to know how to*)
je	peux	dois	veux	sais
tu	peux	dois	veux	sais
il/elle/on	peut	doit	veut	sait
nous	pouvons	devons	voulons	savons
vous	pouvez	devez	voulez	savez
ils/elles	peuvent	doivent	veulent	savent

When modal verbs are followed by another verb, the latter is in the infinitive:

On doit accepter… We have to accept…
Tu peux regarder… You can watch…
Ils savent nager. They know how to swim.

7.2 The perfect tense

Use the perfect tense to express completed actions in the past, e.g. 'I played' or 'I have played'.

To form the perfect tense you need two parts: an auxiliary (a present tense form of *avoir* or *être*) and a past participle. Past participles are explained in 7.3.

Verbs which take *avoir*

Most verbs use the present tense of *avoir* (*j'ai, tu as, il a, nous avons, vous avez, ils ont*) to form the perfect tense.

*La délinquance **a diminué**.* Crime has diminished.

*Ils **ont résolu** le problème.* They solved the problem.

*Nous **avons pris** le train.* We took the train.

Verbs which take *être*

Some common verbs use the present tense of *être* to form the perfect tense instead (*je suis, tu es, il est, nous sommes, vous êtes, ils sont*).

*Je **suis allé** en ville.* I went to town.

*Il **est né** en 1890.* He was born in 1890.

You need to memorise which verbs take *être*; they are connected with movement or a change of state, and it can help to learn them in pairs as in the table below.

aller	*to go*	venir	*to come*
arriver	*to arrive*	partir	*to leave*
entrer	*to enter, to go in*	sortir	*to go out*
monter	*to go up*	descendre	*to go down*
naître	*to be born*	mourir	*to die*
retourner	*to return*	rentrer	*to go home*
rester	*to stay*	tomber	*to fall*
devenir	*to become*	revenir	*to come back*

Also all **reflexive verbs** form the perfect tense with *être*.

*Je **me suis** peu **intéressé** aux études.* I wasn't very interested in studying.

*Ils **se sont intégrés** facilement.* They fitted in easily.

With all these *être* verbs, the past participle must agree with the subject of the verb, adding a final *-e* for a feminine subject, *-s* for plural, *-es* for feminine plural.

*Les inégalités **sont devenues** plus évidentes.* The inequalities have become more obvious.

je suis parti/parti**e**	nous sommes parti**s**/
tu es parti/parti**e**	parti**es**
il est parti	vous êtes parti/parti**e**/
elle est parti**e**	parti**s**/parti**es**
on est parti/parti**e**/parti**s**/	ils sont parti**s**
parti**es**	elles sont parti**es**

7.3 The past participle

The past participle is a key element of compound tenses such as the perfect tense (see 7.2), the pluperfect (7.8), the future perfect (7.9) and the perfect infinitive (7.24).

For regular verbs it is formed as follows:

-er verbs – **é**	-ir verbs – **i**	-re verbs – **u**
trouver – **trouvé**	finir – **fini**	vendre – **vendu**

Some past participles are irregular and need to be learned:

English	infinitive	past participle
to have	avoir	**eu**
to drink	boire	**bu**
to know	connaître	**connu**
to run	courir	**couru**
to have to	devoir	**dû**
to say	dire	**dit**
to write	écrire	**écrit**
to be	être	**été**
to do	faire	**fait**
to read	lire	**lu**
to put	mettre	**mis**
to die	mourir	**mort**
to be born	naître	**né**
to open	ouvrir	**ouvert**
to be able	pouvoir	**pu**
to take	prendre	**pris**
to receive	recevoir	**reçu**
to know how to	savoir	**su**
to come	venir	**venu**
to live	vivre	**vécu**
to see	voir	**vu**
to want	vouloir	**voulu**

Past participles have an additional final *-e*, *-s* or *-es* to agree with the subject when *être* is the auxiliary used to form the perfect tense.

When *avoir* is the auxiliary, normally the past participle does not change... unless there is a direct object which comes before the verb. When this happens in the sentence, the past participle has to agree with the object (called a 'preceding direct object').

In the sentence below, *la Convention* is the direct object, represented by the pronoun *l'* which comes before the perfect tense of *signer*:

*On a élaboré la Convention de Genève et aujourd'hui près de 150 Etats **l'ont signée**.*
The Geneva Convention was drawn up and today nearly 150 states have signed it.

The past participle *signé* needs to be feminine, *signée*. (Note that *élaboré* does not need the feminine ending! It has a direct object, but not a preceding direct object.)

Another example:

*Où sont mes chaussures? Je **les ai mises** dans ta chambre.*
Where are my shoes? I put them in your bedroom.

Les is a direct object pronoun standing for *les chaussures* which are feminine plural, so the past participle has to agree. (Note that in this case the ending affects pronunciation: *mis* has a silent *s*, but *mise/mises* ends with a *z* sound.)

7.4 The imperfect tense

The imperfect tense is used for:

- a general description in the past, to translate 'she felt sad' or 'it was good'.

- a continuous or interrupted action in the past, to say 'I was watching TV (when…)'

- a repeated or habitual action in the past, e.g. 'I used to play netball' or 'I would play netball'.

See below (1–5) for other uses.

To form the imperfect tense, take the stem, which is the *nous* form of the present tense without the *-ons*, and add the endings shown in the table below.

avoir: nous avons ⟶ ***av-***

faire: nous faisons ⟶ ***fais-***

finir: nous finissons ⟶ ***finiss-***

attendre: nous attendons ⟶ ***attend-***

Exception: *être* ⟶ ***ét-***

	endings	example: faire
je	**-ais**	je faisais
tu	**-ais**	tu faisais
il/elle/on	**-ait**	il/elle/on faisait
nous	**-ions**	nous faisions
vous	**-iez**	vous faisiez
ils/elles	**-aient**	ils/elles faisaient

Further uses of the imperfect tense

1 The imperfect of *être en train de* + infinitive:

*J'**étais** en train de me lever quand on a sonné à la porte.*
I was just (in the middle of) getting up when the bell rang.

2 With *depuis*, meaning 'had been doing' (see 7.26):

*Ils **attendaient** depuis une heure quand le train est arrivé.*
They had been waiting for an hour when the train arrived.

3 The imperfect of *venir de* + infinitive to say 'had just done' (see 7.26):

*Nous **venions** d'arriver lorsqu'il a cessé de pleuvoir.*
We had just arrived when it stopped raining.

4 After *si* when the main verb is in the conditional:

*Si j'**avais** assez d'argent, je passerais mes vacances au Sénégal.*
If I had enough money, I would spend my holidays in Senegal.

5 After *si* when making a suggestion:

*Si on **sortait** ce soir?*
What if we went out this evening?

7.5 The immediate future

Use the immediate future to talk about the near future: to say something 'is going to' happen.

*Je **vais télécharger** cette chanson.*
I'm going to download this song.

It is made up of two parts: the present tense of *aller* (*je vais, tu vas, il va, nous allons, vous allez, ils vont*) and an infinitive.

7.6 The future tense

Use the future tense to make predictions and statements about the future: to say something 'will' happen.

*Ce projet **entraînera** des problèmes.*
This project will bring problems.

*On **finira** par comprendre.*
We will end up understanding.

*Les Américains **feront** beaucoup.*
The Americans will do a lot.

*On **devra** continuer la production.*
We will have to continue production.

Most verbs have a regular future tense. The future endings are the same for all three regular groups, and are added to the stem which is the same as the infinitive (for *-re* verbs remove the final *e* first).

	endings	regarder	choisir	répondre
je	**-ai**	regarderai	choisirai	répondrai
tu	**-as**	regarderas	choisiras	répondras
il/elle/on	**-a**	regardera	choisira	répondra
nous	**-ons**	regarderons	choisirons	répondrons
vous	**-ez**	regarderez	choisirez	répondrez
ils/elles	**-ont**	regarderont	choisiront	répondront

Irregular verbs

Some key verbs have an irregular future stem, so you need to learn these, but the endings are still regular.

aller	ir-	j'**ir**ai
avoir	aur-	j'**aur**ai
devoir	devr-	je **devr**ai
envoyer	enverr-	j'**enverr**ai
être	ser-	je **ser**ai
faire	fer-	je **fer**ai
pouvoir	pourr-	je **pourr**ai
savoir	saur-	je **saur**ai
venir	viendr-	je **viendr**ai
voir	verr-	je **verr**ai
vouloir	voudr-	je **voudr**ai
falloir	faudr-	(il) **faudr**a

7.7 The conditional

Use the conditional (strictly speaking, a 'mood' not a 'tense') to convey 'would', 'could' or 'should', i.e. to talk about what would happen or how something would be.

*Quel message **laisseriez**-vous?*
What message **would** you **leave**?

*Ce **serait** triste si tout le monde se ressemblait.*
It **would be** sad if we were all the same.

The conditional is also used (e.g. in journalism) to allege an unproven statement:
*Les Roms **seraient** entre deux et trois mille.*
There are said to be between two and three thousand Gypsies.

To form it, start with the future tense stem (see 7.6), and add the conditional endings, which are identical to the imperfect endings (see 7.4).

	endings	regarder	choisir	répondre
je	**-ais**	regarderais	choisirais	répondrais
tu	**-ais**	regarderais	choisirais	répondrais
il/elle/on	**-ait**	regarderait	choisirait	répondrait
nous	**-ions**	regarderions	choisirions	répondrions
vous	**-iez**	regarderiez	choisiriez	répondriez
ils/elles	**-aient**	regarderaient	choisiraient	répondraient

Because the conditional uses the same stem as the future tense, the irregular stems are exactly the same as for the future – see list in 7.6.

Modal verbs

The conditional forms of modal verbs are particularly useful and worth learning.

Devoir in the conditional + infinitive = should/ought to do
*On **devrait** trier les déchets.*
We should sort our refuse.

Pouvoir in the conditional + infinitive = could/might do
*Vous **pourriez** faire un don.*
You could make a donation.

Vouloir in the conditional + infinitive = would like to do
***Voudriez**-vous nous aider?*
Would you like to help us?

Il faut becomes *il faudrait* in the conditional = it should be necessary, we should do
*Il **faudrait** réduire nos besoins.*
We would have to reduce our needs.

Il vaut becomes *il vaudrait* = it would be worth, it would be better to
*Il **vaudrait** mieux résoudre ce problème.*
It would be better to solve this problem.

7.8 The pluperfect tense

As in English, the pluperfect is a compound tense used to talk about what 'had happened'.

*Il a dit qu'il **avait commencé** à jouer au handball à l'école.*
He said that he **had started** to play handball at school.

*Elle a expliqué qu'elle **était arrivée** trop tard.*
She explained that she **had arrived** too late.

The pluperfect is made up of two parts: the imperfect of *avoir* or *être* and a past participle. Past participles are explained in 7.3. As with the perfect tense, with *être* verbs, the past participle must agree with the subject.

avoir verbs e.g. faire	être verbs e.g. aller
j'avais fait	j'étais allé(e)
tu avais fait	tu étais allé(e)
il/elle/on avait fait	il/elle/on était allé(e)(s)
nous avions fait	nous étions allé(e)s
vous aviez fait	vous étiez allé(e)(s)
ils/elles avaient fait	ils/elles étaient allé(e)s

7.9 The future perfect tense

The future perfect expresses what 'will have happened' before another event or by a certain time in the future. It is formed from the future of *avoir* or *être* and a past participle.

*Dans une semaine, j'**aurai déposé** mes papiers.*
In a week, I **will have handed in** my papers.

*Demain, à cette heure, mon frère **sera arrivé**.*
By this time tomorrow, my brother **will have arrived**.

It is used after expressions such as *quand, dès que, après que, une fois que, aussitôt que, lorsque* when the verb in the main clause is in the future. (NB. This is different from English: see the first example below, where the English is not 'he will have arrived'.)

*Il m'appellera dès qu'il **sera arrivé**.*
He will phone me as soon as he **has arrived**.

It can express a supposition or a threat:

*Il **aura** encore **oublié**.* He'll have forgotten again.

*Tu l'**auras cherché**!*
You will have earned it!/It'll be your fault!

avoir verbs e.g. perdre	être verbs e.g. partir
j'aurai perdu *I will have lost*	je serai parti(e) *I will have left*
tu auras perdu	tu seras parti(e)
il/elle/on aura perdu	il/elle/on sera parti(e)(s)
nous aurons perdu	nous serons parti(e)s
vous aurez perdu	vous serez parti(e)(s)
ils/elles auront perdu	ils/elles seront parti(e)s

7.10 The conditional perfect

The conditional perfect expresses what 'would have happened'. It is formed from the <u>conditional</u> of *avoir* or *être* and a past participle.

*Il **aurait travaillé** un peu plus, si...*
He **would have worked** a bit more, if...

*Mathieu n'**aurait** pas **partagé** sa fortune, parce que...*
Mathieu **would**n't **have shared** his fortune, because...

*Il ne **serait** pas **devenu** footballeur professionnel.*
He **would**n't **have become** a professional footballer.

With *être*, remember to make the past participle agree with the subject, as in the perfect tense:

*A ce moment-là **elle** serait parti**e**.*
She would have left by then.

Note the useful conditional perfect forms of *devoir* and *pouvoir*, which express that something 'should have happened' and 'could have happened':

*Elle **aurait dû** partir plus tôt.*
She **should have** left earlier.

*Les immigrés **auraient pu** faire leur demande avant.*
The immigrants **could have** made their request before.

When there is an 'if' clause as well as a main clause in the conditional perfect, the 'if' clause is in the <u>pluperfect</u> tense, as in English:

*Il ne **serait** pas **devenu** footballeur s'il n'<u>avait</u> pas <u>eu</u> la chance d'être sportif.*
He **would**n't **have become** a footballer, if he <u>had</u>n't <u>had</u> the luck to be a sportsman.

avoir verbs e.g. perdre	être verbs e.g. partir
j'aurais perdu	je serais parti(e)
I would have lost	*I would have left*
tu aurais perdu	tu serais parti(e)
il/elle/on aurait perdu	il/elle/on serait parti(e)(s)
nous aurions perdu	nous serions parti(e)s
vous auriez perdu	vous seriez parti(e)(s)
ils/elles auraient perdu	ils/elles seraient parti(e)s

7.11 The past historic

The past historic (*le passé simple*) is the literary equivalent of the perfect tense. It is used only in <u>formal</u> writing (e.g. historical writing, novels and newspaper articles). You will hardly ever need to use it yourself, but it is important to be able to recognise and understand it.

*Le conflit algérien **provoqua** une crise morale.*
The Algerian conflict provoked a moral crisis.

*Il **reçut** une lettre.* He received a letter.

*La réputation de la France **souffrit**.*
France's reputation suffered.

All -*er* verbs (including *aller*) follow the pattern shown for *regarder* in the table. Regular -*ir* and -*re* verbs have the endings shown for *répondre*. Many irregular verbs have the endings shown for *recevoir*.

	regarder	répondre	recevoir
je	regard**ai**	répond**is**	reç**us**
tu	regard**as**	répond**is**	reç**us**
il/elle/on	regard**a**	répond**it**	reç**ut**
nous	regard**âmes**	répond**îmes**	reç**ûmes**
vous	regard**âtes**	répond**îtes**	reç**ûtes**
ils/elles	regard**èrent**	répond**irent**	reç**urent**

Note these irregular verbs:

avoir	j'eus, il eut, ils eurent
être	je fus, il fut, ils furent
faire	je fis, il fit, ils firent
voir	je vis, il vit, ils virent
venir	je vins, il vint, ils vinrent

7.12 The subjunctive mood

The subjunctive and indicative parts of the verb are known as <u>moods</u> of the verb, not tenses; they convey the speaker's attitude to the action described.

The subjunctive is nearly always used in a subordinate clause, i.e. the second part of a sentence, introduced by *que*. It is used when statements are not to be taken as pure fact, but more as a matter of judgement or attitude.

1   It is used after conjunctions including these:
    avant que before
    après que after
    bien que although
    quoique although
    afin que so that
    pour que so that
    de façon que in such a way that
    sans que without
    *... **avant qu'il** ne **soit** trop tard.*
    ... before it is too late. (Formal French adds *ne*.)
    *Il faut transformer les véhicules **pour qu'ils soient** moins gourmands en énergie.*
    We have to transform vehicles so that they consume less energy.

2   It is used after impersonal verbs including these:
    il faut que
    il est nécessaire/impératif/essentiel que
    *Il est important **que nous changions** nos véhicules...* It's important that we change our vehicles...

3 It is used after expressions of wish, doubt, fear, uncertainty, regret:

je veux que

je voudrais que

je ne pense pas que

pensez-vous que… ?

on craint que

il est possible que

il se peut que

je regrette que

je suis désolé(e) que

j'ai honte que

*Je ne pense pas **que cela soit** possible.*
I don't think that is possible.

NB. It is <u>not</u> used after expressions of probability (where there is little doubt), so the following require a verb in the indicative ('normal' not subjunctive): *il est probable que, il est certain que, il me paraît que, il me semble que*.

4 It is used after words with a sense of the superlative, followed by *qui* or *que*:

le seul, l'unique, le premier, le dernier, le meilleur

*C'est **la seule** espèce **qui puisse** résister.*
It's the only species that can resist.

7.13 The present subjunctive

For most regular verbs, the present subjunctive is formed from the stem – the *ils/elles* form of the present tense minus the final *-ent* – plus the endings *-e, -es, -e, -ions, -iez, -ent*.

Example: *finir*
present tense: *ils finissent*
stem *finiss-*
present subjunctive: *je finisse, tu finisses, il finisse, nous finissions, vous finissiez, ils finissent*

Note that the *nous* and *vous* forms are the same as the imperfect (indicative) tense.

Irregular forms worth learning:

aller	aille, ailles, aille, allions, alliez, aillent
avoir	aie, aies, ait, ayons, ayez, aient
être	sois, sois, soit, soyons, soyez, soient
faire	fasse, fasses, fasse, fassions, fassiez, fassent
falloir	il faille
pouvoir	puisse, puisses, puisse, puissions, puissiez, puissent
savoir	sache, saches, sache, sachions, sachiez, sachent
vouloir	veuille, veuilles, veuille, voulions, vouliez, veuillent

7.14 The perfect subjunctive

In sentences that need the subjunctive, it may be necessary to use the perfect subjunctive, not the present subjunctive. This is when it expresses something that happened in the past, before the verb in the main clause. The perfect subjunctive is formed from *avoir* or *être* in the subjunctive and a past participle.

*Bien qu'elle **ait perdu** 15 kilos,...*
Although she has lost 15 kg,...

*Je suis désolé que mon fils **ait agressé** ce garçon.*
I'm sorry that my son attacked this boy.

*Cette production est la meilleure que je **aie** jamais **vue**.* This production is the best I've ever seen.

*Il se peut qu'**elle soit** déjà **partie**.*
It's possible that she has already left.

*Je regrette que cet incident **se soit passé**.*
I'm sorry this incident has taken place.

avoir verbs e.g. voir	être verbs e.g. aller
j'aie vu	je sois allé(e)
tu aies vu	tu sois allé(e)
il/elle/on ait vu	il/elle/on soit allé(e)(s)
nous ayons vu	nous soyons allé(e)s
vous ayez vu	vous soyez allé(e)(s)
ils/elles aient vu	ils/elles soient allé(e)s

7.15 The imperfect subjunctive

This is used in literature and formal writing; you need to be able to recognise and understand it. It is formed by adding the endings shown in the table below to the stem; the stem is the *il/elle* part of the past historic (see 7.11), without any final *t*.

	endings	example: parler (il parla)	example: finir (il finit)
je	-sse	je parlasse	je finisse
tu	-sses	tu parlasses	tu finisses
il/elle/on	-^t	il/elle/on parlât	il/elle/on finît
nous	-ssions	nous parlassions	nous finissions
vous	-ssiez	vous parlassiez	vous finissiez
ils/elles	-ssent	ils/elles parlassent	ils/elles finissent

7.16 The passive voice

The passive voice describes an event without necessarily mentioning who is responsible for it: I <u>was attacked</u>; that car <u>has been sold</u>; the building <u>had been closed</u>. (To specify who or what the action has been done by, add *par...* as in some of the examples below.)

They contrast with verbs in the <u>active</u> voice, where the subject carries out the action in the verb: I <u>attacked</u> the task; they <u>have sold</u> that car; someone <u>had closed</u> the building.

Use an appropriate form of *être* plus a past participle (see 7.3) which must agree with the subject. *Etre* can be in any tense; see the underlined words in the examples.

- present: *Les océans **sont pollués** par les accidents de pétroliers.* The oceans are polluted by oil tanker accidents.

- perfect: *La récolte **a été détruite**.* The harvest has been destroyed.

- imperfect: *Il **était** toujours **surpris** par les chiffres.* He was always surprised by the figures.

- pluperfect: *Des candidats **avaient été exclus**.* Candidates had been excluded.

- future: *Des coopérations **seront organisées**.* Joint operations will be organised.

Avoiding the passive

The passive is used less often in French than in English. It's usually better to avoid it in French, and use instead an expression with *on* or a reflexive verb.

***On** m'a agressé(e).* I was attacked.

***On** avait exclu des candidats.* Candidates had been excluded.

*Les produits **se vendent** sur Internet.* The products are sold on the internet.

Note that, in particular, the passive cannot be used to translate English phrases such as 'I was asked...' and 'they were given...' In French these would need to be reworded to use *on*:

On m'a demandé... On leur a offert...

7.17 The imperative

The imperative is used to give instructions and commands. They are positive ('do...') or negative ('don't...'). They can be informal (*tu* form) or formal (*vous* form), or a suggestion (*nous* form).

All you have to do is remove the subject pronoun from the <u>present</u> tense. With -*er* verbs, for the *tu* form, remove the final *s*.

present tense	imperative
-er verbs	
tu regardes	**Regarde** la télé. *Watch TV.*
nous regardons	**Regardons** le film. *Let's watch the film.*
vous regardez	**Regardez** les spots. *Watch the ads.*
-ir verbs	
tu choisis	**Choisis** un produit. *Choose a product.*
nous choisissons	**Choisissons** un cadeau. *Let's choose a gift.*
vous choisissez	**Choisissez** une émission. *Choose a programme.*
-re verbs	
tu prends	**Prends** une photo. *Take a photo.*
nous prenons	**Prenons** une glace. *Let's have an ice cream.*
vous prenez	**Prenez** de l'argent. *Take some money.*

A few verbs have irregular imperatives and need to be learned separately.

avoir	aie, ayons, ayez
être	sois, soyons, soyez
savoir	sache, sachons, sachez
vouloir	veuille, veuillons, veuillez

The *tu* form of *aller* is *va*, except in the expression *vas-y!* (go on!) where the *s* is pronounced like a *z*.

Reflexive verbs always require the extra reflexive pronoun, placed after the verb:

se dépêcher to hurry (up)
dépêche-toi, dépêchons-nous, dépêchez-vous

7.18 Present participles

The present participle can by used by itself, at the beginning of a sentence, to express the idea of 'because' or 'since':

***Croyant** qu'il s'était trompé de chemin, il a fait demi-tour.* Thinking that he'd taken the wrong route, he turned round.

It can also be used after the preposition ***en***:

*... **en faisant** éclater les frontières culturelles* ... while breaking down cultural barriers

***En se connectant**, on peut accéder à tout.* By going online, you can access everything.

It is formed from the *nous* form of the present tense, changing the -*ons* to -*ant*.

faire → *nous faisons* → *en faisant*

connecter → *nous connectons* → *en connectant*

For reflexive verbs, use a reflexive pronoun appropriate to the context: *en me connectant, je peux...*

7.19 Direct and indirect speech

Direct speech is used for the actual words being said; they often appear within speech marks.

Il a dit: « Il y a des problèmes de logement. »
He said: 'There are housing problems.'

Indirect speech is when someone's words are reported by the speaker or someone else.

Il a dit qu'il y avait des problèmes de logement.
He said there were housing problems.

Verb tenses have to change when you use **indirect speech** – see examples in the grid below.

direct speech	indirect speech
Je **suis** paresseux. *present*	Il a dit qu'il **était** paresseux. *imperfect*
Je **ferai** plus attention la prochaine fois. *future*	Il a dit qu'il **ferait** plus attention la prochaine fois. *conditional*
J'**ai commencé** à jouer à l'école. *perfect*	Il a dit qu'il **avait commencé** à l'école. *pluperfect*
Demain, j'**aurai préparé** mes affaires. *future perfect*	Il a dit que le lendemain, il **aurait préparé** ses affaires. *conditional perfect*

Pronouns and possessive adjectives may also need to change, from first to third person: *je* becomes *il* or *elle*, *mes affaires* becomes *ses affaires*, and so on.

In text containing **direct speech**, the verb and subject are inverted after the words spoken, so *il a dit* becomes *a-t-il dit* or *a dit + nom*. (See page 121.)

« J'ai appris à jouer à l'âge de onze ans », a dit le prof.

« J'en suis devenue accro », a-t-elle dit.

7.20 Reflexive verbs

Reflexive verbs are conjugated in the same way as other verbs, but have a reflexive pronoun between subject and verb: *me, te, se, nous, vous, se*.

*Je **m'intéresse** à la communication.*
I'm interested in communicating.

s'intéresser to be interested	
je m'intéresse	nous **nous** intéressons
tu **t'**intéresses	vous **vous** intéressez
il/elle/on **s'**intéresse	ils/elles **s'**intéressent

In the perfect tense, reflexive verbs take *être* and the past participle agrees with the subject:

*On s'est bien entendu**s**/entendu**es**.*
We (masc./fem.) got on well.

The infinitive usually begins with *se* or *s'*, but when it is used in a sentence the pronoun changes to agree with the subject of the main verb:

*Je voudrais **me doucher**.* I'd like to have a shower.

In a positive command, the reflexive pronoun is attached to the end of the imperative:

*Asseyez-**vous**!* Sit down!

But in a negative command, the reflexive pronoun stays in its usual place in front of the verb:

*Ne **vous** asseyez pas!* Don't sit down!

7.21 Impersonal verbs

As well as *il y a* (there is/are) and *il reste* (there's... left), there are other impersonal verbs used only in the *il* form, the third person singular.

il est trois heures, il pleut, il fait mauvais – and other time and weather phrases

il faut... it is necessary to...

il vaut mieux... it's worth...

il est + adjectif (clair/important/essentiel, etc.) + de/que

They can be used in other tenses:

Il y aura *plus de prisons engorgées.*

Il était évident que *le taux de criminalité avait chuté.*

7.22 Infinitive constructions

You often need to use the infinitive form of a verb, particularly when it follows another verb or a preposition. The lists below give some instances.

Verbs followed by the infinitive with no preposition between

aimer	*to like to*
croire	*to believe*
devoir	*to have to*
espérer	*to hope*
faire	*to make, to do*
falloir	*to be necessary*
laisser	*to let*
oser	*to dare*
penser	*to think*
pouvoir	*to be able*
préférer	*to prefer*
savoir	*to know how to*
vouloir	*to want to*

*J'espère **finir** bientôt.* I hope to finish soon.

*Il **faut comprendre** que...*
You have to understand that...

*On **peut faire** de la publicité en ligne.*
You can advertise on line.

Verbs followed by *à* + infinitive

aider à	*to help to*
apprendre à	*to learn to*
arriver à	*to manage to*
chercher à	*to try to*
commencer à	*to begin to*
continuer à	*to continue to*
encourager à	*to encourage to*
hésiter à	*to hesitate to*
penser à	*to think of*
réussir à	*to succeed in*

On **commence à prendre** conscience du déclin.
We're beginning to take note of the decline.

Verbs followed by *de* + infinitive

accepter de	*to agree to*
s'arrêter de	*to stop*
avoir envie de	*to feel like*
avoir le droit de	*to have the right to*
avoir peur de	*to be afraid to*
cesser de	*to stop*
choisir de	*to choose*
décider de	*to decide*
empêcher de	*to prevent*
essayer de	*to try*
éviter de	*to avoid*
finir de	*to finish*
oublier de	*to forget*
refuser de	*to refuse*
rêver de	*to dream of*
risquer de	*to be likely to*
venir de	*to have just*

J'ai **décidé de cesser de fumer** l'année dernière.
I decided to stop smoking last year.

Prepositions + infinitive

au lieu de	*instead of*
afin de	*so as to*
avant de	*before*
par	*by*
pour	*in order to*
sans	*without*
sur le point de	*about to*

afin d'apaiser les banlieues... in order to appease the suburbs...
sans compter le coût... without counting the cost...

7.23 Dependent infinitives

Faire + infinitive indicates that the subject 'causes' an action to be done by someone or something else. Compare the following examples:

Je répare la douche. I'm repairing the shower (myself).

Je fais réparer la douche. I'm getting the shower repaired, i.e. I'm getting someone round to repair the shower.

Faire may be used in any tense, for example:

Je vais faire réparer la douche.
I'm going to get the shower repaired.

J'ai fait réparer la douche.
I've had the shower repaired.

Other examples:

faire construire to have something built

faire penser: *Cela me fait penser à...*
That makes me think of...

faire comprendre: *Cela nous a fait comprendre que...*
It has made us understand that...

se faire + infinitive
This indicates that the subject gets something done to or for himself/herself.

se faire embaucher: *Il s'est fait embaucher dans une usine.*
He got a job/got himself employed in a factory.

se faire renvoyer: *Je me suis fait renvoyer.*
I got myself sacked.

se faire faire: *Je me suis fait faire un petit potager.*
I had a little vegetable garden made for me.

7.24 Perfect infinitives

The perfect infinitive is used after *après* to convey 'after doing' or 'after having done' something. (The French structure is more like 'after to have done...'.) Use the infinitive of *avoir* or *être* and a past participle. The normal rules about past participle agreement apply.

*Après **avoir réfléchi**, je pars quand même.*
After reflecting, I'm leaving all the same.

*Après **être arrivée**, elle a défait ses valises.*
After arriving, she unpacked her cases.

*Après **avoir eu** des problèmes avec les agences, je veux voyager à ma guise.* Having had problems with travel agencies, I like to travel under my own steam.

7.25 Negatives

To say you don't do something, simply put *ne* before the verb (or in a compound tense, before the auxiliary verb) and *pas* after it.

*Je **ne** fais **pas** de sport.* I don't do any sport.

*Je **n'**ai **pas** fait de sport hier.*
I didn't do any sport yesterday.

*Je **ne** suis **pas** allé(e) au centre sportif.*
I didn't go to the sports centre.

Other negative expressions:

ne… plus	no more/no longer	Je ne fume plus.
ne… jamais	never	Je ne joue jamais au rugby.
ne… rien	nothing	Ils ne font rien.
ne… personne	no-one, nobody	Elle n'aime personne.
ne… que	only	Il n'en reste que deux.
ne… aucun(e)	not any	Il n'en reste aucun.
ne… nulle part	nowhere	On ne va nulle part.
ne… ni… ni…	neither… nor…	Je n'aime ni le tennis ni le cricket.

In the perfect tense, the negative expression goes around *avoir* or *être*, except *ne… personne/aucun/que* where it goes round both parts of the verb:

*Je **n'ai jamais** joué au handball.*
I've never played handball.

*Il **n'a vu personne**.* He did not see anyone.

*Je **n'**en **ai acheté que** cinq.*
I've bought only five of them.

If you want to make an infinitive negative, the negative expression comes before the infinitive:

*Il a décidé de **ne plus jouer** au tennis.*
He decided to not play tennis any more.

*Il est important de **ne rien déranger**.*
It is important not to disturb anything.

7.26 Using *depuis* and *venir de*

depuis

Depuis means 'since' or 'for (a time)' in the past. If the action is still going on, use it with the present tense:

*Je **vais** à la pêche depuis l'âge de huit ans.*
I've been going fishing since I was eight.

*Elle **apprend** le français depuis six mois.*
She's been learning French for six months.

If the action lasted for some time but is now over, use *depuis* with the imperfect tense:

*J'**attendais** le bus depuis dix minutes.*
I had been waiting for the bus for 10 minutes.

venir de

Venir de in the present tense is used to convey the idea of something that has just happened:

*Je **viens** d'arriver.* I've **just** arrived.

*Elle **vient** de me le dire.* She's just told me.

*Nous **venons** d'apprendre la nouvelle.*
We've just heard the news.

Use the imperfect tense of *venir de* to say something had just happened:

*Je **venais** de finir mon dîner, quand…*
I had just finished my dinner, when…

8 Prepositions

8.1 *à, de*

Remember that when *à* or *de* come before a definite article (*le, la, l', les*), they may need to change:

	masc.	fem.	before vowel or silent h	masc. plural	fem. plural
à	au	à la	à l'	aux	aux
de	du	de la	de l'	des	des

*Je vais **au cinéma** une fois par mois.*
I go to the cinema once a month.

*J'adore aller **aux magasins** le week-end.*
I love going to the shops at the weekend.

*Le lycée se trouve en face **de l'hôtel**.*
The school is opposite the hotel.

*J'habite tout près **des magasins**.*
I live right near the shops.

8.2 Other prepositions

après	after
avant	before
avec	with
chez	at the house of
dans	in
depuis	for / since
derrière	behind
devant	in front of
en face de	opposite
en	in / by / on / to
entre	between
par	by / per
pendant	during
pour	for
près de	near
sans	without
sous	under
sur	on
vers	about / towards

Certain prepositions in French are used in the same way as their English equivalents:

*J'aime mieux partir **en** vacances **avec** mes copains.*
I prefer to go **on** holiday **with** my friends.

*Il est arrivé **à** l'aéroport **sans** passeport.*
He arrived **at** the airport **without** a passport.

However, in many cases, the choice of the correct preposition needs some thought, and a good dictionary can help here.

dans le train on the train; *sous la pluie* in the rain; *à la télévision* on the television

For holiday destinations, note the following:

- feminine countries require *en* for to/in:
en France, en Hollande
- masculine countries take *au*:
au Japon, au Canada
- masculine plurals take *aux*:
aux Etats-Unis, aux Pays-Bas
- towns and islands take *à*:
à Paris, à Madagascar

9 Conjunctions

Conjunctions (also called connectives) link parts of sentences. Some common ones are listed below.

mais	but
au contraire	on the contrary
par contre	on the other hand
pourtant, cependant, quand même	however
néanmoins, tout de même	nevertheless
car, comme, parce que, puisque	for, since, because
vu que	seeing that
d'autant plus que	all the more since
dans la mesure où	insofar as
d'ailleurs, de plus	besides, moreover
donc, alors, par conséquent	and so, therefore
en fait, en effet	in fact
bien sûr	of course
certes	certainly
d'abord	first of all
puis, ensuite	then
enfin	finally
de toute façon, en tout cas	in any case

10 Interrogatives

To ask a 'yes/no' question, you can:

- use rising intonation (*Vous aimez cette musique?*)
- start with *est-ce que* (*Est-ce que vous aimez cette musique?*)
- invert pronoun and verb (*Aimez-vous cette musique?*).

To ask for other information, you need an interrogative adverb, pronoun or adjective, as listed below.

quand	when	Quand est-ce qu'il arrive?
où	where	Où es-tu allé en vacances?
comment	how	Comment va-t-elle voyager?
combien	how many / how much	Combien de pages y a-t-il?
pourquoi	why	Pourquoi est-ce que tu fais ça?
qui	who	Qui va en ville?
que	what	Que dit-il?
quoi	what (after a preposition)	Avec quoi?
quel	which, what	Quels fruits aimez-vous?
lequel	which one(s)	Lequel préférez-vous?

Asking about people: 'who?'

Qui or *Qui est-ce qui* is used to ask about the subject of the verb:

Qui parle? Qui est-ce qui parle? Who's speaking?

Qui or *Qui est-ce que* is used to ask about the object of the verb:

Qui as-tu appelé? Qui est-ce que tu as appelé? Who did you call?

Asking about things: 'what?'

Qu'est-ce qui is used to ask about the subject of the verb:

Qu'est-ce qui est biodégradable? What is biodegradable?

Que or *Qu'est-ce que* is used to ask about the object of the verb:

Que faites-vous des déchets?/Qu'est-ce que vous faites des déchets?
What do you do with the rubbish?

Use *quoi* when the object of the sentence is preceded by a preposition:

*Vous le faites **avec quoi**?* What do you do that with?

Quoi is also used in *C'est quoi?* (What is it?), an informal alternative to *Qu'est-ce que c'est?*

Asking 'which?'

Quel is an adjective and must agree with the noun it qualifies: *quel, quelle, quels, quelles.*

A quelle heure...? At what time...?
En quelle année est-il né? In which year was he born?
Quels sports faites-vous? Which sports do you do?

Asking 'which one?'

Lequel must agree with the noun it represents: *lequel, laquelle, lesquels, lesquelles*.

Je cherche une auberge. Laquelle recommandez-vous? Which one do you recommend?

When *lequel* etc. follow *à* or *de*, they contract: see grid for *lequel* as a relative pronoun, page 108.

11 Word order: inversion of subject and verb

In French, the normal word order is: <u>subject</u> (a noun or pronoun) followed by <u>verb</u>:

<u>On</u> <u>va</u> en ville. We're going to town.

With some **question** forms, and following quotations in **direct speech**, there is inversion, i.e. the subject and the verb swap places. Between two vowels, add a *t* with hyphens:

« *Où <u>va-t-on</u>?* » *<u>demanda-t-il</u>.*
'Where are we going?' he asked.

« *En ville* » *<u>répondit-elle</u>.* 'To town,' she replied.

Some **adverbs** and **adverbial phrases** at the beginning of a clause trigger <u>subject-verb inversion</u>.

Toujours *<u>est-il</u> qu'on risque de laisser des empreintes électroniques en se connectant.*
Nevertheless, the fact remains that you might leave electronic fingerprints when you log on.

C'est risqué: ***du moins*** *<u>peut-on</u> se protéger des virus.*
It's risky – at least you can protect yourself against viruses.

En vain *<u>s'oppose-t-on</u> à la technologie.*
In vain people are opposed to technology.

(Alternatively, you can often keep normal word order by placing the adverb later in the sentence: *On s'oppose* ***en vain*** *à la technologie.*)

In longer sentences, the subject may be repeated as a pronoun (*il/elle*, etc.) and that is inverted with the verb rather than the full subject:

Rarement *les automobilistes <u>peuvent-ils</u> excéder la vitesse sans surveillance.*
Motorists are rarely able to break the speed limit without being watched by cameras.

Aussi *les systèmes de navigation par satellite en voiture <u>sont-ils</u> dangereux.*
Therefore, satellite navigation systems in cars are dangerous.

With *peut-être* (perhaps) and *sans doute* (no doubt, of course) you have to either use inversion or add *que* and use normal word order. So in the following pairs, both sentences are correct:

Peut-être **augmenteront-ils** *la surveillance.*
Peut-être **qu'ils augmenteront** *la surveillance.*
Perhaps they'll increase surveillance.

Sans doute les avances **comportent-elles** *des problèmes aussi.*
Sans doute **que les avances comportent** *des problèmes aussi.*
No doubt, advances also bring problems.

12 Verb tables

		present	perfect	imperfect	future	conditional	subjunctive
REGULAR VERBS							
-er verbs **jouer** *to play*	je/j'	joue	ai joué	jouais	jouerai	jouerais	joue
	tu	joues	as joué	jouais	joueras	jouerais	joues
	il/elle/on	joue	a joué	jouait	jouera	jouerait	joue
	nous	jouons	avons joué	jouions	jouerons	jouerions	jouions
	vous	jouez	avez joué	jouiez	jouerez	joueriez	jouiez
	ils/elles	jouent	ont joué	jouaient	joueront	joueraient	jouent
-ir verbs **finir** *to finish*	je/j'	finis	ai fini	finissais	finirai	finirais	finisse
	tu	finis	as fini	finissais	finiras	finirais	finisses
	il/elle/on	finit	a fini	finissait	finira	finirait	finisse
	nous	finissons	avons fini	finissions	finirons	finirions	finissions
	vous	finissez	avez fini	finissiez	finirez	finiriez	finissiez
	ils/elles	finissent	ont fini	finissaient	finiront	finiraient	finissent
-re verbs **vendre** *to sell*	je/j'	vends	ai vendu	vendais	vendrai	vendrais	vende
	tu	vends	as vendu	vendais	vendras	vendrais	vendes
	il/elle/on	vend	a vendu	vendait	vendra	vendrait	vende
	nous	vendons	avons vendu	vendions	vendrons	vendrions	vendions
	vous	vendez	avez vendu	vendiez	vendrez	vendriez	vendiez
	ils/elles	vendent	ont vendu	vendaient	vendront	vendraient	vendent
reflexive verbs **s'amuser** *to enjoy yourself*	je	m'amuse	me suis amusé(e)	m'amusais	m'amuserai	m'amuserais	m'amuse
	tu	t'amuses	t'es amusé(e)	t'amusais	t'amuseras	t'amuserais	t'amuses
	il/elle/on	s'amuse	s'est amusé(e)(s)	s'amusait	s'amusera	s'amuserait	s'amuse
	nous	nous amusons	nous sommes amusé(e)s	nous amusions	nous amuserons	nous amuserions	nous amusions
	vous	vous amusez	vous êtes amusé(e)(s)	vous amusiez	vous amuserez	vous amuseriez	vous amusiez
	ils/elles	s'amusent	se sont amusé(e)s	s'amusaient	s'amuseront	s'amuseraient	s'amusent
IRREGULAR VERBS							
aller *to go*	je/j'	vais	suis allé(e)	allais	irai	irais	aille
	tu	vas	es allé(e)	allais	iras	irais	ailles
	il/elle/on	va	est allé(e)(s)	allait	ira	irait	aille
	nous	allons	sommes allé(e)s	allions	irons	irions	allions
	vous	allez	êtes allé(e)(s)	alliez	irez	iriez	alliez
	ils/elles	vont	sont allé(e)s	allaient	iront	iraient	aillent
avoir *to have*	je/j'	ai	ai eu	avais	aurai	aurais	aie
	tu	as	as eu	avais	auras	aurais	aies
	il/elle/on	a	a eu	avait	aura	aurait	ait
	nous	avons	avons eu	avions	aurons	aurions	ayons
	vous	avez	avez eu	aviez	aurez	auriez	ayez
	ils/elles	ont	ont eu	avaient	auront	auraient	aient
devoir *to have to / must*	je/j'	dois	ai dû	devais	devrai	devrais	doive
	tu	dois	as dû	devais	devras	devrais	doives
	il/elle/on	doit	a dû	devait	devra	devrait	doive
	nous	devons	avons dû	devions	devrons	devrions	devions
	vous	devez	avez dû	deviez	devrez	devriez	deviez
	ils/elles	doivent	ont dû	devaient	devront	devraient	doivent
dire *to say / to tell*	je/j'	dis	ai dit	disais	dirai	dirais	dise
	tu	dis	as dit	disais	diras	dirais	dises
	il/elle/on	dit	a dit	disait	dira	dirait	dise
	nous	disons	avons dit	disions	dirons	dirions	disions
	vous	dites	avez dit	disiez	direz	diriez	disiez
	ils/elles	disent	ont dit	disaient	diront	diraient	disent

		present	perfect	imperfect	future	conditional	subjunctive
être *to be*	je/j'	suis	ai été	étais	serai	serais	sois
	tu	es	as été	étais	seras	serais	sois
	il/elle/on	est	a été	était	sera	serait	soit
	nous	sommes	avons été	étions	serons	serions	soyons
	vous	êtes	avez été	étiez	serez	seriez	soyez
	ils/elles	sont	ont été	étaient	seront	seraient	soient
faire *to do / to* *make*	je/j'	fais	ai fait	faisais	ferai	ferais	fasse
	tu	fais	as fait	faisais	feras	ferais	fasses
	il/elle/on	fait	a fait	faisait	fera	ferait	fasse
	nous	faisons	avons fait	faisions	ferons	ferions	fassions
	vous	faites	avez fait	faisiez	ferez	feriez	fassiez
	ils/elles	font	ont fait	faisaient	feront	feraient	fassent
mettre *to put*	je/j'	mets	ai mis	mettais	mettrai	mettrais	mette
	tu	mets	as mis	mettais	mettras	mettrais	mettes
	il/elle/on	met	a mis	mettait	mettra	mettrait	mette
	nous	mettons	avons mis	mettions	mettrons	mettrions	mettions
	vous	mettez	avez mis	mettiez	mettrez	mettriez	mettiez
	ils/elles	mettent	ont mis	mettaient	mettront	mettraient	mettent
pouvoir *to be able to* */ can*	je/j'	peux	ai pu	pouvais	pourrai	pourrais	puisse
	tu	peux	as pu	pouvais	pourras	pourrais	puisses
	il/elle/on	peut	a pu	pouvait	pourra	pourrait	puisse
	nous	pouvons	avons pu	pouvions	pourrons	pourrions	puissions
	vous	pouvez	avez pu	pouviez	pourrez	pourriez	puissiez
	ils/elles	peuvent	ont pu	pouvaient	pourront	pourraient	puissent
prendre *to take*	je/j'	prends	ai pris	prenais	prendrai	prendrais	prenne
	tu	prends	as pris	prenais	prendras	prendrais	prennes
	il/elle/on	prend	a pris	prenait	prendra	prendrait	prenne
	nous	prenons	avons pris	prenions	prendrons	prendrions	prenions
	vous	prenez	avez pris	preniez	prendrez	prendriez	preniez
	ils/elles	prennent	ont pris	prenaient	prendront	prendraient	prennent
sortir *to go out*	je	sors	suis sorti(e)	sortais	sortirai	sortirais	sorte
	tu	sors	es sorti(e)	sortais	sortiras	sortirais	sortes
	il/elle/on	sort	est sorti(e)(s)	sortait	sortira	sortirait	sorte
	nous	sortons	sommes sorti(e)s	sortions	sortirons	sortirions	sortions
	vous	sortez	êtes sorti(e)(s)	sortiez	sortirez	sortiriez	sortiez
	ils/elles	sortent	sont sorti(e)s	sortaient	sortiront	sortiraient	sortent
venir *to come*	je	viens	suis venu(e)	venais	viendrai	viendrais	vienne
	tu	viens	es venu(e)	venais	viendras	viendrais	viennes
	il/elle/on	vient	est venu(e)(s)	venait	viendra	viendrait	vienne
	nous	venons	sommes venu(e)s	venions	viendrons	viendrions	venions
	vous	venez	êtes venu(e)(s)	veniez	viendrez	viendriez	veniez
	ils/elles	viennent	sont venu(e)s	venaient	viendront	viendraient	viennent
vouloir *to want*	je/j'	veux	ai voulu	voulais	voudrai	voudrais	veuille
	tu	veux	as voulu	voulais	voudras	voudrais	veuilles
	il/elle/on	veut	a voulu	voulait	voudra	voudrait	veuille
	nous	voulons	avons voulu	voulions	voudrons	voudrions	voulions
	vous	voulez	avez voulu	vouliez	voudrez	voudriez	vouliez
	ils/elles	veulent	ont voulu	voulaient	voudront	voudraient	veuillent

Glossaire

A

à son insu *without him/her knowing*

aboutir *to end up*

accepter de *to agree to*

accorder *to grant, to allow*

l' accueil (m) *reception, welcome*

accusé *accused*

actif *(of) working (age)*

actuel *topical*

un adhérent *member*

adhérer à *to join, to be a member of*

affamé *starving*

une agence d'intérim *temping agency*

alimenter *to feed*

alléger *to lessen, relieve*

un amant *lover*

améliorer *to improve*

une amende *fine*

une animatrice *sales / promotion staff*

apaiser *to quell, to appease*

arriver à *to manage to*

un asile *asylum*

une association caritative *charitable foundation, charity*

atteigne: *subj. of* atteindre *reach*

atteindre *to reach*

atteint *affected*

une atteinte *attempt, attack*

augmenter *to increase*

l' automobiliste (m/f) *motorist*

l' avidité (f) *greed*

avoir du mal à *to have dificulty in*

avoir la cote (fam.) *to be very popular / highly rated*

un ayant droit *a person entitled to something*

B

la balade *a walk*

la banlieue *suburb*

bannir *to banish*

le barrage *dam*

le/la bénévole *volunteer*

le beur *2nd generation North African living in France*

le bidonville *shanty town*

les biens (mpl) *goods, property*

biodégradable *biodegradable*

bosser (fam.) *to work*

le bouc émissaire *scapegoat*

bouleverser *to upset*

le brevet *certificate, diploma*

brûlé *burnt*

le BTS: Brevet de technicien supérieur *vocational training certificate taken after the age of 18*

C

le cadre *setting*

le cambriolage *burglary*

caritatif *charitable*

le CDD: contrat à durée déterminée *fixed-term contract*

le CDI: contrat à durée indéterminée *permanent contract*

cependant *however*

le charbon *coal*

la chasse *hunting*

chasser *to drive out*

le châtiment *punishment*

le chef de rayon *department supervisor*

le chiffon *rag*

le chiffre *figure*

le chômage *unemployment*

le chômeur *an unemployed person*

la chute d'eau *waterfall*

la cible *target*

ciblé sur *targeted at*

la circulation routière *road traffic*

citer *to quote*

le citoyen *citizen*

la citoyenneté *citizenship*

le clochard *tramp*

se coincer *to get stuck*

commencer par *to start by*

commettre *to commit*

compte tenu de *considering, in view of*

D

la conduite *driving*

confier *to entrust*

connu *well known*

consacré à *dedicated to*

la couche d'ozone *the ozone layer*

coupable *guilty*

le/la coupable *guilty person*

la cour d'appel *court of appeal*

la coutume *custom*

les crapules (fpl) *scum, riffraff*

la critique *criticism*

la croissance *growth*

croître *to grow*

la croix gammée *swastika*

davantage *more*

déboiser *to deforest*

la décennie *decade*

décevoir (pp. déçu) *to disappoint*

la déchéance *decline*

les déchets (mpl) *waste, refuse*

la déchetterie *rubbish tip*

le déchirement *tear, breakdown*

déclencher *to trigger*

le décryptage du génome *decoding of the human genome*

la défaite *defeat*

le défaut *fault*

défavorisé *underprivileged*

se défendre *to defend oneself*

la dégradation *worsening*

la délinquance *crime, criminality*

la délinquance juvénile *juvenile delinquency*

le délit *offence*

déménager *to move house*

le dénouement *outcome*

dépendant de *dependent on*

le déplacement *travel*

déprimant *depressing*

déranger *to disturb*

le déroulement *development*

désespéré *in despair*

désormais *from now on*

la détente *relaxation*

le discours *speech*

disloqué *disembodied*

disparaître *disappear*

disposer de *to have*

le dispositif *measure, arrangement*

dissuader *to deter*

diversifier *to diversify*

diviser *to divide*

le domicile *home*

les dommages et intérêts (mpl) *damages*

le/la dramaturge *dramatist, playwright*

les droits de l'homme (mpl) *human rights*

dû/due à *due to*

la durabilité *sustainability*

le durcissement *hardening*

la durée *period of time*

la durée déterminée *fixed term*

E

les eaux douces (fpl) *fresh water, lakes*

un écart *gap, difference*

une échelle *scale*

un écrivain *writer*

efficace *useful, efficient, effective*

s' efforcer d'apporter *to strive to provide*

un égout *sewer*

s' égrener *to range from*

élaborer *to set out*

s' éloigner *to move away*

émanant *emanating*

l' emballage (m) *packaging*

l' embarras (m) *problem, dilemma*

une embauche *employment, start, job*

(se faire) embaucher *to (get) employ(ment)*

un embouteillage *traffic jam*

embrasser *to kiss*

une émeute *riot*

émouvant *moving*

une empreinte écologique *carbon footprint*

s' empresser de *to be anxious to, to hasten to*

un emprunt *loan; borrowing*

s' en prendre à *to take it out on, to attack*

en proie à *victim of*

à l' encontre de *in the path of*

l' énergie éolienne (f) *wind power*

un engin *man-made device*

engorgé *overcrowded*

l' enjeu (m) *issue, stake*

l' ennui (m) *boredom*

s' enraciner *to take root*

enregistré *recorded*

entamer *to open up*

entraîner *to lead to, to bring about, to entail*

envahir *to invade*

envahissant *invading*

une éolienne *turbine*

l' épuisement (m) *exhaustion, running out*

épuiser *to use up*

une équipe *team*

équitable *fair*

l' ère industrielle (f) *industrial era*

l' esclavage (m) *slavery*

une espèce *species*

un espoir *hope*

étendu *spread out*

être à l'abri de *to be safe from*

être contraint de *to be forced to*

être déclenché *to be triggered off*

être prié de *to be requested to*

être pris à parti *to be picked on*

être soumis à *to be subject to*

éviter *to avoid*

en exil *in exile*

s' exprimer *to be expressed*

expulser *to expel*

F

le fabricant *manufacturer*

la faiblesse *weakness*

la faiblesse de leurs revenus *their low income*

se faire agresser *to be attacked*

faire bondir *to enrage*

faire grand bruit *to cause an outcry*

faire l'objet de *to be the subject of*

ferroviaire *using rail, railway (adj.)*

se ficher de (fam.) *not to give a damn about*

le fichier *file, data file*

fier / fière de *proud of*

la flambée des prix *price hike*

le fleuve *river*

fluvial *using rivers*

la fonction publique *public service*

la fonte des calottes glaciaires *melting of the ice caps*

les forces (fpl) de l'ordre *the police*

la foule *crowd*

fournir *to provide*

les frais (mpl) *expenses*

le frein *brake*

la fuite *escape*

G

le gamin *kid*

le gaspillage *waste*

gaspiller *to waste*

la génétique *genetics*

le genre *kind*

gérer *to manage, to conduct*

la gestion *management*

le goudron *tar*

gourmand *greedy*

la grande distribution *(chains of) supermarkets*

la grande surface *hypermarket*

le Grenelle *"round table" to bring organisations together*

grimper *to climb*

la guérison *cure*

H

s' habituer à *to get used to*

la haine *hatred*

héberger quelqu'un *to put someone up*

se heurter à *to bump into, to come up against*

hors *except for, apart from*

I

il en est de même pour *the same applies to*

il le vaut bien *he deserves it, he's worth it*

l' immédiateté (f) *immediacy*

important *significant*

s' imposer *to be assertive/ convincing*

les inactifs (mpl) *the numbers unemployed*

inadmissible *unacceptable*

l' inconnu (m) *the unknown*

inciter *to stir up*

inégalement *unequally*

l' inégalité (f) *inequality*

inépuisable *inexhaustible*
une infraction *breach, infringement*
l' inondation (f) *flood*
inscrire *to write*
l' inspection (f) du travail *occupational health and safety*
s' installer *to settle*
insuffisant *insufficient*
s' intégrer *to fit in*
l' interdiction de (f) *ban on, banning of*
l' interprétation (f) *performance*
l' intolérance (f) *intolerance*
l' intrigue (f) *plot*
à l' inverse *on the contrary*
l' issue (f) (à la dette) *the solution (to debt)*

J

jetable *disposable*
juif/juive *Jewish*

L

la licence *(university) degree; licence*
le licenciement *redundancy*
lié *linked*
le lieu *place*
le lieu de travail *workplace*
le littoral *shore, coast*
le/la locataire *tenant*
le logement *housing, accommodation*
la loi *law*
lointain *far away*
la longévité *long life*
le loup *wolf*
la lutte *struggle, fight*
lutter *to fight, to struggle*

M

malgré tout *in spite of everything*
le mammifère *mammal*
la manifestation *demonstration*
manifester *to protest*
la marche arrière *reverse (gear)*
la marée *tide*
marginaliser *to exclude from society*
le massif *mountain*
la méfiance *distrust*
à la même enseigne *in the same boat*

le mendiant *beggar*
mendier *to beg*
mépriser *to despise*
le metteur en scène *director (film, play)*
se mettre à *to start to*
mettre en place *to set up, to put in place*
le milieu *environment, setting*
le milliard *billion, thousand million*
la mise en œuvre *construction*
la mise en veille *putting on standby*
la mise en scène *production*
miser sur *to bank on, to count on*
la misère *extreme poverty*
le moindre déplacement *the least movement*
le/la musulman(e) *Muslim*

N

le naufrage *shipwreck*
le navire *ship*
négliger de *to neglect to*
négocier *to negotiate*
nuisible *harmful*

O

obsédé *obsessed*
s' occuper de *to deal with*
une ONG: organisation non gouvernementale *NGO, humanitarian organisation*
or *well, but, now*
s' opposer à *to oppose*
opprimer *to oppress*
l' ordre public (m) *law and order*
les ordures ménagères (fpl) *household waste*
un ours *bear*
un ouvrier *worker*

P

le paludisme *malaria*
le panneau *panel*
partager *to share*
parvenir *to succeed*
parvenir à *to manage to*
le patrimoine *heritage*
la pauvreté *poverty*
à peine *only just, barely, hardly*
la peine *punishment; sorrow*

percevoir *to earn*
périscolaire *outside school*
au petit matin *early in the morning*
le pétrole *oil, petroleum*
le personnage *character*
peuplé *populated*
la pièce (de théâtre) *play*
la plaisanterie *joke*
plus élevé *higher*
le point de repère *landmark*
la politique énergétique *energy policy*
la population active *active population*
les pourparlers (mpl) *talks, negotiations*
précaire *precarious, unsound*
préconiser *to recommend*
le préjugé *prejudice*
les pressions sociales (fpl) *social pressures*
la prestation sociale *social security benefit*
prévoir *to plan*
primordial *very important, fundamental*
aux prises avec *struggling against*
prison avec sursis *suspended sentence*
privé *private*
privé de *deprived of*
prôner *to preach*
les propos (mpl) haineux *hateful things/remarks*
proposer de *to suggest*
provenir: proviendra *to come from: will come from*
puiser *to draw from*
puissant *powerful*
putrescible *biodegradable*

Q

quant à *as for*
le quartier *area, neighbourhood*
quasiment *almost*
quotidien *daily*

R

la racine *root*
à rallonge *never-ending*
le rapport *relationship*
la raréfaction *scarcity*
ratifier *to ratify, to endorse*

le/la réalisateur/trice *(film) director*
le réchauffement *warming*
la récidive *reoffending*
récidiver *to reoffend*
la récolte *harvest*
réduire en morceaux *to smash to pieces*
le régime nutritionnel *diet*
en règle *in order*
le rejet *rejection*
rejeter *to throw away, to reject*
relever le défi *to raise the challenge*
remonter à *to reach*
renoncer à *to give up*
renouvelable *renewable*
répandu *widespread*
réparti *shared out*
le repatriement *repatriation*
le répit *respite, rest*
reporter sur *to transfer to*
la répression *punishment*
réprimer *to crack down on*
le/la responsable *manager, person in charge*
se ressembler *to resemble each other, to be the same*
rétablir *to restore*
la réunion *the meeting*
la réussite *success*
le révélateur *indicator*
le revenu *income*
les richesses (fpl) *wealth*
le robinet *tap*
le roman *novel*
rompre *to break, to upset*
les Roms *gypsies*

S

sache: *subj. of savoir know*
le sans-papiers *illegal immigrant*
scolariser *to educate*
le SDF: sans domicile fixe *homeless person*
la sécheresse *drought*
le semestre *term (of six months)*
sensible *aware, sensitive*
la serre *greenhouse*
servir à *to be used for / as*
le seuil *threshold*
le seuil de pauvreté *poverty line*
sévir *to be rife/rampant*
la sidérurgie *steel, steel industry*
soi *oneself*

souligner *to stress*
souscrire *to subscribe*
surgir *to arise*
supprimer *to do away with*
surmonter *to overcome*
surpeuplé *overcrowded*

T

taguer *to graffiti*
la taille *size*
le taux d'élucidation *clear-up rate*
le taux de chômage *unemployment rate*
téléguider *to remote control*
témoigner de *to indicate*
à temps partiel *part-time*
tenter *to attempt*
le terrain vague *waste land*
le théâtre *theatre; the scene*
le titre de séjour *residence permit*
touché par *affected by*
toucher *to earn*
d'une traite *without stopping on the way*
traité de racaille *branded as scum*
traiter de *to deal with*
la travée *aisle*
la trêve *truce*
trier *to sort, to separate out*
triste *sad*
le/la tsigane *gypsy*
tuer *to kill*

U

l' ubiquité (f) *being/going everywhere*

V

la vague *wave*
la veille *the night before*
en veille *in sleep / standby mode*
véritable *real*
la viande Halal *Halal meat*
le videur *bouncer*
viser *to aim at*
viser à *to aim / intend to*
la voie de dépassement *overtaking lane*
la voie publique *public highway*
voire *indeed, even*
le vol à la tire *pickpocketing*
vraisemblable *realistic*

Z

la zone frontalière *border zone*

Acknowledgements

The authors and publisher would like to thank the following for permission to reproduce material:

pp10, 18, 20 © Extracts from *Ecologuide de A à Z*, 2004, Fondation Nicolas Hulot pour la Nature et l'Homme, www.fnh.org; p10 www.ecologie.gouv.fr/IMG/pdf/charte_environnement-2.pdf; pp11, 12 © Greenpeace, www.greenpeace.fr; p15 Thanks to LCI.fr, http://tf1.lci.fr/infos/sciences/environnement/0,,3470555,00-voitures-ecolo-libre-service-paris-.html, March 2007; p22 Article by Sciama, Y. and Delbecq, S. in *Science et vie Hors 240*, Mondadori France; p26 Association Passerelle Éco d'Éducation à l'Écologie Pratique, http://www.passerelleco.info/article.php?id_article=314, source: http://empreinte.kiosq.info, 2007; p28 © WWF, http://www.wwf.fr/s_informer/nos_missions/especes_menacees, 2007; p30 © AFP, www.jeunesdumaroc.com/breve6733.html, 2007; p34 based on INSEE, www.insee.fr/fr/ffc/docs_ffc/IP1042.pdf; p35 (centre) Courtesy of UNHCR, (top) Courtesy of France Terre d'Asile; p36 www.lepost.fr, 18 Sept 2007; p38 www.legrandsoir.info, 11 Nov 2007; p42 www.lexpress.fr, 17 Nov 2005; p46 Insee Première, No. 1042, Sept. 2005; p52 Platat, S. from www.liberation.fr © Libération, 6 July 2007; p54 Based on article by Falila Gbadamassi, www.afrik.com/article10762.html, 2007; pp60, 66, 69, 74, 78 Mermet, G., *Francoscopie 2007*, © Larousse 2006; p60 (rates of unemployment) Perspectives de l'emploi de L'OCDE - Edition 2008, OECD 2008, www.oecd.org/els/emploi/perspectives; p62 (top left) © Phillippe Bécquelin, DACS 2008, (top right) Courtesy of UNICEF, (centre) Courtesy of Médecins Sans Frontières, (bottom) Courtesy of Oxfam; p62 Unicef France, http://www.unicef.fr/accueil/decouvrir/unicef-france/qui-sommes-nous-/var/lang/FR/rub/593.html, 2007; p62 Médecins sans frontières, http://notes1.msf.fr/site/site.nsf/pages/decouvrir, 2007; p62 www.oxfamfrance.org, 2007; pp68, 70 Premier ministre - service d'information du Gouvernement, http://www.premier-ministre.gouv.fr/acteurs/gouvernement/conseils_ministres_35/conseil_ministres_23_janvier_1261/les_resultats_lutte_delinquance_59000.html, 2007; p70 http://www.linternaute.com/actualite/interviews/07/jean-philippe-arlaud-delinquance/jean-philippe-arlaud-cout-de-la-delinquance.shtml

pp18, 28, 70,76 (top), 77 © Stephen Elford Illustration

Front cover photograph courtesy of Photolibrary/ Digital Vision

Photographs:
p6 Getty Images; p9 (top & p16) © lazortech. Image from BigStockPhoto.com, (bottom) © Thaut Images – Fotolia.com; p10 © iStockphoto.com / salihguler; p11 (top) © Leslee Miller. Image from BigStockPhoto.com, (left) © REUTERS/Tomas Bravo, (right) © REUTERS/STRINGER Mexico; p12 (top left) © Norman Pogson – Fotolia.com, (top right) © FlemishDreams – Fotolia.com, (bottom left) © Carl Durocher. Image from BigStockPhoto.com, (bottom right) © Valentin Mosichev – Fotolia.com; p13 (far left) © Anyka – Fotolia.com, (left) © iStockphoto.com / Guillaume Dubé, (right) © iStockphoto.com / Patryk Galka, (far right) © Brian Weed. Image from BigStockPhoto.com; p14 © Michael Wilkens – Fotolia.com; p15 (top) © iStockphoto.com / Tony Kwan, (bottom) © Art Kowalsky / Alamy; p17 (top) © iStockphoto.com / Svetlana Tebenkova, (bottom) © Jason Smith. Image from BigStockPhoto.com; p19 (left) © iStockphoto.com / Kevin Russ, (centre) © iStockphoto.com / RichVintage, (right) © iStockphoto.com / Tom Marvin; p20 (left) © iStockphoto.com / Kathy Steen, (right) © iStockphoto.com / Alexander Hafemann; p21 © iStockphoto.com / Dorota Michalec; p22 (p8 & p24) © Marzanna Syncerz – Fotolia.com, (left) © Ashley Cooper / Alamy; p23 © iStockphoto.com / Peter Eckhardt; © iStockphoto.com / Svetlana Tebenkova; p25 (top & p32) © iStockphoto.com / Domenico Pellegriti, (bottom) © Tatiana Markow / Sygma / Corbis; p28 (top) © iStockphoto.com / Damien Richard, (bottom) © Goos_Lar – Fotolia.com; p29 ©

iStockphoto.com / Alex Rowland; p30 © Liu Liqun / Corbis; p31 © Ralph Loesche. Image from BigStockPhoto.com; pp33 & 40 © David R. Frazier Photolibrary, Inc. / Alamy; p34 © iStockphoto.com / Catherine Yeulet; p35 (bottom) © Jean Ayissi / AFP / Getty Images; p36 © SOS Racisme; p37 (top) © iStockphoto.com / Sarah Howling, (left) © iStockphoto.com / Lewis Wright, (right) © tose – Fotolia.com; p38 © Olivier Laban-Mattei / AFP / Getty Images; p39 (top) Courtesy of Paul Watson, (bottom) © iStockphoto.com / Vladimir Mucibabic; p41 (top & p48) © Michael Thompson. Image from BigStockPhoto.com, (bottom) © iStockphoto.com / Aldo Murillo; p42 © David Turnley / Corbis; p43 (A) © Reuters / Benoit Tessier, (B) © Emmanuel Dunand / AFP / Getty Image, (C) © Sipa Press / Rex Features; p44 © Sipa Press / Rex Features; p45 © Martin Bureau / AFP / Getty Images; p46 © iStockphoto.com / Bonnie Jacobs; p47 Courtesy of Réseau Éducation Sans Frontières; pp49 and 56 © Reuters / Eric Gaillard; p50 © iStockphoto.com / Don Bayley; p51 © iStockphoto.com / Chris Schmidt; p52 © Alix / Phanie / Rex Features; p53 (left) © Mehmet Dilsiz. Image from BigStockPhoto.com, (right) © iStockphoto.com / Lisa Kyle Young; p54 (left) © LICRA, (right) courtesy of Olivier Fellmann; p55 © iStockphoto.com / Loic Bernard; pp57 & 64 © Mike Goldwater / Alamy; p58 © iStockphoto.com / Leon Bonaventura; p59 © Jacques Brinon / AP / PA Photos; p61 (top left) © iStockphoto.com / bobbieo, (top right) © iStockphoto.com / Dianne Maire, (bottom) © Paul Prescott; p63 © UN Photo / Eskinder Debebe; p65 (top & p72) © iStockphoto.com / Douglas Kim, (bottom) © 2008 Jupiterimages Corporation; p67 © iStockphoto.com / René Mansi; p68 (top) © Reuters / Stringer France, (middle left) © LanaK – Fotolia.com, (bottom) © ChristianSchwier.de – Fotolia.com; p69 © iStockphoto.com / Andrejs Zemdega; p70 © Sipa Press / Rex Features; p71 (top) © iStockphoto.com / Luke Daniek, (middle right) © iStockphoto.com / Anna Bryukhanova, (bottom) © Gianni Muratore / Alamy; p73 (top & p80) © rgbspace – Fotolia.com, (bottom) © ESA; p75 © iStockphoto.com / Chris Schmidt; p79 © iStockphoto.com / Joseph Luoman; p81 (top) © Martine Coquilleau – Fotolia.com, (background) © iStockphoto.com / Robert Hill, (right) © The Gallery Collection / Corbis, (middle) © iStockphoto.com / Liza McCorkle; p82 (top left) © Valery Hache / AFP / Getty Images, (top right) © iStockphoto.com / Arpad Benedek, (bottom left) © 2008 123RF Limited, (bottom right) © Marc Rigaud – Fotolia.com; p83 (top) © iStockphoto.com / Andreas Karelias, (bottom) © F1online digitale Bildagentur GmbH / Alamy; p84 (top) © Patrice Collet. Image from BigStockPhoto.com, (background) © Richard Bouhet / AFP / Getty Images; p85 © Michael Klinec / Alamy; p86 (top) © Alain Nogues / Corbis Sygma, (centre) © Popperfoto / Getty Images, (bottom) © Bettmann / Corbis; p87 © Interfoto Pressebildagentur / Alamy; p88 (top) © Photos 12 / Alamy, (centre) © Dusan Ponist. Image from BigStockPhoto.com, (bottom) © iStockphoto.com / Dana Ceclan; p89 (top) © AFP/Getty Images, (right) © Phil Date. Image from BigStockPhoto.com; p90 (top right) © Lipnitzki / Roger Viollet / Getty Images, (lower right) © Popperfoto / Getty Images, (bottom) © Ulf Andersen / Getty Images, (top left) © ullsteinbild / TopFoto; p91 © Warner Bros. / The Kobal Collection / Calvo, Bruno; p92 © AFP / Getty Images; p93 (top) © AFP / Getty Images, (lower) © Harcourt Publishers; p94 (top) © Morell Jacques / Corbis KIPA, (centre) © Popperfoto / Getty Images, (bottom) © Josch / AFP / Getty Images; p95 (top) © Dominique Faget / AFP / Getty Images, (bottom) © Fethi Belaid / AFP / Getty Images; p96 (top) © Lipnitzki / Roger Viollet / Getty Images, (bottom) © Mary Evans Picture Library / Alamy; p97 (top) © AFP / Getty Images, (bottom) © iStockphoto.com / René Mansi, (right) © Pimentel Jean / Collection Corbis KIPA; p98 (top) © Humberto Olarte Cupas / Alamy, (bottom) © Roger Viollet / Getty Images; p99 (top) © Philippe Wojazer / AFP / Getty Images, (bottom) © Rene Drouyer. Image from BigStockPhoto.com; p100 (top) © Christian Jakubaszek / Getty Images, (bottom) © Thierry Zoccolan / AFP / Getty Images; p101 (left) © Tim Clary / AFP / Getty Images, (right) © National Gallery of Scotland / Getty Images